Lifetime Physical Fitness And Wellness

A Personalized Program

SECOND EDITION

Werner W. K. Hoeger
Boise State University

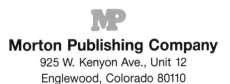

Morton Publishing Company
925 W. Kenyon Ave., Unit 12
Englewood, Colorado 80110

To my precious wife and beautiful children. My wife's input, assistance, constant support, and my children's patience and encouragement made this work possible.

Printed in the United States of America

ISBN:0-89582-191-5

Preface

The current American way of life no longer provides the human body with sufficient physical exercise to maintain adequate health. Furthermore, many present lifestyle patterns are such a serious threat to our health that they actually increase the deterioration rate of the human body and often lead to premature illness and mortality.

Although people in the United States are firm believers in the benefits of physical activity and positive lifestyle habits as a means to promote better health, most do not reap these benefits because they simply do not know how to implement a sound physical fitness and wellness program that will indeed yield the desired results.

Scientific evidence has clearly shown that improving the quality and most likely the longevity of our lives is a matter of personal choice. The biggest challenge that we are faced with at the end of this century is to teach individuals how to take control of their personal health habits to ensure a better, healthier, happier, and more productive life. The information presented in this book has been written with this objective in mind — providing you with the opportunity to initiate your own positive health and lifestyle program.

As you work through the chapters in this book, you will be able to develop and regularly update your own lifetime program to improve the various components of physical fitness and wellness. The emphasis throughout is on teaching you how to take control of your personal health and lifestyle habits so you can make a constant and deliberate effort to stay healthy and realize your highest potential for well-being.

New Features Of The Second Edition

Most of the chapters in this edition of *Lifetime Physical Fitness & Wellness* have been updated to include recent information reported in the literature. In addition, the following changes have been made in this second edition:

- The previous Chapter 11, "Relevant Questions Related to Fitness and Wellness . . . and the Answers," has been replaced by a new chapter, "Addictive Behavior and Prevention of Sexually Transmitted Diseases." This chapter has been incorporated to discuss these two wellness components, which are current health issues that may directly affect your state of health and well-being. All of the information previously contained in Chapter 11 has been disseminated throughout the other ten chapters in the book.
- A twelfth chapter, "Charting Your Future Path to Wellness," has been added to this new edition. In this chapter you can conduct a self-evaluation of the objectives accomplished during the course. You also are taught how to write fitness and wellness objectives to help you chart and implement a personal wellness program following completion of this course.

- Several changes were made to Chapter 6, "Nutrition for Weight Control and Wellness." A more thorough description of the macronutrients, information on vitamin and mineral supplementation, an introduction to eating disorders, and tips to help change behavior and adhere to a lifetime weight control program have been added to the chapter. In addition, the list of the nutritive value of selected foods contained in Appendix B has been expanded to 322 foods.
- A circumference measurements technique to assess percent body fat has been added to the chapter on body composition (Chapter 5).
- Guidelines for preventing additional cancer sites have been included in Chapter 8.
- New software has been developed for the IBM and Macintosh® computers. The Apple version has been updated. An exercise log and a nutrient analysis are features recently added to the software package.
- All new color photography is used throughout the textbook.

Acknowledgements

I wish to express gratitude to my friends and colleagues throughout the country for their support and contributions in the preparation of this text. Special thanks go to the faculty of Physical Education at Boise State University for their valuable assistance and to the students who served as models for the photographs in this new edition.

Contents

List of Figures

List of Tables

Introduction to Lifetime Physical Fitness and Wellness

Movement and physical activity are basic functions for which the human organism was created. Advances in modern technology, however, have almost completely eliminated the need for physical activity in most everyone's daily life. Exercise is no longer a natural part of our existence. We now live in an automated society, where most of the activities that used to require strenuous physical exertion can be accomplished by machines with the simple pull of a handle or push of a button. The available scientific evidence shows that physical inactivity and sedentary lifestyle have become a serious threat to our health and significantly increase the deterioration rate of the human body.

With the new developments in technology, three additional factors — nutrition, stress, and environment — have significantly changed our lives and have had a negative effect on human health. Fatty foods, sweets, alcohol, tobacco, excessive stress (distress), and pollution in general have detrimental effects on people.

At the beginning of the century, the most common health problems in the United States were infectious diseases such as tuberculosis, diphtheria, influenza, kidney disease, polio, and other diseases common in infancy and childhood. Progress in the field of medicine led to elimination of these diseases, but as the American lifestyle changed, a parallel increase was seen in chronic diseases such as hypertension, atherosclerosis, coronary disease, strokes, diabetes, cancer, emphysema, and cirrhosis of the liver.

As the incidence of chronic diseases increased, it became obvious that prevention was the best medicine when dealing with these new health problems. Estimates indicate that over 50 percent of all disease is self-controlled, 64 percent of the factors contributing to mortality are caused by lifestyle (48 percent) and environmental (16 percent) factors, and 83 percent of all deaths in the United States prior to age sixty-five are preventable. Most Americans are threatened by the very lives they lead today.

LEADING CAUSES OF DEATH IN THE UNITED STATES

The leading causes of death in the country today are basically lifestyle-related (see Table 1.1). About 70 percent of all deaths are caused by cardiovascular disease (includes heart disease and cerebrovascular diseases) and cancer. Approximately 80 percent of these could be prevented through a positive lifestyle program. Accidents comprise the third leading cause of death. Although not all accidents are preventable, many are. A significant number of fatal accidents stems from alcohol use and lack of use of seat belts. The fourth cause of death, chronic obstructive pulmonary disease, is related largely to tobacco use.

Cardiovascular Disease

The most prevalent degenerative diseases in the United States are those of the cardiovascular system. Close to one-half of all deaths in the country result from cardiovascular disease. According to the American Heart Association, heart and blood vessel disease costs were in excess of $83.7 billion in 1985. Heart attacks alone cost American

Table 1.1.
Leading Causes of Death in the United States: 1987

Cause	Total Number of Deaths	Percent of Total Deaths
1. Major cardiovascular diseases	966,400	45.4
2. Cancer	477,190	22.4
3. Accidents	94,840	4.5
4. Chronic obstructive pulmonary disease	78,270	3.7
5. All other causes	510,300	24.0

Source: National Center for Health Statistics, U.S. Public Health Service, DHHS.

industry 132 million workdays annually, including $12.4 billion in lost productivity because of physical and emotional disability. The 1985 estimates by the American Heart Association showed that:

- 64,890,000 Americans were affected by cardiovascular disease
- 59,130,000 had high blood pressure (one in four adults)
- 4,870,000 were afflicted with coronary heart disease
- 2,150,000 had rheumatic heart disease
- 1,990,000 suffered strokes
- 1,500,000 suffered heart attacks, and more than half a million died as a direct result of them

About 50 percent of the time, the first symptom of coronary heart disease is a heart attack itself, and 40 percent of the people who suffer a first heart attack die within the first twenty-four hours. In one of every five cardiovascular deaths, sudden death is the initial symptom. Close to 200,000 of those who die are persons in their most productive years, between ages thirty and sixty-five. Additionally, the American Heart Association estimates that over $700 million a year are spent in replacing employees who are recovering from heart attacks. Oddly enough, most coronary heart disease risk factors are reversible and can be controlled by the individuals themselves through appropriate lifestyle modifications.

Even though cardiovascular disease is still the leading cause of death in the country, the mortality rates for this disease have been decreasing in the last two decades. In the last few years approximately 200,000 people who were expected to die as a direct result of heart and blood vessel disease were saved each year. This reduction is attributed primarily to prevention

programs dealing with risk factor management and to better health care. A comprehensive discussion on the leading risk factors for cardiovascular disease, and recommended guidelines to implement a risk reduction program, are found in Chapter 7.

Cancer

Cancer is defined as an uncontrolled growth and spread of abnormal cells in the body. Some cells grow into a mass of tissue called a tumor, which can be either benign or malignant. A malignant tumor would be considered a "cancer." If the spread of cells is not controlled, death ensues. Over 22 percent of all deaths in the United States are a result of cancer. About 494,000 people died of this disease in 1988, and an estimated 985,000 new cases were expected the same year. Table 1.2 shows the 1988 estimated figures by the American

Table 1.2.
Estimated New Cases and Deaths for Major Sites of Cancer: 1988

Site	New Cases	Deaths
Lung	152,000	139,000
Colon-Rectum	147,000	61,500
Breast (women)	135,000	42,300
Prostate	99,000	28,000
Pancreas	27,000	24,500
Leukemia	26,900	18,100
Ovary	19,000	12,000
Bladder	46,000	10,400
Oral	30,000	9,100
Skin	27,000[a]	7,800
Uterus	47,000[b]	7,000

From *Cancer Facts and Figures*. American Cancer Society, 1988.
[a] Estimates are over 500,000 if new cases on nonmelanoma are included.
[b] New cases total over 100,000 if carcinoma in situ is included.

Cancer Society for major sites of cancer, excluding nonmelanoma skin cancer and carcinoma in situ.

Scientific evidence and testing procedures for early detection of cancer are continuously changing and improving. Cancer now is viewed as the most curable of all chronic diseases. Over 5 million Americans with a history of cancer are still alive, and nearly 3 million of them are considered cured. Evidence now indicates that as much as 80 percent of all human cancer can be prevented through positive lifestyle modifications. The basic recommendations include a diet high in cabbage-family vegetables, high in fiber, high in vitamins A and C, and low in fat. Alcohol and salt-cured, smoked, and nitrite-cured foods should be used in moderation. Cigarette smoking and tobacco use in general should be eliminated, and obesity should be avoided. Additional guidelines for your own cancer prevention program are given in Chapter 8.

Accidents

Most people do not perceive accidents as being a health problem, but accidents are the third leading cause of death in the United States, affecting the total well-being of millions of Americans each year. Accident prevention and personal safety are also part of a health enhancement program aimed at achieving a higher quality of life. Proper nutrition, exercise, abstinence from cigarette smoking, and stress management are of little help if the person is involved in a disabling or fatal accident resulting from distraction, a single reckless decision, or not properly wearing safety seat belts.

Accidents do not just happen. We cause accidents, and we are victims of accidents. Although some factors in life are completely beyond our control, such as earthquakes, tornadoes, or airplane crashes, more often than not, personal safety and accident prevention are a matter of common sense. Most accidents are the result of poor judgment and confused mental states. Accidents frequently happen when we are upset, not paying attention to the task with which we are involved, or by abusing alcohol and other drugs.

Alcohol abuse is the number one cause of all accidents. Statistics clearly show that alcohol intoxication is the leading cause in fatal automobile accidents. Other drugs commonly abused in society alter feelings and perceptions, lead to mental confusion, and impair judgment and coordination, thereby greatly enhancing the risk for accidental morbidity and mortality.

To help improve your personal safety, you are encouraged to fill out the "Health Protection Plan for Environmental Hazards, Crime Prevention, and Personal Safety," given in Appendix C. Keep in mind that you control most actions in your life. By following the recommendations given in this questionnaire, you can further enhance your personal safety and well-being.

Chronic Obstructive Pulmonary Disease

Chronic obstructive pulmonary disease (COPD) is a term used to describe an air flow limiting disease that includes chronic bronchitis, emphysema, and a reactive airway component similar to that of asthma. The incidence of COPD increases proportionately with cigarette smoking (or other forms of tobacco use) and exposure to certain types of industrial pollution. In the case of emphysema, genetic factors also may play a role.

WHAT IS PHYSICAL FITNESS?

Physical fitness has been defined in many different ways. A physician may define it as the absence of disease. Some athletes may rate fitness according to the amount of musculature developed. Other individuals perceive fitness as the ability to perform certain sports skills. The President's Council on Physical Fitness and Sports has stated that physical fitness is the measure of the body's strength, stamina, and flexibility. Perhaps the most comprehensive definition has been given by the American Medical Association, which defines physical fitness as the general capacity to adapt and respond favorably to physical effort. This implies that individuals are physically fit when they can meet the ordinary as well as the unusual demands of daily life safely and effectively without being overly fatigued, and still have energy left for leisure and recreational activities.

Physical fitness can be classified into two categories: health-related fitness and motor skill-related fitness. Most authorities agree that, from a health point of view, total physical fitness involves four basic components that are separate but interrelated: cardiovascular endurance, muscular strength and endurance, muscular flexibility, and body composition (ideal body weight and fat percentage). These are depicted in Figure 1.1. To improve the overall fitness level, an individual has to participate in specific programs to improve each of the four basic components. Nevertheless, after the initial fitness boom swept across the country in the 1970s, it became clear that just

improving the four components of physical fitness alone would not always decrease the risk for disease and ensure better health. As a result, a new concept developed in the 1980s that goes beyond the basic components of fitness. This new concept is referred to as *wellness* and will be discussed later in this chapter.

The motor skill-related aspects of fitness are of greater significance in athletics. In addition to the four components just mentioned, motor skill-related fitness includes agility, balance, coordination, power, reaction time, and speed. Although these components are important in achieving success in athletics, they are not crucial for developing better health. Therefore, this book discusses only the health-related components of fitness.

THE WELLNESS CONCEPT

Wellness can be defined as the constant and deliberate effort to stay healthy and achieve the highest potential for total well-being. The concept of wellness incorporates many components in addition to those associated with physical fitness. These include proper nutrition, smoking cessation, stress management, alcohol and drug abuse control, regular physical examinations, health education counseling, and environmental support, as shown in Figure 1.2. The difference

Figure 1.1. *Health-related components of physical fitness.*

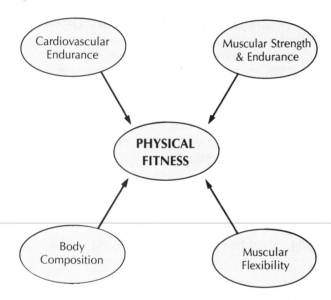

Figure 1.2. *Wellness components*

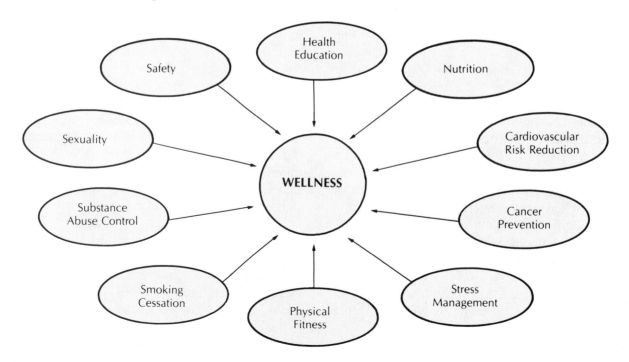

between physical fitness and wellness is illustrated clearly in the wellness continuum of Figure 1.3. For example, an individual who is running three miles a day, lifting weights regularly, participating in stretching exercises, and maintaining ideal body weight can be easily classified in the good or excellent category for each of the fitness components. Nevertheless, if this person suffers from high blood pressure, smokes, consumes alcohol, eats a diet high in fatty foods, or some combination of these, the individual probably is developing several risk factors for cardiovascular disease and may not be aware of it. (A risk factor is defined as an asymptomatic state that a person has that may lead to disease.)

One of the best examples that good physical fitness is not always a risk-free guarantee for a healthy, productive life was the tragic death in 1984 of Jim Fixx, author of *The Complete Book of Running*. At the time of his death by heart attack, Fixx was fifty-two years old. He had been running between sixty and eighty miles per week and had believed that anyone in his type of condition would not die from heart disease. At age thirty-six, Jim Fixx smoked two packs of cigarettes per day, weighed about 215 pounds, did not engage in regular cardiovascular exercise, and had a family history of heart disease. His father had experienced a first heart attack at age thirty-five and later died at age forty-three. Perhaps in an effort to decrease his risk of heart disease, Fixx began to increase his fitness level. He started to jog, lost fifty pounds, and quit cigarette smoking. Nevertheless, on several occasions Fixx declined to take an exercise electrocardiogram (stress ECG) test, which most likely would have revealed his cardiovascular problem. This unfortunate death is a good example that exercise programs by themselves will not make high-risk people immune to heart disease — other than possibly delaying the onset of a serious or fatal problem.

THE RELATIONSHIP BETWEEN FITNESS/WELLNESS AND HEALTH

A most inspiring story illustrating what fitness can do for a person's health was reported in the March, 1983, issue of *Runner's World* magazine. George Snell from Sandy, Utah, was forty-five at Christmas 1981 and weighed approximately 400 pounds. His blood pressure was 220/180, he had become blind because of diabetes that he did not know he had, and his blood glucose level was 487. Snell started a walking/jogging program in January of 1982. After only eight months he had lost almost 200 pounds, his eyesight had returned, his glucose level was down to 67, and he was taken off medication. That same year in October, less than ten months after initiating his personal exercise program, he completed his first marathon, a running course of 26.2 miles.

Although many benefits can be enjoyed as a result of participating in a regular physical fitness and wellness program, the greatest benefit of all is that individuals enjoy a better quality of life. Even though there are some indications that they also will live a longer life, statistically this is difficult to prove because of the many factors that can have an effect on our health and well-being. Tables 1.3 and 1.4 are examples of scientific research that has shown an inverse relationship between exercise and premature mortality rates. When it comes to quality of life, however,

Figure 1.3. *Wellness continuum*

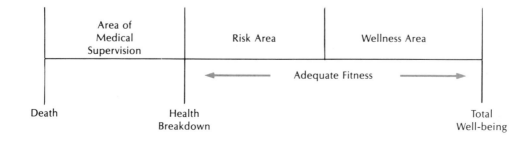

{

Table 1.3.
Cause-Specific Death Rates[a] per 10,000 Man-Years of Observation
Among 16,936 Harvard Alumni, 1982 to 1978, by Physical Activity Index

Cause of Death (n = 1,413)	% of Total Deaths	Physical Activity Index, Kcal/week		
		<500	500-1,999	2,000+
Cardiovascular Diseases	45.3	39.5	30.8	21.4
Cancer	31.6	25.7	19.2	19.0
Accidents	5.5	3.6	3.9	3.0
Suicides	4.8	5.1	3.2	2.9
Respiratory Diseases	4.3	6.0	3.2	1.5

From Paffenbarger, R. S., R. T. Hyde, A. L. Wing, and C. H. Steinmetz. "A Natural History of Athleticism and Cardiovascular Health." *JAMA* 252(4): 491-495, 1984. Copyright 1985, American Medical Association.

[a]Adjusted for differences in age, cigarette smoking, and hypertension.

Table 1.4.
Deaths from Coronary Heart Disease per 100 Men and Women by Amount of Physical Exertion

Sex	Age	Degree of Exercise			
		None	Slight	Moderate	Heavy
Men	40-49	1.46	1.17	1.12	1.00
	50-59	1.43	1.17	1.06	1.00
	60-69	1.91	1.64	1.19	1.00
	70-79	2.91	2.03	1.45	1.00
Women	40-49	—	1.29	1.07	1.00
	50-59	—	1.21	1.06	1.00
	60-69	2.01	1.86	1.11	1.00
	70-79	3.15	2.30	1.33	1.00

From Hammond, E. C., and L. Garfinkel. "Coronary Heart Disease, Stroke, and Aortic Aneurysm." *Archives of Environmental Health* 19(8):174, 1979. A publication of the Helen Dwight Reid Educational Foundation. (Table based on data of more than 1 million men and women studied over a period of six years).

physically fit individuals who lead a positive lifestyle unquestionably live a better and healthier life. These people can enjoy life to its fullest potential, with a lot fewer health problems than inactive individuals who also may be indulging in negative lifestyle patterns. Although it is difficult to compile an all-inclusive list of the benefits of physical fitness and wellness, Figure 1.4 provides a summary of many of these benefits.

As the need for physical exertion steadily decreased in the last century, the nation's health expenditures dramatically increased (see Figure 1.5.). Total medical expenditures in the United States in 1950 were $12 billion. In 1960 this figure reached $26.9 billion, by 1970 it increased to $75 billion, and by 1980 health care costs accounted for $243.4 billion. At the present rate this figure is estimated to exceed $500 billion by the end of the decade, which is in excess of ten percent of the Gross National Product. Over half of this cost is being absorbed by American business and industry.

A clear example of the benefits derived from fitness and wellness is seen among many corporations in our country that are now offering health promotion programs to their employees. Many companies are now finding out that it costs less to keep employees healthy than treating them once they are sick. The following list of facts and figures points out the need, as well as economical

Figure 1.4. *Benefits derived through participation in a comprehensive fitness and wellness program*

1. Improves and strengthens the cardiovascular system (improved oxygen supply to all parts of the body, including the heart, the muscles, and the brain)

2. Maintains better muscle tone, muscular strength, and endurance

3. Improves muscular flexibility

4. Helps maintain ideal body weight

5. Improves posture and physical appearance

6. Decreases risk for chronic diseases and illness (heart disease, cancer, strokes, high blood pressure, pulmonary disease, arthritis, etc.)

7. Decreases mortality rate from chronic diseases

8. Decreases risk and mortality rates from accidents

9. Relieves tension and helps in coping with stresses of life

10. Increases levels of energy and job productivity

11. Slows down the aging process

12. Improves self-image and morale and aids in fighting depression

13. Motivates toward positive lifestyle changes (better nutrition, smoking cessation, alcohol and drug abuse control)

14. Decreases recovery time following physical exertion

15. Speeds up recovery following injury and/or disease

16. Eases the process of childbearing and childbirth

17. Regulates and improves overall body functions

18. Improves quality of life; makes people feel and live better

Figure 1.5. *U.S. health care cost increments in the last four decades*

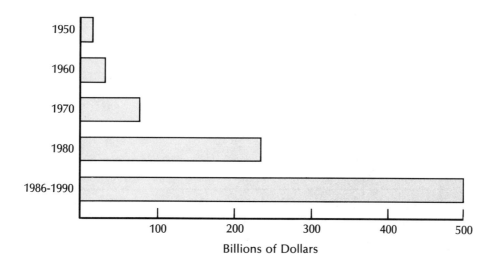

and health benefits to organizations providing wellness programs:

1. The cost of insurance premiums to American industry continues to increase each year. For some corporations, such as Kimberly-Clark, the cost of insurance premiums increased by 75 percent in a span of only four years. At the Ford Motor Company, health benefits are the most expensive fringe benefit, increasing in cost from $450 million in 1977 to $600 million in 1979. Similarly, since 1975 General Motors has been spending more for health benefits than for steel used in building automobiles.

2. The backache syndrome, usually the result of physical degeneration (inelastic and weak muscles), cost American industry over $1 billion annually in lost productivity and services alone. An additional $225 million are spent in workmen's compensation. The Adolph Coors Company, Golden, Colorado, which initiated a wellness program in 1981 for employees and their families, reported savings of more than $319,000 in 1983 alone through a preventive and rehabilitative back injury program.

3. A 1981 survey of the 1,500 largest employers in the United States showed that organizations offering prevention/health promotion programs to their employees had an average annual health care cost per employee of $806.

This compared with the average per-employee cost of $1,015 for all companies, representing a $209 saving per employee per year (an approximate 20 percent difference).

4. The Prudential Insurance Company of Houston conducted a study of its 1,300 employees. Those who participated for at least one year in the company's fitness program averaged 3.5 days of disability, as compared to 8.6 days for nonparticipants. The study estimated the direct savings from salary paid out during sickness at $204 per employee, and three to four times that amount in indirect costs due to replacements, productivity loss, overtime, and the like.

5. The Mesa Petroleum Company, Amarillo, Texas, has been offering an on-site fitness program since 1979 to its 350 employees and their family members (64 percent of the employees use the fitness center on a regular basis). A 1982 survey showed an average of $434 per person in medical costs for the nonparticipating group in the company, while the participating group averaged only $173 per person per year (see Figure 1.6). This represents a yearly reduction of $200,000 in medical expenses. Sick leave time was also significantly less for the physically active group — twenty-seven hours per year as compared to forty-four for the inactive group.

Figure 1.6. *Relationship between medical claims and exercise participation (expressed in kilocalories burned per kilogram of body weight per week) at the Mesa Petroleum Company, Amarillo, Texas (1982).*

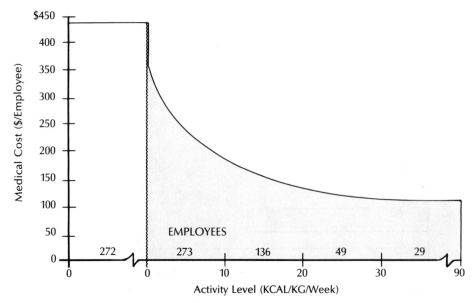

From "Reduced Costs, Increased Production are Rationale for Tax-Favored Corporate Fitness Plans." *Employee Benefit Plan Review* 20-22, November, 1983.

6. Data analysis conducted by Tenneco Incorporated in Houston in 1982 and 1983 showed a significant reduction in medical care costs for men and women who participated in an exercise program. Annual medical care costs for male and female exercisers were $562 and $639 respectively. For the nonexercising group, the costs were reported at $1,004 for the men and $1,536 for the women. Sick leave also was reduced in both the men and women participants. The greatest difference was seen between female exercisers and nonexercisers — 22.5 fewer hours for the exercisers. The difference between men exercisers and nonexercisers was 5.5 fewer hours for the exercising group. Furthermore, a survey of the more than 3,000 employees indicated that job productivity is related to fitness. The company reported that individuals with high ratings of job performance also rated high in exercise participation.

7. In 1980, the New York Telephone Company spent $2.84 million on wellness and prevention programs for 80,000 of its employees. As a direct result of the program, however, the company saved $5.54 million in employee absence and treatment costs. This represented a health care cost reduction of $69.25 per employee.

8. An independent research project of the Canadian government in 1981 documented an $84 per employee saving in health care costs for Canada Life Assurance Company in the first year of its wellness program. An additional $210 per employee saving in absenteeism and turnover also was calculated. The results were obtained by comparing figures with the North American Life Company, which offered no fitness or lifestyle programs.

In addition to these benefits, many corporations now are using fitness and wellness as an incentive to attract, hire, and retain their employees. Organizations devote resources to these programs because they know they can expect less absenteeism, hospitalization, disability, job turnover rates, premature death, and health costs, as well as increased morale and job productivity. Many companies now are taking a hard look at the fitness level of potential employees and seriously using this information in their screening process. Some organizations even refuse to hire smokers or overweight individuals.

Many executives believe that an on-site health promotion program is the best fringe benefit they can enjoy at their company. Young executives also are looking for such organizations, not only for the added health benefits but also because they suggest an attitude of concern and care by corporate officials.

THE WELLNESS CHALLENGE

With such impressive information now available on the benefits of fitness and wellness, improving the quality and, possibly, longevity of our lives clearly is a matter of personal choice. A better, healthier life is something that every person needs to strive to attain. The biggest challenge for the 1990s is to teach individuals how to take control of their personal health habits by practicing positive lifestyle activities that will decrease the risk of illness and help achieve total well-being.

Researchers also have indicated that practicing eight simple lifestyle habits can significantly increase longevity:

1. Sleeping seven to eight hours each night.
2. Eating breakfast every day.
3. Not eating between meals.
4. Eating less sweets and fat.
5. Maintaining ideal body weight.
6. Exercising regularly.
7. Drinking only moderate amounts of alcohol (or none at all).
8. Not smoking cigarettes.

As a result of current scientific data and the fitness and wellness movement of the past two decades, most people in the country now see a need to participate in such programs to improve and maintain adequate health. Many people, however, are still not participating because they are unaware of the basic principles for safe and effective exercise participation. Others are exercising erroneously and therefore do not reap the full benefits of their program. Although almost half of the adult population in the United States claims to participate in some sort of physical activity, a 1986 report by the U.S. Public Health Service indicated that only 10 to 20 percent exercised vigorously enough to develop the cardiovascular system. Because cardiovascular activities are the most popular form of exercise, perhaps an even lower percentage of the population engages in or derives benefits from strength and flexibility programs. In addition, at least half of the adult population in the country is estimated to have a weight problem.

A PERSONALIZED APPROACH

Because fitness and wellness needs vary significantly from one person to the other, exercise and wellness prescriptions should be individualized to obtain optimal results. The information presented in this book has been developed to provide the reader with the necessary information to write a personalized lifetime program to improve physical fitness and to promote preventive health care and personal wellness. In the ensuing chapters you will learn how to:

1. Determine whether medical clearance is required for safe exercise participation.
2. Assess and improve your current level of cardiovascular endurance, muscular strength and endurance, muscular flexibility, and body composition.
3. Conduct your own nutrient analysis, follow the recommendations for adequate nutrition, and develop a sound weight control program.
4. Determine your potential risk for cardiovascular disease and cancer, and implement the recommended guidelines for a risk reduction program.
5. Assess your level of tension and stress and implement a stress management program.
6. Implement programs for accident prevention, substance abuse control (including smoking cessation), and prevention of sexually transmitted diseases.
7. Write behavioral objectives to help chart your personal wellness program for the future.
8. Discern between myths and facts of exercise and health-related concepts.

YOUR PERSONAL FITNESS AND WELLNESS PROFILE

As you work through the various chapters in this book, you will be able to develop a personal fitness and wellness profile. When you obtain the information pertaining to each component of fitness and wellness, you may enter your results on the profile found in Appendix A. You also may obtain a computerized printout by using the software available with this book. Once the results for each component have been established, either with the help of your instructor or using your own judgement, set the target goals to achieve over the next ten to fourteen weeks. During the first two or three weeks, pay particular attention to the components of physical fitness. You should first determine the fitness components of the profile so that you may proceed with your exercise program and allow sufficient time to retest each fitness component within eight to twelve weeks of the initial assessment.

A WORD OF CAUTION BEFORE YOU START

In recent years several tragic deaths have occurred while some prominent national figures were participating in physical activity. These unfortunate events raised some questions as to the safety involved in exercise participation. Therefore, before you start an exercise program or participate in any exercise testing, fill out the questionnaire given in Figure 1.8. If your answer to any of the questions is positive, you should consult a physician before participating in a fitness program. Exercise testing and participation is contraindicated under some of the conditions listed in this questionnaire and may require a stress electrocardiogram (stress ECG) test, pictured in Figure 1.7. If you have any questions regarding your current health status, consult your doctor before initiating, continuing, or increasing your level of physical activity.

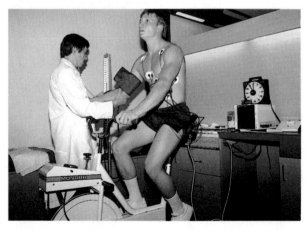

Figure 1.7. *Exercise Tolerance Test with twelve-lead electrocardiographic monitoring (stress ECG).*

Bibliography

Allsen, P. E., J. M. Harrison, and B. Vance. *Fitness for Life: An Individualized Approach.* Dubuque, IA: Wm. C. Brown, 1984.

American Cancer Society. *1988 Cancer Facts and Figures.* New York: ACS, 1988.

American College of Sports Medicine. *Guidelines for Graded Exercise Testing and Exercise Prescription.* Philadelphia: Lea and Febiger, 1986.

"America's Fitness Binge." *U.S. News and World Report* 58-61, May 3, 1982.

American Heart Association. *1988 Heart Facts.* Dallas, TX: AHA, 1988.

Duncan, D. F., and R. S. Gold. "Reflections: Health Promotion — What Is It?" *Health Values* 10(3):47-48, 1986.

Gettman, L. R. "Cost/Benefit Analysis of a Corporate Fitness Program." *Fitness in Business* 1(1):11-17, 1986.

Hammond, E. C., and L. Garfinkel. "Coronary Heart Disease, Stroke, and Aortic Aneurysm." *Archives of Environmental Health* 19(8):174, 1979.

Hoeger, W. W. K. *Principles and Laboratories for Physical Fitness & Wellness.* Englewood, CO: Morton Publishing, 1988.

Hoeger, W. W. K. *The Complete Guide for the Development & Implementation of Health Promotion Programs.* Englewood, CO: Morton Publishing, 1987.

Kaufman, J. E. "State of the Art: Physical Fitness in Corporations." *Employee Services Management* 26(1):8-9, 26-27, 1983.

Marcotte, B., and J. H. Price. "The Status of Health Promotion Programs at the Worksite, A Review." *Health Education* pp. 4-8, July/August, 1983.

"New Fitness Data Verifies: Employees Who Exercise Are Also More Productive." *Athletic Business* 8(12):24-30, 1984.

Paffenbarger, R. S., R. T. Hyde, A. L. Wing, and C. H. Steinmetz. "A Natural History of Athleticism and Cardiovascular Health." *JAMA* 252(4):491-495, 1984.

President's Council on Physical Fitness and Sports. *Physical Fitness in Business and Industry.* Washington, DC: Council, 1972.

"Reduced Costs, Increased Production are Rationale for Tax-Favored Corporate Fitness Plans." *Employee Benefit Plan Review* 20-22, November, 1983.

Shilstone, S. "The Fitness Renaissance: Will It Stand the Test of Time?" *Sunbelt Executive:* 54-56, 1984.

Smith, L. K. "Cost-Effectiveness of Health Promotion Programs." *Fitness Management* 2(3):12-15, 1986.

Sorochan, W. D. *Promoting Your Health.* New York: John Wiley & Sons, 1981.

Van Camp, S. P. "The Fixx Tragedy: A Cardiologist's Perspective." *Physician and Sports Medicine* 12(9): 153-155, 1984.

Wright, C. C. "Cost Containment Through Health Promotion Programs." *Journal of Occupational Medicine* 22:36-39, 1980.

Figure 1.8. *Health history questionnaire*

Although exercise testing and exercise participation is relatively safe for most apparently healthy individuals under age forty-five, the reaction of the cardiovascular system to increased levels of physical activity cannot allways be totally predicted. Consequently, there is a small but real risk of certain changes occurring during exercise testing or participation. Some of these changes may include abnormal blood pressure, irregular heart rhythm, fainting, and, in rare instances, a heart attack or cardiac arrest.

Therefore, it is imperative that you provide honest answers to this questionnaire. Exercise may be contraindicated under some of the conditions listed below; others may simply require special consideration. **If any of the conditions apply, consult your physician before you participate in an exercise program.** Also, promptly report to your instructor any exercise-related abnormalities that you may experience during regular exercise participation.

A. Have you ever had or do you now have any of the following conditions:
- [ ] 1. A myocardial infarction
- [ ] 2. Coronary artery disease
- [ ] 3. Congestive heart failure
- [ ] 4. Elevated blood lipids (cholesterol and triglycerides)
- [ ] 5. Chest pain at rest or during exertion
- [ ] 6. Shortness of breath
- [ ] 7. An abnormal resting or stress electrocardiogram
- [ ] 8. Uneven, irregular, or skipped heartbeats (including a racing or fluttering heart)
- [ ] 9. A blood embolism
- [ ] 10. Thrombophlebitis
- [ ] 11. Rheumatic heart fever
- [ ] 12. Elevated blood pressure
- [ ] 13. A stroke
- [ ] 14. Diabetes
- [ ] 15. A family history of coronary heart disease, syncope, or sudden death before age sixty
- [ ] 16. Any other heart problem that makes exercise unsafe

B. Do you suffer from any of the following conditions:
- [ ] 1. Arthritis, rheumatism, or gout
- [ ] 2. Chronic low back pain
- [ ] 3. Any other joint, bone, or muscle problems
- [ ] 4. Any respiratory problems
- [ ] 5. Obesity (more than 30 percent overweight)
- [ ] 6. Anorexia
- [ ] 7. Bulimia
- [ ] 8. Mononucleosis
- [ ] 9. Any physical disability that could interfere with safe exercise participation

C. Do any of the following conditions apply:
- [ ] 1. Do you smoke cigarettes?
- [ ] 2. Are you taking any prescription medication?
- [ ] 3. Are you forty-five years or older?

D. Do you have any other concern regarding your ability to safely participate in an exercise program? If so, explain:

_____

_____

Student's Signature: _____ Date: _____

Cardiovascular Endurance Assessment And Prescription Techniques

Cardiovascular endurance has been defined as the ability of the lungs, heart, and blood vessels to deliver adequate amounts of oxygen and nutrients to the cells to meet the demands of prolonged physical activity. As a person breathes, part of the oxygen contained in ambient air is taken up in the lungs and transported in the blood to the heart. The heart is then responsible for pumping the oxygenated blood through the circulatory system to all organs and tissues of the body. At the cellular level, oxygen is used to convert food substrates, primarily carbohydrates and fats, into energy necessary to conduct body functions and maintain a constant internal equilibrium.

During physical exertion a greater amount of energy is needed to carry out the work. As a result, the heart, lungs, and blood vessels have to deliver more oxygen to the cells to supply the required energy to accomplish the task. During prolonged physical activity, an individual with a high level of cardiovascular endurance is able to deliver the required amount of oxygen to the tissues with relative ease. The cardiovascular system of a person with a low level of endurance has to work much harder, because the heart has to pump more often to supply the same amount of oxygen to the tissues, and consequently fatigues faster. Hence, a higher capacity to deliver and utilize oxygen (oxygen uptake) indicates a more efficient cardiovascular system.

Cardiovascular endurance activities are also frequently referred to as *aerobic* exercises. The word "aerobic" means "with oxygen." Whenever an activity requires the utilization of oxygen to produce energy, it is considered an aerobic exercise. Examples of cardiovascular or aerobic exercises are walking, jogging, swimming, cycling, cross-country skiing, rope skipping, and aerobic dancing.

Anaerobic activities, on the other hand, are carried out without oxygen. The intensity of anaerobic exercise is so high that oxygen cannot be utilized to produce energy. Because energy production is very limited in the absence of oxygen, these activities can be carried out only for short periods of time. The higher the intensity, the shorter the duration. Activities such as the 100, 200, and 400 meters in track and field, the 100 meters in swimming, gymnastics routines, and weight training are good examples of anaerobic activities. Only aerobic activities will help increase cardiovascular endurance. Anaerobic activities will not significantly contribute toward development of the cardiovascular system.

Physical activity is no longer a natural part of our existence. We live in an automated world, where most of the activities that used to require strenuous physical exertion can be accomplished by machines with the simple pull of a handle or push of a button. For instance, if there is a need to go to a store that may be only a couple of blocks away, most people drive their automobiles and then spend several minutes driving around the parking lot in an effort to find a spot ten yards closer to the store's entrance. The groceries do not even have to be carried out any more. They are usually taken out in a cart and placed in the vehicle by a youngster working at the store.

Similarly, during a normal visit to a multi-level shopping mall, it can be easily observed that almost everyone chooses to ride the escalators

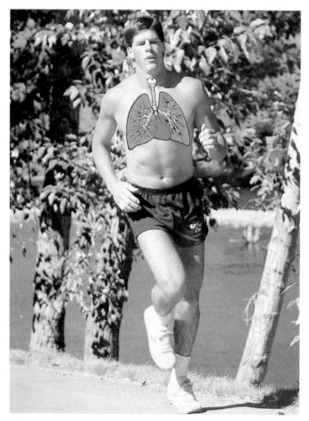

Figure 2.1. *Cardiovascular endurance: The ability of the lungs, heart, and blood vessels to deliver adequate amounts of oxygen to the cells to meet the demands of prolonged physical activity.*

IMPORTANCE OF CARDIOVASCULAR ENDURANCE

A sound cardiovascular endurance program greatly contributes toward the enhancement and maintenance of good health. Of the four components of physical fitness, cardiovascular endurance is the single most important factor. Certain amounts of muscular strength and flexibility are necessary in daily activities to lead a normal life. A person can get away without large amounts of strength and flexibility but cannot do so without a good cardiovascular system.

As was discussed in Chapter 1, the typical American is not exactly a good role model when it comes to physical fitness. According to the U.S. Public Health Service, only 10 to 20 percent of the adult population exercises vigorously enough to develop the cardiovascular system. Aerobic exercise is especially important in the prevention of diseases associated with the cardiovascular system.

A poorly conditioned heart, which has to pump more often just to keep a person alive, is subject to more wear-and-tear than a well-conditioned heart. In situations in which strenuous demands are placed on the heart, such as doing yard work, lifting heavy objects or weights, or running to catch a train, the unconditioned heart may not be able to sustain the strain. Additionally, regular participation in cardiovascular endurance activities help you achieve and maintain ideal body weight — the fourth component of physical fitness.

BENEFITS OF CARDIOVASCULAR ENDURANCE TRAINING

Every individual who initiates a cardiovascular or aerobic exercise program can expect a number of physiological adaptations that result from training. Among these benefits are:

1. A decrease in resting heart rate and an increase in cardiac muscle strength. During resting conditions the heart ejects between five and six quarts of blood per minute. This amount of blood is sufficient to meet the energy demands in the resting state. Like any other muscle, the heart responds to training by increasing in strength and size. As the heart gets stronger, the muscle can produce a more

instead of taking the stairs. Automobiles, elevators, escalators, telephones, intercoms, remote controls, and electric garage door openers are all modern-day commodities that minimize the amount of movement and effort required by the human body.

One of the most significant detrimental effects of modern-day technology has been an increase in chronic conditions that are related to a lack of physical activity (e.g., hypertension, heart disease, chronic low back pain, and obesity). These conditions are also referred to as *hypokinetic diseases.* The term "hypo" implies low or little, and "kinetic" implies motion. Lack of vigorous physical activity is a fact of modern life that most people can no longer avoid, but if we want to enjoy many of the twentieth-century commodities and still expect to live life to its fullest, a lifetime cardiovascular exercise program must become a part of daily living.

forceful contraction that causes a greater ejection of blood with each beat (stroke volume), yielding a decreased heart rate. This reduction in heart rate also allows the heart to rest longer between beats. Resting heart rates are frequently decreased by ten to twenty beats per minute (bpm) after only six to eight weeks of training. A reduction of twenty bpm would save the heart about 10,483,200 beats per year. The average heart beats between seventy and eighty bpm, but in highly trained athletes, resting heart rates frequently are around forty bpm.

2. A lower heart rate at given work loads. When compared with untrained individuals, a trained person has a lower heart-rate response to a given task. This is because of the increased efficiency of the cardiovascular system. Individuals are also surprised to find that following several weeks of training, a given work load (let's say a ten-minute mile) elicits a much lower heart rate as compared to the initial response when training first started.

3. A decrease in recovery time. Trained individuals enjoy a quicker recovery to resting values following an exercise bout. A fit system is able to restore at a greater speed any internal equilibrium that was disrupted during exercise.

4. An increase in the number of functional capillaries. These smaller vessels supply nutrients to the working muscles and allow for the exchange of oxygen and carbon dioxide between the blood and the cells. As more vessels open up, more nutrients can be delivered and a greater amount of gas exchange can take place, therefore decreasing the onset of fatigue during prolonged exercise. This increase in capillaries also speeds up the rate at which waste products of cell metabolism can be removed. This increased capillarization is also seen in the heart, which enhances the oxygen delivery capacity to the heart muscle itself.

5. An increase in the number and size of the mitochondria, along with an increase in their ability to burn fat during aerobic exercise. All energy necessary for cell function during cardiovascular exercise is produced in the mitochondria. As the size and number increase with training, so does the potential to

produce energy for muscular work. Additionally, there is a potential twofold increase in mitochondrial (aerobic) enzymes. This increase, along with the enhanced capillarization, increases the muscles' capability to mobilize and burn fat during aerobic exercise.

6. An increase in the oxygen-carrying capacity in the body. With aerobic training there is an increase in the red blood cell count, which contains hemoglobin that is responsible for transporting oxygen in the blood.

7. A higher maximal oxygen uptake, which improves aerobic capacity. The amount of oxygen that the body is able to utilize during cardiovascular exercise is significantly enhanced. Changes in maximal oxygen uptake have been observed within three weeks of aerobic training. It can rise by 15 to 30 percent in three months and as much as 50 percent in two years. This physiological adaptation allows the individual to exercise longer and at a higher rate before becoming fatigued.

8. A decrease in blood lipids. A regular aerobic exercise program will cause a reduction in blood fats such as cholesterol and triglycerides, both of which have been linked to the formation of the atherosclerotic plaque that obstructs the arteries (see Figures 7.4 and 7.5 in Chapter 7). This reduction decreases the risk of cardiovascular disease.

9. A decrease in resting blood pressure. On the average, cardiovascularly fit individuals have lower blood pressures than unfit people. Perhaps of greater significance is the role of aerobic exercise in the treatment of hypertensive patients. Several well-documented studies have shown that nearly 90 percent of hypertensive patients who initiate an aerobic exercise program can expect a significant decrease in blood pressure after only a few months of training. These changes, however, are not maintained if aerobic exercise is discontinued.

RELEVANT QUESTIONS RELATED TO CARDIOVASCULAR TRAINING — AND THE ANSWERS

In addition to the previously stated physiological adaptations, several other benefits can be enjoyed as a result of a cardiovascular exercise program. These benefits have not always been completely clear, have been somewhat controversial, or are sometimes used to misinform fitness and wellness participants. Let's examine some of these issues:

Does aerobic exercise make a person immune to heart and blood vessel disease? Although aerobically fit individuals have a low incidence of cardiovascular disease, a regular aerobic exercise program by itself is not an absolute guarantee against cardiovascular disease. Many other factors may increase the person's risk, including genetic predisposition. Overall risk factor management is the best guideline to minimize the risk for cardiovascular disease, but your chances of surviving a heart attack are much greater if you have been exercising regularly.

Scientific evidence does indicate, however, that a regular aerobic exercise program helps decrease the risk for cardiovascular disease. To obtain a certain degree of protection against cardiovascular disease, approximately 300 calories should be expended on a daily basis through aerobic exercise. Dr. Thomas K. Cureton, in his book *The Physiological Effects of Exercise Programs Upon Adults,* reports that 300 calories per exercise session provide the necessary stimuli to control blood lipids, which constitute a primary risk factor for atherosclerosis, coronary heart disease, and strokes.

Dr. Ralph Paffenbarger and his co-researchers (see Chapter 1, Table 1.3) showed that 2,000 calories expended per week as a result of physical activity yielded the lowest risk for cardiovascular disease among a group of almost 17,000 Harvard alumni. Two thousand calories per week represents about 300 calories per daily exercise session.

Do people experience a "physical high" during aerobic exercise? During vigorous exercise, morphine-like substances called *endorphines* are released from the pituitary gland in the brain. These act not only as a pain killer, but they also can induce feelings of euphoria and natural well-being. Increased levels of endorphines are commonly seen as a result of aerobic endurance activities and may remain elevated for as long as thirty to sixty minutes following exercise. Many experts now believe that these higher levels explain the so-called physical high that people experience during and after prolonged exercise participation.

Endorphine levels have also been shown to be elevated during pregnancy and delivery. Because endorphines act as pain killers, these higher levels could explain a woman's increased tolerance to the pain and discomfort experienced during natural childbirth and the pleasant feelings experienced shortly after the birth of the baby. Very possibly, well-conditioned women may achieve higher endorphine levels during delivery, making childbirth less traumatic than that of untrained women.

What causes muscle soreness and stiffness? Muscle soreness and stiffness are very common among individuals who initiate an exercise program or participate after a prolonged layoff from exercise. The acute soreness experienced the first few hours after exercise is thought to be related to a lack of blood (oxygen) flow and general fatigue of the exercised muscles. The delayed soreness that appears several hours after exercise (usually twelve hours later) and lasts for two to four days may be related to actual minute tears in muscle tissue, muscle spasms that increase fluid retention stimulating the pain nerve endings, and overstretching or tearing of connective tissue in and around muscles and joints.

The best way to prevent soreness and stiffness is by stretching adequately before and after exercise and gradually progressing into your exercise program. Do not attempt to do too much too quickly. If you experience soreness and stiffness, mild stretching, low-intensity exercise to stimulate blood flow, and a warm bath can help relieve the pain.

How should acute sport injuries be treated? The best treatment has always been prevention itself. If a given activity is causing unusual discomfort or chronic irritation, you need to treat the cause by decreasing the intensity, switching activities, or using better equipment such as suitable and proper-fitting shoes.

If an acute injury has occurred, the standard method of treatment is cold application, compression, and/or splinting, and elevation of the affected body part. Cold should be applied three to five times a day for fifteen to twenty minutes during the first twenty-four to thirty-six hours. Cold can be applied by submerging the injured area in cold water, by using an ice bag, or by applying ice massage to the affected part. Compression can be applied with an elastic bandage or wrap. Elevation, whenever possible, is used to decrease blood flow to the injured part.

The purpose of these three treatment modalities is to minimize swelling in the area, which significantly increases the time of recovery. After the initial twenty-four to thirty-six hours, heat can be used if there is no further swelling or inflammation. If you have doubts regarding the nature or seriousness of the injury (such as suspected fracture), however, you should seek a medical evaluation.

Whenever there is obvious deformity such as in fractures, dislocations, or partial dislocations; splinting, cold application with an ice bag, and medical attention are required. Never try to reset any of these conditions by yourself, as greater damage to muscles, ligaments, and nerves is possible. Treatment of these injuries should always be left to specialized medical personnel.

Is it safe to exercise during pregnancy? There is no reason why women should not exercise during pregnancy. If anything, it is desirable that women do so to strengthen the body and prepare for delivery. Physically fit women experience easier delivery and faster recovery than unfit women. Among Indian tribes pregnant women typically continue to carry out all of their hard labor chores up to the very day of delivery; and a few hours after the birth of the baby, they resume their normal activities. There have also been several women athletes who have competed in different sports during the early stages of pregnancy. At the 1952 Olympic Games, a pregnant woman won a bronze medal in track and field. Nevertheless, the final decision for exercise participation should be made by the woman and her personal physician.

Experts have recommended that women who have been exercising regularly continue to carry out the same activity through the fifth month of pregnancy, but they should take care not to exceed a working heart rate of 140 beats per minute. After the fifth month, walking, stationary cycling, and/or moderate swimming are indicated in conjunction with some light strengthening exercises. For women who have not exercised regularly, twenty to thirty minutes of daily walking and light strengthening exercises are recommended throughout the entire pregnancy.

Does exercise help relieve dysmenorrhea (painful menstruation)? Exercise has not been shown to either cure or aggravate painful menstruation,

but it has been shown to relieve menstrual cramps because of improved circulation to the uterus. The decrease in menstrual cramps could also be related to increased levels of endorphines produced during prolonged physical activity, which may counteract pain.

Does exercise participation hinder menstruation? In some instances, highly trained athletes may develop amenorrhea (cessation of menstruation) during training and competition. This condition is frequently seen in extremely lean individuals who also engage in sports that require very strenuous physical effort over a sustained period of time, but it is by no means irreversible. At present it is unknown whether the condition is caused by physical or emotional stress related to high-intensity training, excessively low body fat, or other factors.

Although, on the average, women experience a decrease in physical capacity during menstruation, medical surveys at the Olympic Games have verified that women have broken Olympic and world records at all stages of the menstrual cycle. Menstruation should not keep a woman from participating in athletics; nor will it necessarily have a negative impact on performance.

Does exercise decrease the risk of osteoporosis? Osteoporosis has been defined as the softening, deterioration, or loss of total body bone. Bones become so weak and brittle that fractures, primarily of the hip, wrist, and spine, occur very readily. About 1.3 million fractures are attributed to this condition each year. Osteoporosis slowly begins in the third and fourth decade of life, and women are especially susceptible after menopause. This results primarily from estrogen loss following menopause, which increases the rate at which bone mass is broken down.

Prevention of osteoporosis begins early in life by including adequate amounts of calcium in the diet (the recommended dietary allowance is 800 to 1200 mg per day) and regularly participating in an exercise program. Weight-bearing activities such as walking, jogging, and weight training are especially helpful. Not only do they tone up muscles, but they also develop stronger and thicker bones. Following menopause, maintenance of calcium intake, adequate physical exercise, and personal evaluation by a physician for possible estrogen therapy are recommended to prevent osteoporosis. In conjunction with adequate calcium intake, there may be a need for more vitamin D, which is necessary for optimal calcium absorption.

Does exercise offset the detrimental effects of cigarette smoking? Physical exercise often motivates toward smoking cessation but does not offset any ill-effects of smoking. If anything, smoking greatly decreases the ability of the blood to transport oxygen to working muscles. Oxygen is carried in the circulatory system by hemoglobin, the iron-containing pigment of the red blood cells. Carbon monoxide, a by-product of cigarette smoke, has 210 to 250 times greater affinity for hemoglobin than does oxygen. Consequently, carbon monoxide combines much faster with hemoglobin, decreasing the oxygen-carrying capacity of the blood. Chronic smoking also increases airway resistance, requiring the respiratory muscles to work much harder and consume more oxygen just to ventilate a given amount of air. If you quit smoking, exercise does help increase the functional capacity of the pulmonary system.

How long should a person wait after a meal before engaging in strenuous physical exercise? The length of time that an individual should wait before exercising after a meal depends on the amount of food consumed. On the average, after a regular meal the person should wait about two to three hours before participating in strenuous physical activity. However, there is no reason why the individual should not be able to take a walk or do some other light physical activity following a meal. If anything, such practice helps burn extra calories and may help the body metabolize fats more efficiently.

CARDIOVASCULAR ENDURANCE ASSESSMENT

Cardiovascular endurance, cardiovascular fitness, or aerobic capacity is determined by the maximal amount of oxygen that the human body is able to utilize per minute of physical activity. This value can be expressed in liters per minute (L/min) or milliliters per kilogram per minute (ml/kg/min). The latter is most frequently used because it takes into consideration total body mass (weight). When comparing two individuals with the same absolute value, the one with the lesser body mass will have a higher relative value, indicating that a greater amount of oxygen is available to each kilogram (2.2 pounds) of body weight. Because all tissues and organs of the body

utilize oxygen to function, a higher amount of oxygen consumption indicates a more efficient cardiovascular system.

The most precise way to determine maximal oxygen uptake is through direct gas analysis. This is done using a metabolic cart through which the amount of oxygen consumption can be directly measured. This technique is very sophisticated, however, and the test requires costly equipment that is not readily available in most health/fitness centers. As a result, several alternative methods of estimating maximal oxygen uptake using limited equipment have been developed.

Even though most cardiovascular endurance tests are probably safe to administer to apparently healthy individuals (those with no major coronary risk factors), the American College of Sports Medicine recommends that a physician be present for all maximal exercise tests on individuals over the age of thirty-five (regardless of state of health). A maximal test can be described as any test that requires an all-out effort, to the point of complete fatigue, on the part of the participant. For submaximal tests, a physician should be present when testing higher risk/asymptomatic individuals over the age of thirty-five or any symptomatic or diseased people regardless of age.

CARDIOVASCULAR FITNESS TESTS

In this chapter three common techniques used in assessing cardiovascular endurance will be explained. You will have to select only one of these three tests to determine your current cardiovascular fitness level.

Although most healthy individuals are able to perform any of these tests, before you choose one of them, read the following introduction and possible contraindications to each test. Make sure that you have carefully filled out the questionnaire in Figure 1.8 in Chapter 1. If medical clearance is necessary, check with a physician before you take any of the tests. Your choice of test should also be based on the physical facilities and equipment available to you. After selecting a test, you may go directly to the description of the test procedures and prepare to take your test. Keep in mind that these are three different testing protocols and that each test will not necessarily yield the same results. Therefore, to make valid comparisons, the same test should be used when doing pre- and post-assessments.

1. **The 1.5-mile Run Test.** This test is most frequently used to determine cardiovascular fitness according to the time it takes to run/walk a 1.5-mile course. Maximal oxygen uptake is estimated based on the time it takes to cover the distance (see Figure 2.2 and Table 2.1).

The only equipment necessary to conduct this test is a stopwatch and a track or premeasured 1.5-mile course. It is perhaps the easiest test to administer, but caution should be taken when conducting the test. Because the objective of the test is to cover the distance in the shortest period of time, it can be considered to be a maximal exercise test. The use of this test should be limited to conditioned individuals who have been cleared for exercise. It is contraindicated for unconditioned beginners (you should have at least six weeks of aerobic training), symptomatic individuals, and those with known cardiovascular disease or heart disease risk factors.

Figure 2.2. *Procedure for the 1.5-Mile Run Test*

1. Make sure that you qualify for this test. This test is contraindicated for unconditioned beginners, individuals with symptoms of heart disease, and those with known heart disease or risk factors.

2. Select the testing site. Find a school track (each lap is ¼ of a mile) or a premeasured 1.5-mile course.

3. Have a stopwatch available to determine your time.

4. Conduct a few warm-up exercises prior to the test. Do some stretching exercises, some walking, and slow jogging.

5. Initiate the test and try to cover the distance in the fastest time possible (walking or jogging). Time yourself during the run to see how fast you have covered the distance. If any unusual symptoms arise during the test, do not continue. Stop immediately and retake the test after another six weeks of aerobic training.

6. At the end of the test, cool down by walking or jogging slowly for another three to five minutes. Do not sit or lie down after the test.

7. According to your performance time, look up your estimated maximal oxygen uptake in Table 2.1.

8. Example: A twenty-year-old female runs the 1.5-mile course in 12 minutes and 40 seconds. Table 2.1 shows a maximal oxygen uptake of 39.8 ml/kg/min for a time of 12:40. According to Table 2.6, this maximal oxygen uptake would place her in the good cardiovascular fitness category.

Table 2.1.
Estimated Maximal Oxygen Uptake (Max VO$_2$) in ml/kg/min for the 1.5-Mile Run Test

Time	Max VO$_2$	Time	Max VO$_2$	Time	Max VO$_2$	Time	Max VO$_2$	Time	Max VO$_2$
6:10	80.0	8:50	59.1	11:30	44.4	14:10	35.5	16:50	29.1
6:20	79.0	9:00	58.1	11:40	43.7	14:20	35.1	17:00	28.9
6:30	77.9	9:10	56.9	11:50	43.2	14:30	34.7	17:10	28.5
6:40	76.7	9:20	55.9	12:00	42.3	14:40	34.3	17:20	28.3
6:50	75.5	9:30	54.7	12:10	41.7	14:50	34.0	17:30	28.0
7:00	74.0	9:40	53.5	12:20	41.0	15:00	33.6	17:40	27.7
7:10	72.6	9:50	52.3	12:30	40.4	15:10	33.1	17:50	27.4
7:20	71.3	10:00	51.1	12:40	39.8	15:20	32.7	18:00	27.1
7:30	69.9	10:10	50.4	12:50	39.2	15:30	32.2	18:10	26.8
7:40	68.3	10:20	49.5	13:00	38.6	15:40	31.8	18:20	26.6
7:50	66.8	10:30	48.6	13:10	38.1	15:50	31.4	18:30	26.3
8:00	65.2	10:40	48.0	13:20	37.8	16:00	30.9	18:40	26.0
8:10	63.9	10:50	47.4	13:30	37.2	16:10	30.5	18:50	25.7
8:20	62.5	11:00	46.6	13:40	36.8	16:20	30.2	19:00	25.4
8:30	61.2	11:10	45.8	13:50	36.3	16:30	29.8		
8:40	60.2	11:20	45.1	14:00	35.9	16:40	29.5		

Adapted from Cooper, K. H. "A Means of Assessing Maximal Oxygen Intake." *JAMA* 203:201-204, 1968; Pollock, M. L. et al. *Health and Fitness Through Physical Activity.* New York: John Wiley and Sons, 1978; Wilmore, J. H. *Training for Sport and Activity.* Boston: Allyn and Bacon, 1982.

2. **The Step Test.** This test requires little time and equipment and can be administered to almost everyone, because submaximal workloads are used to estimate maximal oxygen uptake. This test should not be administered to symptomatic and diseased individuals, or to those at high risk (no symptoms) over age thirty-five. Significantly overweight individuals and those with joint problems in the lower extremities may have a difficult time performing the test.

The actual step test (see Figure 2.3) takes only three minutes. A fifteen-second recovery heart rate is taken between five and twenty seconds following the test. The equipment required is a bench or gymnasium bleacher 16¼ inches high, a stopwatch, and a metronome.

You will need to know how to take your heart rate by counting your pulse. This can be done on the wrist by placing two or three fingers over the radial artery (on the side of the thumb) or over the carotid artery in the neck just below the jaw next to your voice box (see Figures 2.4 and 2.5). If individuals are

Figure 2.3. *Procedure for the Step Test*

1. The test is conducted with a bench or gymnasium bleacher 16¼ inches high.

2. The stepping cycle is performed to a four-step cadence (up-up-down-down). Men should perform twenty-four complete step-ups per minute, regulated with a metronome set at 96 beats per minute. Women perform twenty-two step-ups per minute, or 88 beats per minute on the metronome.

3. Allow a brief practice period of five to ten seconds to familiarize yourself with the stepping cadence.

4. Begin the test and perform the step-ups for exactly three minutes.

5. Upon completion of the three minutes, remain standing and take your heart rate for a fifteen-second interval from five to twenty seconds into recovery. Convert recovery heart rate to beats per minute (multiply 15-second heart rate by 4).

6. Maximal oxygen uptake in ml/kg/min is estimated according to the following equations:

   Men:
   maximal oxygen uptake = 111.33 − (0.42 × recovery heart rate in bpm)

   Women:
   maximal oxygen uptake = 65.81 − (0.1847 × recovery heart rate in bpm)

7. Example: The recovery fifteen-second heart rate for a male subject following the three-minute step test is found to be 39 beats. Maximal oxygen uptake is estimated as follows:

   Fifteen-second heart rate = 39 beats
   Minute heart rate = 39 × 4 = 156 bpm

   Maximal oxygen uptake = 111.33 − (0.42 × 156) = 45.81 ml/kg/min

8. Maximal oxygen uptake also can be obtained according to recovery heart rates in Table 2.2.

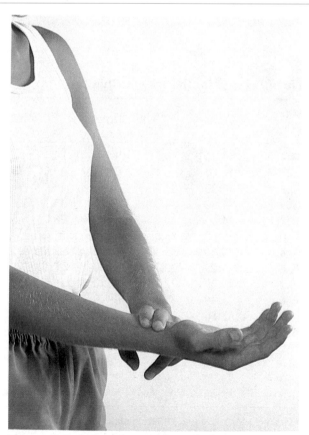

Figure 2.4. *Pulse taken at the radial artery.*

From McArdle, W. D., et al. *Exercise Physiology: Energy, Nutrition, and Human Performance.* Philadelphia: Lea & Febiger, 1986.

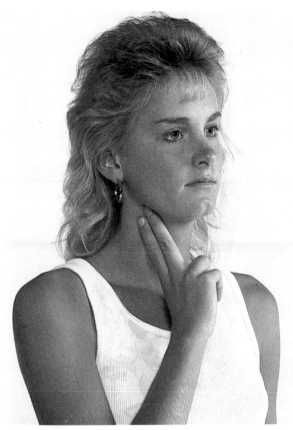

Figure 2.5. *Pulse taken at the carotid artery*

Table 2.2.
Predicted Maximal Oxygen Uptake (Max VO$_2$)
for the Three-Minute Step Test in ml/kg/min

15-Sec HR[a]	HR-bpm[b]	Max VO$_2$ Men	Max VO$_2$ Women
30	120	60.9	43.6
31	124	59.3	42.9
32	128	57.6	42.2
33	132	55.9	41.4
34	136	54.2	40.7
35	140	52.5	40.0
36	144	50.9	39.2
37	148	49.2	38.5
38	152	47.5	37.7
39	156	45.8	37.0
40	160	44.1	36.3
41	164	42.5	35.5
42	168	40.8	34.8
43	172	39.1	34.0
44	176	37.4	33.3
45	180	35.7	32.6
46	184	34.1	31.8
47	188	32.4	31.1
48	192	30.7	30.3
49	196	29.0	29.6
50	200	27.3	28.9

[a] heart rate
[b] beats per minute

taught to take their own heart rate, a large group of people can be tested at once when using gymnasium bleachers.

In recent years there has been some controversy regarding carotid artery palpation as a means to assess exercise heart rate. The controversy is based on research conducted in the late 1970s that showed a decrease in heart rate when monitored through carotid artery palpation. Strong external pressure or massaging receptors located in the carotid artery can produce a slower heart rate in some individuals, particularly those with certain types of vascular problems. Nevertheless, several studies conducted in the 1980s have shown that carotid artery palpation causes small or no changes at all in healthy individuals or cardiac patients. The best recommendation at this point is that individuals who cannot readily feel the carotid pulse (those who have to exert strong pressure or keep moving the fingers around to find the pulse) should use radial artery palpation to monitor exercise heart rate.

3. **Astrand-Ryhming Test.** Because of its simplicity and practicality, the Astrand-Ryhming test has become one of the most common protocols used when estimating maximal oxygen uptake in the laboratory setting. The test is conducted on a bicycle ergometer, and, similar to the step test, it requires only a submaximal workload and little time to administer. The contraindications given for the step test also apply for the Astrand-Ryhming test. Nevertheless, because the participant does not have to support his/her own body weight while riding the bicycle, the test can be used with overweight individuals and those with limited joint problems in the lower extremities.

The bicycle ergometer to be used on this test should allow for the regulation of workloads (see test procedures using Figure 2.6). Besides the bicycle ergometer, a stopwatch and an additional technician are needed to perform the test. The duration of the test is six minutes, and the heart rate is taken every minute (see Figure 2.7). At the end of the test, the heart rate should be in the range given for each workload in Table 2.3 (primarily between 120 and 170 beats per minute).

Good judgement is essential when administering the test to older people. Low workloads should be used, because if the higher heart rates (150 to 170 bpm) are reached these individuals could be working near or at their maximal capacity, making it an unsafe test to perform without adequate medical supervision. When choosing workloads for older people, final exercise heart rates should not exceed 130 to 140 bpm.

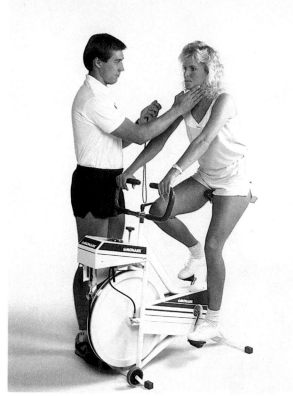

Figure 2.7. *Monitoring heart rate on the carotid artery during the Astrand-Ryhming Test*

Figure 2.6. *Procedure for the Astrand-Ryhming Test*

1. Adjust the bike seat so that the knees are almost completely extended as the foot goes through the bottom of the pedaling cycle.

2. During the test, keep the speed constant at fifty revolutions per minute. Test duration is six minutes.

3. Select the appropriate work load for the bike based on age, weight, health, and estimated fitness level. For unconditioned individuals: women, use 300 kpm (kilopounds per meter) or 450 kpm; men, 300 kpm or 600 kpm. Conditioned adults: women, 450 kpm or 600 kpm; men, 600 kpm or 900 kpm.[a]

4. Ride the bike for six minutes and check the heart rate every minute, during the last ten seconds of each minute. Determine heart rate by recording the time it takes to count thirty pulse beats, and then converting to beats per minute using Table 2.3.

5. Average the final two heart rates (fifth and sixth minutes). If these two heart rates are not within five beats per minute of each other, continue the test for another few minutes until this is accomplished. If the heart rate continues to climb significantly after the sixth minute, stop the test and rest for fifteen to twenty minutes. You may then retest, preferably at a lower work load. The final average heart rate should also fall between the ranges given for each work load in Table 2.4 (e.g., men: 300 kpm = 120 to 140 beats per minute; 600 kpm = 120 to 170 beats per minute).

6. Based on the average heart rate of the final two minutes and your work load, look up the maximal oxygen uptake in Table 2.4 (e.g., men: 600 kpm and average heart rate = 145, maximal oxygen uptake = 2.4 liters/minute).

7. Correct maximal oxygen uptake using the correction factors found in Table 2.5 (e.g., maximal oxygen uptake = 2.4 and age thirty-five, correction factor = .870. Multiply 2.4 × .870 and final corrected maximal oxygen uptake = 2.09 liters/minute).

8. To obtain maximal oxygen uptake in ml/kg/min, multiply the maximal oxygen uptake by 1,000 (to convert liters to milliliters) and divide by body weight in kilograms (to obtain kilograms, divide your body weight in pounds by 2.2046).

9. Example:

   Corrected maximal oxygen uptake = 2.09 liters/minute
   Body weight = 132 pounds or 60 kilograms (132 ÷ 2.2046 = 60)

   Maximal oxygen uptake in ml/kg/min = 2.09 × 1,000 = 2,090
   2,090 divided by 60 = 34.8 ml/kg/min

[a] On the Monarch bicycle ergometer when riding at a speed of fifty revolutions per minute, a load of 1 kp = 300 kpm, 1.5 kp = 450, 2 kp = 600 kpm, and so forth, with increases of 150 kpm to each ½ kp.

Table 2.3.
Conversion of the Time for 30 Pulse Beats to Pulse Rate Per Minute

Sec.	bpm	Sec.	bpm	Sec.	bpm
22.0	82	17.3	104	12.6	143
21.9	82	17.2	105	12.5	144
21.8	83	17.1	105	12.4	145
21.7	83	17.0	106	12.3	146
21.6	83	16.9	107	12.2	148
21.5	84	16.8	107	12.1	149
21.4	84	16.7	108	12.0	150
21.3	85	16.6	108	11.9	151
21.2	85	16.5	109	11.8	153
21.1	85	16.4	110	11.7	154
21.0	86	16.3	110	11.6	155
20.9	86	16.2	111	11.5	157
20.8	87	16.1	112	11.4	158
20.7	87	16.0	113	11.3	159
20.6	87	15.9	113	11.2	161
20.5	88	15.8	114	11.1	162
20.4	88	15.7	115	11.0	164
20.3	89	15.6	115	10.9	165
20.2	89	15.5	116	10.8	167
20.1	90	15.4	117	10.7	168
20.0	90	15.3	118	10.6	170
19.9	90	15.2	118	10.5	171
19.8	91	15.1	119	10.4	173
19.7	91	15.0	120	10.3	175
19.6	92	14.9	121	10.2	176
19.5	92	14.8	122	10.1	178
19.4	93	14.7	122	10.0	180
19.3	93	14.6	123	9.9	182
19.2	94	14.5	124	9.8	184
19.1	94	14.4	125	9.7	186
19.0	95	14.3	126	9.6	188
18.9	95	14.2	127	9.5	189
18.8	96	14.1	128	9.4	191
18.7	96	14.0	129	9.3	194
18.6	97	13.9	129	9.2	196
18.5	97	13.8	130	9.1	198
18.4	98	13.7	131	9.0	200
18.3	98	13.6	132	8.9	202
18.2	99	13.5	133	8.8	205
18.1	99	13.4	134	8.7	207
18.0	100	13.3	135	8.6	209
17.9	101	13.2	136	8.5	212
17.8	101	13.1	137	8.4	214
17.7	102	13.0	138	8.3	217
17.6	102	12.9	140	8.2	220
17.5	103	12.8	141	8.1	222
17.4	103	12.7	142	8.0	225

Table 2.4.
Maximal Oxygen Uptake Estimates for the Astrand-Ryhming Test in Liters Per Minute (L/min)

	Work Load (kpm/min)									
	Men					Women				
Heart Rate	300	600	900	1200	1500	300	450	600	750	900
120	2.2	3.4	4.8			2.6	3.4	4.1	4.8	
121	2.2	3.4	4.7			2.5	3.3	4.0	4.8	
122	2.2	3.4	4.6			2.5	3.2	3.9	4.7	
123	2.1	3.4	4.6			2.4	3.1	3.9	4.6	
124	2.1	3.3	4.5	6.0		2.4	3.1	3.8	4.5	
125	2.0	3.2	4.4	5.9		2.3	3.0	3.7	4.4	
126	2.0	3.2	4.4	5.8		2.3	3.0	3.6	4.3	
127	2.0	3.1	4.3	5.7		2.2	2.9	3.5	4.2	
128	2.0	3.1	4.2	5.6		2.2	2.8	3.5	4.2	4.8
129	1.9	3.0	4.2	5.6		2.2	2.8	3.4	4.1	4.8
130	1.9	3.0	4.1	5.5		2.1	2.7	3.4	4.0	4.7
131	1.9	2.9	4.0	5.4		2.1	2.7	3.4	4.0	4.6
132	1.8	2.9	4.0	5.3		2.0	2.7	3.3	3.9	4.5
133	1.8	2.8	3.9	5.3		2.0	2.6	3.2	3.8	4.4
134	1.8	2.8	3.9	5.2		2.0	2.6	3.2	3.8	4.4
135	1.7	2.8	3.8	5.1		2.0	2.6	3.1	3.7	4.3
136	1.7	2.7	3.8	5.0		1.9	2.5	3.1	3.6	4.2
137	1.7	2.7	3.7	5.0		1.9	2.5	3.0	3.6	4.2
138	1.6	2.7	3.7	4.9		1.8	2.4	3.0	3.5	4.1
139	1.6	2.6	3.6	4.8		1.8	2.4	2.9	3.5	4.0
140	1.6	2.6	3.6	4.8	6.0	1.8	2.4	2.8	3.4	4.0
141		2.6	3.5	4.7	5.9	1.8	2.3	2.8	3.4	3.9
142		2.5	3.5	4.6	5.8	1.7	2.3	2.8	3.3	3.9
143		2.5	3.4	4.6	5.7	1.7	2.2	2.7	3.3	3.8
144		2.5	3.4	4.5	5.7	1.7	2.2	2.7	3.2	3.8
145		2.4	3.4	4.5	5.6	1.6	2.2	2.7	3.2	3.7
146		2.4	3.3	4.4	5.6	1.6	2.2	2.6	3.2	3.7
147		2.4	3.3	4.4	5.5	1.6	2.1	2.6	3.1	3.6
148		2.4	3.2	4.3	5.4	1.6	2.1	2.6	3.1	3.6
149		2.3	3.2	4.3	5.4		2.1	2.6	3.0	3.5
150		2.3	3.2	4.2	5.3		2.0	2.5	3.0	3.5
151		2.3	3.1	4.2	5.2		2.0	2.5	3.0	3.4
152		2.3	3.1	4.1	5.2		2.0	2.5	2.9	3.4
153		2.2	3.0	4.1	5.1		2.0	2.4	2.9	3.3
154		2.2	3.0	4.0	5.1		2.0	2.4	2.8	3.3
155		2.2	3.0	4.0	5.0		1.9	2.4	2.8	3.2
156		2.2	2.9	4.0	5.0		1.9	2.3	2.8	3.2
157		2.1	2.9	3.9	4.9		1.9	2.3	2.7	3.2
158		2.1	2.9	3.9	4.9		1.8	2.3	2.7	3.1
159		2.1	2.8	3.8	4.8		1.8	2.2	2.7	3.1
160		2.1	2.8	3.8	4.8		1.8	2.2	2.6	3.0
161		2.0	2.8	3.7	4.7		1.8	2.2	2.6	3.0
162		2.0	2.8	3.7	4.6		1.8	2.2	2.6	3.0
163		2.0	2.8	3.7	4.6		1.7	2.2	2.6	2.9
164		2.0	2.7	3.6	4.5		1.7	2.1	2.5	2.9
165		2.0	2.7	3.6	4.5		1.7	2.1	2.5	2.9
166		1.9	2.7	3.6	4.5		1.7	2.1	2.5	2.8
167		1.9	2.6	3.5	4.4		1.6	2.1	2.4	2.8
168		1.9	2.6	3.5	4.4		1.6	2.0	2.4	2.8
169		1.9	2.6	3.5	4.3		1.6	2.0	2.4	2.8
170		1.8	2.6	3.4	4.3		1.6	2.0	2.4	2.7

From Astrand, I. *Acta Physiologica Scandinavica* 49(1960). Supplementum 169:45-60.

Table 2.5.
Age-Based Correction Factors for
Maximal Oxygen Uptake (Astrand-Ryhming Test)

Age	Correction Factor	Age	Correction Factor
14	1.11	40	.830
15	1.10	41	.820
16	1.09	42	.810
17	1.08	43	.800
18	1.07	44	.790
19	1.06	45	.780
20	1.05	46	.774
21	1.04	47	.768
22	1.03	48	.762
23	1.02	49	.756
24	1.01	50	.750
25	1.00	51	.742
26	.987	52	.734
27	.974	53	.726
28	.961	54	.718
29	.948	55	.710
30	.935	56	.704
31	.922	57	.698
32	.909	58	.692
33	.896	59	.686
34	.883	60	.680
35	.870	61	.674
36	.862	62	.668
37	.854	63	.662
38	.846	64	.656
39	.838	65	.650

Adapted from Astrand, I. *Acta Physiologica Scandinavica* 49 (1960). Supplementum 169:45-60.

INTERPRETING YOUR MAXIMAL OXYGEN UPTAKE RESULTS

After obtaining your maximal oxygen uptake by taking any of the three cardiovascular endurance tests, you can determine your current level of cardiovascular fitness using Table 2.6. These guidelines have been developed by the American Heart Association. Locate the maximal oxygen uptake in your respective age category, and on the top row you will find your present level of cardiovascular fitness. For example, a nineteen-year-old male with a maximal oxygen uptake of 41 ml/kg/min would be classified in the average cardiovascular fitness category. Once you have established your maximal oxygen uptake and cardiovascular fitness category, record this information in Figure 2.8 in this chapter and Figure A.1 in Appendix A. After you initiate your personal cardiovascular exercise program, you may wish to retest yourself periodically to evaluate your progress.

PRINCIPLES OF CARDIOVASCULAR EXERCISE PRESCRIPTION

All too often, individuals who exercise regularly and then take a cardiovascular endurance test are surprised to find that they are not as conditioned as they thought they were. Although these individuals may be exercising regularly,

Table 2.6.
Cardiovascular Fitness Classification according to Maximal Oxygen Uptake in ml/kg/min

Sex	Age	Fitness Classification				
		Poor	**Fair**	**Average**	**Good**	**Excellent**
Men	<29	<25	25-33	34-42	43-52	53+
	30-39	<23	23-30	31-38	39-48	49+
	40-49	<20	20-26	27-35	36-44	45+
	50-59	<18	18-24	25-33	34-42	43+
	60-69	<16	16-22	23-30	31-40	41+
Women	<29	<24	24-30	31-37	38-48	49+
	30-39	<20	20-27	28-33	34-44	45+
	40-49	<17	17-23	24-30	31-41	42+
	50-59	<15	15-20	21-27	28-37	38+
	60-69	<13	13-17	18-23	24-34	35+

Reproduced with permission. *Exercise Testing and Training of Apparently Healthy Individuals: A Handbook for Physicians.* American Heart Association.

Figure 2.8. *Cardiovascular endurance report.*

Name:		Age:	Sex:
Date	Test Used	Max VO$_2$	Fitness Classification

they most likely are not following the basic principles for cardiovascular exercise prescription; therefore, they do not reap significant benefits.

For a person to develop the cardiovascular system, the heart muscle has to be overloaded like any other muscle in the human body. Just as the biceps muscle in the upper arm is developed by doing some strength-training exercises, the heart muscle also has to be exercised to increase in size, strength, and efficiency. To better understand how the cardiovascular system can be developed, the four basic principles that govern this development will be discussed. These principles are intensity, mode, duration, and frequency of exercise.

Intensity of Exercise

The intensity of exercise is perhaps the most commonly ignored factor when trying to develop the cardiovascular system. This principle refers to how hard a person has to exercise to improve cardiovascular endurance. Muscles have to be overloaded to a given point for them to develop. While the training stimuli to develop the biceps muscle can be accomplished with arm curl-up exercises, the stimuli for the cardiovascular system is provided by making the heart pump at a higher rate for a certain period of time.

Research has shown that cardiovascular development occurs when working at about 60 to

90 percent of the heart's reserve capacity. Many experts, however, prefer to prescribe exercise between 70 and 85 percent of this capacity. This is done to ensure better and faster development (70 percent) and for safety reasons (85 percent), so that unconditioned individuals will not work too close to maximum capacity. The 70 and 85 percentages can be easily calculated, and training can be monitored by checking your pulse. The following steps are used to determine the intensity of exercise or cardiovascular training zone:

1. Estimate your maximal heart rate (Max. HR). The maximal heart rate is dependent on the person's age and can be estimated according to the following formulas:

    Men = 205 minus one-half the age
    $\quad$ (205 − 1/2 age)
    Women = 220 minus age (220 − age)

2. Check your resting heart rate (RHR) sometime after you have been sitting quietly for fifteen to twenty minutes. You may take your pulse for thirty seconds and multiply by 2 or take it for a full minute.

3. Determine the heart rate reserve (HRR). This is done by subtracting the resting heart rate from the maximal heart rate (HRR = Max. HR − RHR). The heart rate reserve indicates the amount of beats available to go from resting conditions to an all-out maximal effort.

4. The cardiovascular training zone is determined by computing the training intensities

(TI) at 70 and 85 percent. Multiply the heart rate reserve by the respective 70 and 85 percentages and then add the resting heart rate to both of these figures (70 percent TI = HRR × .70 + RHR, and 85 percent TI = HRR × .85 + RHR). Your cardiovascular training zone is found between these two target heart rates.

5. *Example.* The cardiovascular training zone for a twenty-year-old female with a resting heart rate of 72 bpm would be:

Max. HR = 220 − 20 = 200 bpm
RHR = 72 bpm
HRR = 200 − 72 = 128 beats
70 Percent TI = (128 × .70) + 72 = 162 bpm
85 Percent TI = (128 × .85) + 72 = 181 bpm
Cardiovascular training zone = 162 to 181 bpm

The cardiovascular training zone indicates that whenever you exercise to improve the cardiovascular system, you have to maintain the heart rate between the 70 and 85 percent training intensities to obtain adequate development. If you have been physically inactive, you may want to use a 60 percent training intensity during the first few weeks of your exercise program. After a few weeks of training, you should also experience a significant reduction in resting heart rate (ten to twenty beats in eight to twelve weeks). Therefore, you should recompute your target zone periodically. Once you have reached an ideal level of cardiovascular endurance, training in the 70 to 85 percent range will allow you to maintain your fitness level.

Exercise heart rate should be monitored regularly during exercise to make sure that you are training in the respective zone. Wait until you are about five minutes into your exercise session before taking your first rate. When you check the heart rate, count your pulse for ten seconds and then multiply by 6 to get the per-minute pulse rate. Exercise heart rate will remain at the same level for about fifteen seconds following exercise. After fifteen seconds, heart rate will drop rapidly. Do not hesitate to stop to check your pulse during your exercise bout. If the rate is too low, increase the intensity of the exercise. If the rate is too high, slow down.

To develop the cardiovascular system, you do not have to exercise above the 85 percent rate. From a health standpoint, training above this percentage will not add any extra benefits and may actually be unsafe for some individuals. For unconditioned adults, it is recommended that cardiovascular training be conducted around the 70 percent rate. This lower rate is recommended to reduce potential problems associated with high-intensity exercise.

Because many people do not check their heart rate during exercise, an alternative method of prescribing intensity of exercise has become more popular in recent years. This method uses a rate of perceived exertion (RPE) scale developed by Gunnar Borg. Using the scale shown in Figure 2.9, a person subjectively rates the perceived exertion or difficulty of exercise when training in the appropriate target zone. The exercise heart rate is then associated with the corresponding RPE value.

For example, if the training intensity requires a heart rate zone between 150 and 170 bpm, the person would associate this with training between "hard" and "very hard." Some individuals, however, may perceive less exertion than others when training in the correct zone. Therefore, associate your own inner perception of the task with the phrases given on the scale. You may then proceed to exercise at that rate of perceived exertion.

It is important that you cross-check your target zone with your perceived exertion in the initial weeks of your exercise program. To help you develop this association, keep a regular record of your activities using the form provided in Figure 2.12 at the end of the chapter. After several weeks of training, you should be able to predict your exercise heart rate just by your own perceived exertion of the exercise session.

Whether you monitor the intensity of exercise by checking your pulse or through rate of

Figure 2.9. *Rate of perceived exertion scale*

6			
7	Very, very light	14	
8		15	Hard
9	Very light	16	
10		17	Very hard
11	Fairly light	18	
12		19	Very, very hard
13	Somewhat hard	20	

From *Borg, G. "Perceived Exertion: A Note on History and Methods." Medicine and Science in Sports and Exercise* 5:90-93, 1983.

perceived exertion, be aware that changes in normal exercise conditions will affect the training zone. For example, exercising on a hot and/or humid day, or at high altitude, increases the heart rate response to a given task. Consequently, make the necessary adjustments in the intensity of your exercise.

Mode of Exercise

Earlier in the chapter, it was mentioned that the type of exercise that develops the cardiovascular system has to be aerobic in nature. Once you have established your cardiovascular training zone, any activity or combination of activities that will get your heart rate up to that training zone and keep it there for as long as you exercise will yield adequate development. Examples of such activities are walking, jogging, aerobic dancing, swimming, cross-country skiing, rope skipping, cycling, racquetball, stair climbing, and stationary running or cycling.

The activity that you choose should be based on your personal preferences, what you enjoy doing best, and your physical limitations. There may be a difference in the amount of strength or flexibility developed through the use of different activities, but as far as the cardiovascular system is concerned, the heart doesn't know whether you are walking, swimming, or cycling. All the heart knows is that it has to pump at a certain rate, and as long as that rate is in the desired range, cardiovascular development will occur.

If the activity that you select to conduct your aerobic exercise program is either swimming or arm exercises only (such as arm ergometry), you will need to decrease your target training zone by 10 beats per minute. For example, if your target zone is 162 to 181 beats per minute, you would need to train only between 152 and 171 beats per minute. Research has shown that maximal heart rates for swimming and arm exercises are lower than those for running. The lower maximal heart rates are attributed to the lesser muscle mass involved (primarily upper body) in these activities, as well as the cooler water temperature and the horizontal body position in swimming.

Duration of Exercise

Regarding the duration of exercise, it is recommended that a person train between fifteen and sixty minutes per session. The duration is based on how intensely a person trains. If the training is done around 85 to 90 percent, fifteen to twenty minutes are sufficient. At the 60 to 70 percent intensity, the person should train for at least thirty minutes. As mentioned earlier, under intensity of training, unconditioned adults should train at the lower percentage; therefore, a minimum of thirty minutes of exercise is required.

As a part of the training session, always include a five-minute warm-up and a five-minute cool-down period. Your warm-up should consist of general calisthenics, stretching exercises, or exercising at a lower intensity level than the actual target zone. To cool down, gradually decrease the intensity of exercise. Do not stop abruptly. This will cause blood to pool in the exercised body parts, thereby diminishing the return of blood to the heart. A decreased blood return can cause dizziness, faintness, or even induce cardiac abnormalities.

Frequency of Exercise

Ideally, a person should engage in aerobic exercise four or five days per week. Research has indicated that to maintain cardiovascular fitness, a training session should be conducted about every forty-eight hours. Three twenty- to thirty-minute training sessions per week, done on nonconsecutive days, will maintain cardiovascular endurance *as long as the heart rate is in the appropriate target zone.*

TIPS FOR IMPLEMENTING AN EXERCISE PROGRAM

Best Time to Exercise

Exercise can be carried out at almost any time of the day with the exception of a period of two to three hours following a heavy meal, or the noon and early afternoon hours on hot and humid days. Many people enjoy exercising early in the morning because it gives them a good boost to start the day. Others prefer the lunch hour for weight control reasons. By exercising at noon, they do not eat as big a lunch, which helps keep daily caloric intake down. Highly stressed people seem to like the evening hours because of the relaxing effects of exercise.

Effects of Temperature and Humidity

Be aware that it is not recommended to exercise in hot and humid conditions. When a person exercises, only 30 to 40 percent of the energy produced in the body is used for mechanical work or movement. The rest of the energy (60-70 percent) is converted into heat. If this heat cannot be properly dissipated because it is either too hot or the relative humidity is too high, body temperature will increase, and in extreme cases death can occur.

The specific heat of body tissue (the heat required to raise the temperature of the body by one degree Centigrade) is .38 calories per pound of body weight per one degree Centigrade (.38 cal/lb/°C). This indicates that if no body heat is dissipated, a 150-pound person would need to burn only 57 calories (150 x .38) to increase total body temperature by 1° C. If this person were to conduct an exercise session requiring 300 calories (about three miles running) without any heat dissipation, inner body temperature would increase by 5.3° C, which is the equivalent of going from 98.6 to 108.1 degrees Fahrenheit (°F)!

The above example clearly illustrates why caution should be used when exercising in hot or humid weather. If the relative humidity is too high, body heat cannot be lost through evaporation because the atmosphere is already saturated with water vapor. In one specific instance, a football casualty occurred at a temperature of only 64° F, but at a relative humidity of 100 percent. Caution must be taken when air temperature is above 90° F and the relative humidity is above 60 percent.

Perhaps the best recommendation is to watch for typical heat-related symptoms. These symptoms usually include cramping, weakness, headaches, dizziness, confusion, hyperventilation, and nausea or vomiting. The sweating mechanism usually stops before severe symptoms occur. If you notice any of these changes when you exercise, stop your work-out, allow yourself to recover in a cool environment, and replace fluids adequately.

The American College of Sports Medicine has recommended that individuals should not engage in strenuous physical activity when the readings of a wet bulb globe thermometer exceed 82.4° F. With this type of thermometer, the wet bulb is cooled by evaporation, and on dry days it will show a lower temperature than the regular (dry) thermometer. On humid days the cooling effect is less because of decreased evaporation; hence the difference between the wet and dry readings is not as great.

In contrast to hot and humid conditions, exercising in the cold usually does not pose a threat to the individual's health because adequate clothing for heat conservation can be worn and exercise itself will increase body heat production. The popular belief that exercising in cold temperatures (32° F and lower) freezes the lungs is totally false, because the air is properly warmed in the air passages before it ever reaches the lungs. It is not cold that poses a threat but, rather, the velocity of the wind that has a great effect on the chill factor.

For example, exercising at a temperature of 25° F with adequate clothing is not too cold, but if the wind is blowing at twenty-five miles per hour, the chill factor reduces the actual temperature to 5° F. This effect is even worse if you are wet and exhausted. Wet clothing loses approximately 90 percent of its insulating properties.

When exercising in the cold, it is important that you protect the face, head, hands, and feet, as they may be subject to frostbite even when the lungs are under no risk. In cold temperatures, about 30 percent of the body's heat is lost through the head's surface area if it is unprotected. Wearing several layers of lightweight clothing is preferable over one single thick layer, because warm air is trapped between layers of clothes, allowing for greater heat conservation.

Importance of Clothing

The type of clothing that you wear during exercise is important. Clothing should fit you comfortably and allow for free movement of the various body parts. You should also select your clothes according to ambient temperature and humidity. Avoid nylon and rubberized materials and tight clothes that will interfere with the cooling mechanism of the human body or obstruct normal blood flow. Proper-fitting shoes, manufactured specifically for your choice of activity, are also recommended to prevent lower limb injuries.

Shin Splints

One of the most common types of injury to the lower limbs is shin splints. This injury is characterized by pain and irritation in the shin region of the leg and is usually the result of one or more of the following: (a) lack of proper and gradual conditioning; (b) conducting physical activities on hard surfaces (wooden floors, hard tracks, cement, and asphalt); (c) fallen arches; (d) chronic overuse; (e) muscle fatigue; (f) faulty posture; (g) inadequate shoes; (h) being excessively overweight and participating in weight-bearing activities.

Shin splints may be managed by: (a) removing or reducing the causing agent (exercising on softer surfaces, wearing better shoes and/or arch supports, or completely stopping exercise until the shin splints heal); (b) doing mild stretching exercises before and after physical activity; (c) use of ice massage for ten to twenty minutes prior to and following physical participation; and (d) applying active heat (whirlpool and hot baths) for fifteen minutes, two to three times a day. In addition, supportive taping during physical activity is helpful. The proper taping technique can be easily learned from a qualified athletic trainer.

Safe Limits

As you initiate your exercise program, be sure to stay within the safe limits for exercise participation. The best method to determine whether you are exercising too strenuously is by checking your heart rate and making sure that it does not exceed the limits of your target zone. Exercising above this target zone may not be safe for unconditioned or high-risk individuals. Keep in mind that you do not need to exercise beyond your target zone to provide the desired benefits for the cardiovascular system.

Signs of Distress

There are several physiological signs that will tell you when you are exceeding functional limitations. A very rapid or irregular heart rate, labored breathing, nausea, vomiting, light-headedness, headaches, dizziness, pale skin, flushness, excessive weakness, lack of energy, shakiness, sore muscles, cramps, and tightness in the chest are all signs of exercise intolerance. One of the basic things that you will need to learn is to listen to your body. If you experience any of these signs, you should seek medical attention before continuing your exercise program.

Your recovery heart rate can also be an indicator of overexertion. To a certain extent, recovery heart rate is related to fitness level. The higher your cardiovascular fitness level, the faster your heart rate will decrease following exercise. As a general rule of thumb, heart rate should be below 120 beats per minute five minutes into recovery. If your heart rate is above 120, you have most likely overexerted yourself or could possibly have some other cardiac abnormality. If you decrease the intensity or duration of exercise, or both, and you still experience a fast heart rate five minutes into recovery, you should consult your physician regarding this condition.

Another sign of distress that sometimes occurs during exercise is side stitch. The exact cause of this sharp pain is unknown. Some experts have suggested that it could be related to a lack of blood flow to the respiratory muscles during strenuous physical exertion. This stitch seems to occur only in unconditioned beginners or trained individuals when they exercise at higher intensities than usual. As you improve your physical condition, this problem will disappear unless you start training at a higher intensity. Whenever you experience this problem, you need to slow down, and if it still persists, stop altogether.

Breathing

Natural breathing during aerobic activity is necessary to prevent the early onset of fatigue. During aerobic work, a greater amount of oxygen is required to produce the energy necessary to do the required task. Therefore, allow your body to freely breathe through your mouth and nose. Do not attempt to regulate your own respiration by consciously altering the natural breathing pattern. The human body will automatically regulate ventilation during exercise. Any attempt on your part to modify this pattern will result in decreased efficiency of the cardiorespiratory system.

Muscle Cramps

Muscle cramps may occur during exercise. Cramps are caused by the body's depletion of essential electrolytes, or a breakdown in the coordination between opposing muscle groups, or a decrease in blood flow to active muscle tissue as a result of tight clothing. If you have a muscle cramp, initially you should attempt to stretch the muscles involved. For example, in the case of the calf muscle, pull your toes up toward the knees. After stretching the muscle, gently rub them down, and finally do some mild exercises that require the use of that particular muscle.

In many instances, and primarily in pregnant and lactating women, muscle cramps are related to a lack of calcium. Women who experience cramps during these periods are given calcium supplements, which usually relieve the problem.

GETTING STARTED AND ENJOYING THE BENEFITS OF A LIFETIME EXERCISE PROGRAM

Having learned the basic principles of cardiovascular exercise prescription, you can proceed to Figure 2.10 and fill out your own prescription. A gradual increase in intensity, duration, and frequency is used in this exercise prescription. Although you could go ahead and attempt to train five or six times per week for thirty minutes at a time, if you have not been exercising regularly, you may find this discouraging and may drop out before getting too far. The reason for this is that as you initiate the program, you will probably develop some muscle soreness and stiffness, and possibly minor injuries.

According to several reports, more than half of those who begin an exercise program drop out in the initial six weeks because of injuries. Muscle soreness, stiffness, and the risk for injuries can be reduced or eliminated by progressively increasing the intensity, duration, and frequency of exercise as outlined in Figure 2.10. You may also want to use the computer software (see Figure 2.11) to obtain a printout of your personalized cardiovascular exercise prescription. Additionally, you can maintain a record of your exercise program by using the cardiovascular exercise record form given in Figure 2.12, or you may create and regularly update a computer file by using the EXLOG computer program available through Morton Publishing Company (see Figure 2.13).

Once you have determined your exercise prescription, the difficult part begins: starting and sticking to a lifetime exercise program. Although you may be motivated after reading the benefits to be derived through physical activity, it takes a lifetime of dedication and perseverance to maintain good fitness. The first few weeks are probably

the most difficult, but "if there is a will, there is a way." Once you begin to see positive changes, it won't be as difficult. Very soon you will develop a habit for exercise that will bring about a deep satisfaction and sense of self-accomplishment. The following suggestions have been used successfully by others.

1. Select aerobic activities that you enjoy doing. Picking an activity that you don't enjoy decreases your chances for exercise adherence. Don't be afraid of trying out a new activity, even if that means learning new skills.

2. Use a combination of activities. You can train by using two or three activities the same week. For some people this decreases the monotony of repeating the same activity every day. Try lifetime sports. Many endurance sports such as racquetball, basketball, soccer, badminton, rollerskating, cross-country skiing, and surfing (paddling the board) provide a nice break from regular workouts.

3. Set aside a regular time for exercise. If you don't plan ahead, it is a lot easier to skip. Holding your exercise hour "sacred" helps you adhere to the program.

4. Obtain adequate equipment for exercise. A poor pair of shoes, for example, can increase the risk for injury, leading to discouragement right from the beginning.

5. Find a friend or group of friends to exercise with. The social interaction will make exercise more fulfilling. Besides, it's harder to skip if someone else is waiting for you.

6. Set goals and share them with others. It is tougher to quit when someone else knows what you are trying to accomplish. When you reach a particular goal, reward yourself with a new pair of shoes or a jogging suit.

7. Don't become a chronic exerciser. Learn to listen to your body. Overexercising can lead to chronic fatigue and injuries. Exercise should be enjoyable, and in the process you should "stop and smell the roses."

8. Exercise in different places and facilities. This practice will add variety to your work-outs.

9. Keep a regular record of your activities. In this manner, you will be able to monitor your progress and compare with previous months and years.

10. Conduct periodic assessments. Improving to a higher fitness category is a reward in itself.

11. See a physician when health problems arise. When in doubt, "it's better to be safe than sorry."

Maintaining Cardiovascular Fitness

To maintain adequate fitness, it is recommended that you maintain a regular exercise program, even during vacations. If you have to interrupt your program for reasons beyond your control, do not attempt to resume your training at the same level you left off, but rather build up gradually again.

The length of time involved in losing the benefits of exercise varies among the different components of physical fitness and also depends on the type of condition achieved prior to cessation. In regard to cardiovascular endurance, it has been estimated that four weeks of aerobic training are completely reversed in two consecutive weeks of physical inactivity. On the other hand, if you have been exercising regularly for months or years, two weeks of inactivity will not hurt you as much as someone who has exercised only a few weeks. As a rule of thumb, after only forty-eight hours of aerobic inactivity, the cardiovascular system starts to lose some of its capacity. (Flexibility can be maintained with two or three stretching sessions per week, and strength is easily maintained with just one maximal training session per week.)

Remember that the benefits of fitness can be maintained only through a regular lifetime program. Exercise is not like putting money in the bank. It does not help to exercise four or five hours on Saturday and not do anything else the rest of the week. If anything, exercising only once a week is unsafe for unconditioned adults. Even the greatest athlete on earth, if he/she stops exercising, after only a few years would be at a similar risk for disease as someone who has never done any physical activity. Staying with a physical fitness program long enough will cause positive physiological and psychological changes, and once you are there, you will not want to have it any other way.

Bibliography

American College of Sports Medicine. *Guidelines for Graded Exercise Testing and Exercise Prescription.* Philadelphia: Lea & Febiger, 1986.

American Heart Association Committee on Exercise. *Exercise Testing and Training of Apparently Healthy Individuals: A Handbook for Physicians.* New York: AHA, 1972.

Arnheim, D. D. *Modern Principles of Athletic Training.* St. Louis: Times Mirror/Mosby College Publishing, 1985.

Astrand, I. *Acta Physiologica Scandinavica* 49, 1960. Supplementum 169:45-60, 1960.

Astrand, P. O., and K. Rodahl. *Textbook of Work Physiology.* New York: McGraw-Hill, 1977.

Borg, G. "Perceived Exertion: A Note on History and Methods." *Medicine and Science in Sports and Exercise* 5:90-93, 1973.

Cooper, K. H. "A Means of Assessing Maximal Oxygen Intake." *JAMA* 203:201-204, 1968.

Cooper, K. H. *The Aerobics Program for Total Well-Being.* New York: Mount Evans and Co., 1982.

Cureton, Thomas K. *The Physiological Effects of Exercise Programs Upon Adults.* New York: Dial Press, Inc., 1965.

Fixx, J. F. *The Complete Book of Running.* New York: Random House, 1977.

Fox, E. L., and D. K. Mathews. *The Physiological Basis of Physical Education and Athletics.* Philadelphia: Saunders College Publishing, 1988.

Hoeger, W. W. K. *Ejercicio, Salud y Vida* [Exercise, Health and Life]. Caracas, Venezuela: Editorial Arte, 1980.

Hoeger, W. W. K. *Principles and Laboratories for Physical Fitness & Wellness.* Englewood, CO: Morton Publishing, 1988.

Karvonen, M. J., E. Kentala, and O. Mustala. "The Effects of Training on the Heart Rate, a Longitudinal Study." *Annales Medicinae Experimetalis et Biologiae Fenniae* 35:307-315, 1957.

McArdle, W. D., F. I. Katch, and V. L. Katch. *Exercise Physiology: Energy, Nutrition and Human Performance.* Philadelphia: Lea & Febiger, 1986.

Pollock, M. L., J. H. Wilmore, and S. M. Fox III. *Health and Fitness Through Physical Activity.* New York: John Wiley & Sons, 1978.

Wilmore, J. H. *Training for Sport and Activity.* Boston: Allyn and Bacon, 1988.

Figure 2.10. *Cardiovascular exercise prescription form*

Name: _____ Date: _____

Intensity of Exercise

1. Estimate your own maximal heart rate (Max. HR). Women use 220 minus age (220 − age), men use 205 minus one-half the age (205 − ½ age).

   Max. HR = _____ − _____ = _____ bpm

2. Determine your resting Heart Rate (RHR) = _____ bpm

3. Heart Rate Reserve (HRR) = Max. HR − RHR

   HRR = _____ − _____ = _____ beats

4. Training Intensities (TI) = HRR × %TI + RHR

TI	=	HRR	×	%TI	+	RHR		

   60 Percent TI   = _____ × .60 + _____ = _____ bpm

   70 Percent TI   = _____ × .70 + _____ = _____ bpm

   85 Percent TI   = _____ × .85 + _____ = _____ bpm

5. Cardiovascular Training Zone. The optimum cardiovascular training zone is found between the 70 and 85 percent training intensities. However, individuals that have been physically inactive or are in the poor or fair cardiovascular fitness categories should use a 60 percent training intensity during the first few weeks of the exercise program.

   Cardiovascular Training Zone: _____ (70% TI) to _____ (85% TI)

   Rate of Perceived Exertion (see Figure 2.9): _____

Mode of Exercise

Select any activity or combination of activities that you enjoy doing. The activity has to be continuous in nature and must get your heart rate up to the cardiovascular training zone and keep it there for as long as you exercise.

Mode(s) of Exercise: _____

Cardiovascular Exercise Prescription

The following is your weekly program for cardiovascular endurance development. If you are in the average, good, or excellent fitness category, you may start at week five. After completing this twelve-week program, in order for you to maintain your fitness level, you should exercise in the 70 to 85 percent training zone for about twenty to thirty minutes, a minimum of three

(continued)

Figure 2.10. *Cardiovascular exercise prescription form (continued)*

times per week, on nonconsecutive days. You should also recompute your target zone period-ically because you will experience a significant reduction in resting heart rate with aerobic train-ing (approximately ten to twenty beats in about eight to twelve weeks).

Week	Duration (min.)	Frequency	Training Intensity	10-Sec. Pulse Count[a]
1	15	3	Approximately 60%	
2	15	4	Approximately 60%	
3	20	4	Approximately 60%	_____ beats
4	20	5	Approximately 60%	
5	20	4	About 70%	
6	20	5	About 70%	
7	30	4	About 70%	_____ beats
8	30	5	About 70%	
9	30	4	Between 70% and 85%	
10	30	5	Between 70% and 85%	
11	30-40	5	Between 70% and 85%	_____ to _____ beats
12	30-40	5-6	Between 70% and 85%	

[a] Fill out your own 10-sec. pulse count under this column.

Figure 2.11. *Sample computerized exercise prescription**

```
       LIFETIME PHYSICAL FITNESS & WELLNESS: A PERSONALIZED PROGRAM
                         by Werner W.K. Hoeger
                       Morton Publishing Company

             PERSONALIZED CARDIOVASCULAR EXERCISE PRESCRIPTION


    Jane Doe                       Age: 20           Date: 02-10-1989
    Maximal heart rate: 200 bpm         Resting heart rate: 76 bpm
    Present cardiovascular fitness level: Fair

    The following is your personal program for cardiovascular fit-
    ness development and/or maintenance.   If you have been exer-
    cising regularly and you are in the average  or good category,
    you may start at week five.   If you are in the excellent cate-
    gory, you can start at week nine.

       Week    Time    Frequency  Training Intensity       Pulse
              (min.)  (per week)  (beats per minute) (10 sec. count)
      -----------------------------------------------------------------
        1      15         3       Approx. 150          25 beats
        2      15         4       Approx. 150          25 beats
        3      20         4       Approx. 150          25 beats
        4      20         5       Approx. 150          25 beats
        5      20         4        About 163           27 beats
        6      20         5        About 163           27 beats
        7      30         4        About 163           27 beats
        8      30         5        About 163           27 beats
        9      30         4       163 to 181           27 to 30
       10      30         5       163 to 181           27 to 30
       11    30--40       5       163 to 181           27 to 30
       12    30--40      5-6      163 to 181           27 to 30
      -----------------------------------------------------------------
    You may participate in any combination of activities which are
    aerobic  and continuous in nature,  such as walking,  jogging,
    swimming,  cross country skiing,  rope skipping,  cycling,  aero-
    bic dancing,  racquetball,  stair climbing,  stationary running
    or cycling, etc. As long as the heart rate reaches the desired
    rate,  and it stays at that level for the period of time indi-
    cated, the cardiovascular system will improve.

    Following the twelve week program,  in order to maintain  your
    fitness level, you should exercise between 163 and 181 bpm for
    about 30 minutes, a minimum of three times per week on noncon-
    secutive days.

    When you exercise, allow about 5 minutes for a gradual warm-up
    period and another  5 for gradual  cool-down.   Also, when you
    check your exercise heart rate,  only count your pulse for  10
    seconds (start counting with 0) and then refer to the above 10
    sec. pulse count.  You may also multiply by  6 to obtain  your
    rate in beats per minute.

    Good cardiovascular fitness will greatly contribute toward the
    enhancement and maintenance of good health.   It is especially
    important in the prevention of coronary heart disease.  We en-
    courage you to be persistent  in your exercise program and  to
    participate regularly.  Best of luck Jane.
```

*Software available through Morton Publishing Company.

Figure 2.12. *Cardiovascular exercise record form*

Name _____

Month _____

Date	Body Weight	Exercise Heart Rate	Type of Exercise	Distance In Miles	Time Hrs/Min	RPE*
1						
2						
3						
4						
5						
6						
7						
8						
9						
10						
11						
12						
13						
14						
15						
16						
17						
18						
19						
20						
21						
22						
23						
24						
25						
26						
27						
28						
29						
30						
31						
Total						

*Rate of perceived exertion.

Month _____

Date	Body Weight	Exercise Heart Rate	Type of Exercise	Distance In Miles	Time Hrs/Min	RPE*
1						
2						
3						
4						
5						
6						
7						
8						
9						
10						
11						
12						
13						
14						
15						
16						
17						
18						
19						
20						
21						
22						
23						
24						
25						
26						
27						
28						
29						
30						
31						
Total						

*Rate of perceived exertion.

Figure 2.12. *Cardiovascular exercise record form (continued)*

Name _____

Month _____

Date	Body Weight	Exercise Heart Rate	Type of Exercise	Distance In Miles	Time Hrs/Min	RPE*
1						
2						
3						
4						
5						
6						
7						
8						
9						
10						
11						
12						
13						
14						
15						
16						
17						
18						
19						
20						
21						
22						
23						
24						
25						
26						
27						
28						
29						
30						
31						
Total						

*Rate of perceived exertion.

Month _____

Date	Body Weight	Exercise Heart Rate	Type of Exercise	Distance In Miles	Time Hrs/Min	RPE*
1						
2						
3						
4						
5						
6						
7						
8						
9						
10						
11						
12						
13						
14						
15						
16						
17						
18						
19						
20						
21						
22						
23						
24						
25						
26						
27						
28						
29						
30						
31						
Total						

*Rate of perceived exertion.

Figure 2.13. *Sample monthly exercise record using the EXLOG (Exercise Log) Computer Program**

LIFETIME PHYSICAL FITNESS & WELLNESS: A PERSONALIZED PROGRAM
By Werner W.K. Hoeger
Morton Publishing Company - Englewood, Colorado

MONTHLY EXERCISE LOG

Jane Anderson
999 North Street
Boise, ID 99999

Month of June 1987

Date	Body Weight	Type of Exercise	Exercise Heart Rate	Duration of Exercise	Distance (miles)	Calories Burned
1	148.0	Jogging 8.5 min/mile	162	27 min.	3.0	360
3	147.5	Jogging 8.5 min/mile	178	15 min.	2.0	199
		Bowling	90	60 min.	0.0	266
5	147.5	Jogging 8.5 min/mile	172	27 min.	3.0	358
6	147.0	Jogging 8.5 min/mile	156	44 min.	5.0	582
		Tennis (competition)	120	45 min.	0.0	423
8	147.0	Jogging 7 min/mile	178	15 min.	2.0	225
11	147.0	Jogging 8.5 min/mile	150	18 min.	2.0	238
13	146.5	Jogging 8.5 min/mile	150	90 min.	10.0	1,187
15	146.0	Racquetball	144	60 min.	0.0	569
16	146.5	Jogging 8.5 min/mile	156	26 min.	3.0	343
17	146.0	Jogging 7 min/mile	178	14 min.	2.0	208
		Basketball (mod)	132	45 min.	0.0	302
19	146.5	Jogging 8.5 min/mile	156	25 min.	3.0	330
20	145.7	Jogging 8.5 min/mile	150	90 min.	10.0	1,180
		Swimming 45 yrds/min	144	30 min.	0.8	249
		Golf	100	100 min.	0.0	437
22	145.5	Jogging 7 min/mile	168	22 min.	3.0	327
24	145.0	Jogging 8.5 min/mile	150	42 min.	5.0	548
25	145.0	Walking (4.5 mph)	100	60 min.	4.0	392
26	144.5	Racquetball	144	60 min.	0.0	564
27	145.2	Jogging 8.5 min/mile	156	88 min.	10.0	1,150
		Golf	100	120 min.	0.0	523
29	145.0	Jogging 8.5 min/mile	156	32 min.	4.0	418
30	144.5	Racquetball	144	60 min.	0.0	564
		Weight Training	120	30 min.	0.0	217

MONTHLY SUMMARY

Average body weight:	146.1 lbs.
Average exercise heart rate:	144 bpm
Total number of days exercised:	19 days
Average exercise time/day:	66 min.
Total number of calories burned:	12,157
Average number of calories per day exercised:	640
Total number of miles run:	67
Total number of miles swum:	1
Total number of miles walked:	4

*Software available through Morton Publishing Company.

Muscular Strength Assessment And Prescription

Many people are still under the impression that muscular strength and endurance are necessary only for athletes and other individuals who hold jobs that require heavy muscular work. Strength and endurance, however, are important components of total physical fitness and have become an integral part of everyone's life.

Adequate levels of strength significantly enhance a person's health and well-being throughout life. A basic component of fitness and wellness, strength is crucial for optimum performance in daily activities such as sitting, walking, running, lifting and carrying objects, doing housework, or even for enjoying recreational activities. Strength is also of great value in improving posture, personal appearance, and self-image; in developing sports skills; and in meeting certain emergencies in life in which strength is necessary to cope effectively. From a health standpoint, strength helps maintain muscle tissue and a higher resting metabolism, decreases the risk for injury, helps prevent and eliminate chronic low back pain, and is an important factor in childbearing.

RELATIONSHIP BETWEEN STRENGTH AND METABOLISM

Perhaps one of the most significant benefits of maintaining a good strength level is its relationship to human metabolism. Metabolism is defined as all energy and material transformations that occur within living cells. A primary result of a strength-training program is an increase in muscle size (lean body mass), known as muscle hypertrophy.

Several studies have shown that there is a direct relationship between oxygen consumption as a result of metabolic activity and amount of lean body mass. Muscle tissue uses energy even at rest, whereas fatty tissue uses very little energy and may be considered metabolically inert from the point of view of caloric use. As muscle size increases, so does the resting metabolism or the amount of energy (expressed in calories) required by an individual during resting conditions to sustain proper cell function. Even small increases in muscle mass increase resting metabolism. Estimates indicate that each additional pound of muscle tissue increases resting metabolism by 50 to 100 calories per day. All other factors being equal, if there are two individuals at 150 pounds with different amounts of muscle mass, let's say five pounds, the one with the greater muscle mass will have a higher resting metabolic rate, allowing this person to eat more calories to maintain the muscle tissue.

Loss of lean tissue is also the main reason for the decrease in metabolism as people grow older. Contrary to some beliefs, metabolism does not slow down with aging. It is not so much that metabolism slows down; it's that we slow down. Lean body mass decreases with sedentary living, which, in turn, slows down the resting metabolic rate. If people continue eating at the same rate, body fat increases. The average decrease in resting metabolism for a sixty-year-old individual is about 360 calories per day as compared to a twenty-six-year-old person. Hence, participating in a strength-training program is an important factor in the prevention and reduction of obesity.

WOMEN AND STRENGTH TRAINING

Because of the increase in muscle mass commonly seen in men who are involved in strength training, many women believe that strength training will make them look muscular and less feminine. Although the quality of muscle in men and women is the same, endocrinological differences will not allow women to achieve the same amount of muscle hypertrophy (size) as men.

The thought that strength training will make women less feminine is as false as to think that playing basketball will turn them into giants. Masculinity and femininity are established by genetic inheritance and not by the amount of physical activity. Variations in the degree of masculinity and femininity are determined by individual differences in hormonal secretions of androgen, testosterone, estrogen, and progesterone. Women with a bigger-than-average build are often inclined to participate in sports because of their natural physical advantage. As a result, many women have associated sports and strength participation with increased masculinity.

As the number of women who participate in sports has steadily increased in the last few years, the myth that strength training masculinizes women has gradually been dissipating. For example, per pound of body weight, women gymnasts are considered to be among the strongest athletes in the world. These athletes engage in very serious strength-training programs and for their body size are most likely twice as strong as the average male. Yet, as illustrated by the athlete in Figure 3.1., women gymnasts are among the most graceful and feminine of all women. In recent years, increased femininity has become the rule rather than the exception for women who participate in strength-training programs.

Even so, you may ask yourself, "If weight training does not masculinize women, why do so many women body builders develop such heavy musculature?" In the sport of body building, the athletes follow intense training routines consisting of two or more hours of constant weight lifting with very short rest intervals between sets. Many times during the training routine, back-to-back exercises requiring the use of the same muscle groups are performed.

The objective of this type of training is to "pump" extra blood into the muscles, which makes the muscles appear much bigger than they really are in resting conditions. Based on the

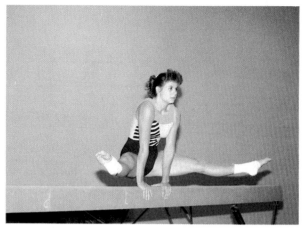

Figure 3.1. *Female gymnast performing a strength skill on the balance beam.*

intensity and the length of the training session, the muscles can remain filled with blood, appearing measurably larger for several hours after completing the training session. Therefore, in real life, these women are not as muscular as they seem when they are "pumped up" for a contest.

In the sport of body building, a big point of controversy is the use of anabolic steroids and human growth hormones, even among women participants. Anabolic steroids are synthetic versions of the male sex hormone testosterone, which promotes muscle development and hypertrophy. The use of these hormones, however, can produce detrimental and undesirable side-effects, which some women deem tolerable (e.g., hypertension, fluid retention, decreased breast size, deepening of the voice, facial whiskers, and body hair growth). The use of these steroids among women is definitely on the increase and, according to Dr. William Taylor, sports medicine physician in Florida, Dr. Robert Kerr, sports medicine physician in Southern California, and Carol Turner, body builder in Los Angeles, about eighty percent of women body builders have used steroids. Furthermore, several women's track-and-field coaches have indicated that as many as ninety-five percent of women athletes in this sport around the world have used anabolic steroids in order to remain competitive at the international level.

There is no doubt that women who take steroids will indeed build heavy musculature like men, and if they are taken long enough, the steroids will have masculinizing effects. As a result, the International Federation of Body Building has instituted a mandatory steroid-testing program among women participating in the Miss Olympia contest.

When drugs are not used to promote development, increased health and femininity are the rule rather than the exception among women who participate in body building, strength training, and sports in general. The use of steroids will masculinize women and destroy the feminine charm that sports participation helps develop.

Another benefit of strength training, which is accentuated even more when combined with aerobic exercise, is a decrease in adipose or fatty tissue around the muscle fibers themselves. Research has shown that in women the decrease in fatty tissue is greater than the amount of muscle hypertrophy. Therefore, it is not at all uncommon to lose inches and yet not lose body weight. Nevertheless, because muscle tissue is more dense than fatty tissue, and in spite of the fact that inches are being lost, women often become discouraged because the results cannot be readily seen on the scale. This discouragement can be easily offset by regularly determining body composition to monitor changes in percent body fat rather than simply measuring total body weight changes. Figure 3.2 compares body composition before and after a combined aerobic- and strength-training program.

MUSCULAR STRENGTH AND ENDURANCE ASSESSMENT

Although muscular strength and endurance are interrelated, a basic difference exists between the two. Strength is defined as the ability to exert maximum force against resistance. Endurance is the ability of a muscle to exert submaximal force repeatedly over a period of time. Muscular endurance depends to a large extent on muscular strength, and to a lesser extent on cardiovascular endurance. Weak muscles cannot repeat an action several times or sustain it for a prolonged period of time. Keeping these two principles in mind, strength tests and training programs have been designed to measure and develop absolute muscular strength, muscular endurance, or a combination of both.

Muscular strength is usually determined by the maximal amount of resistance (one repetition maximum or 1 RM) that an individual is able to lift in a single effort. This assessment gives a good measure of absolute strength, but it does require a considerable amount of time because the 1 RM is determined through trial and error. For example, the strength of the chest muscles is frequently measured with the bench press exercise. If the individual has not trained with weights, he/she may try 100 pounds and find out that this resistance is lifted quite easily. Then fifty pounds are added, but the person fails to lift the resistance. The resistance is then decreased by ten or twenty pounds, and finally, after several trials, the 1 RM is established. Fatigue also becomes a factor, because by the time the 1 RM is established, several maximal or near-maximal attempts have already been performed. Muscular endurance is commonly established by the number of repetitions that an individual can perform against a submaximal resistance or by the length of time that a given contraction can be sustained.

As with cardiovascular endurance assessment, you will be given a choice of three tests to

Figure 3.2. *Graphic illustration of body composition changes as a result of a combined aerobic- and strength-training program*

PRE-TRAINING   POST-TRAINING

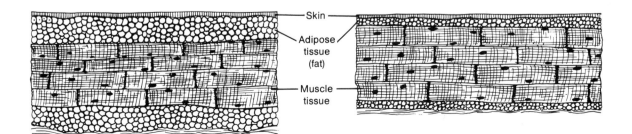

determine your strength and/or endurance levels. Your test selection should be based primarily on the facilities available to you and secondarily on whether you have been on a strength-training program recently. Because there is a small increased risk of injury for individuals attempting a maximal contraction if they have not been lifting regularly, it is perhaps best for these individuals to avoid an absolute strength test.

After you have selected your test, go directly to the procedures that explain the respective test. For safety reasons, always take a friend or group of friends with you whenever you train with weights or conduct any type of strength assessment. Also, because these are three different tests, to make valid comparisons, you should use the same test for pre- and post-assessments.

1. **Muscular Strength and Endurance Test.** In this test (see Figure 3.3), you will lift a submaximal resistance as many times as possible on six different weight-training lifts. The resistance for each lift is determined according to selected percentages of body weight. If you

Figure 3.3. *Procedure for the Muscular Strength and Endurance Test*

1. A sixteen-station, fixed resistance, Universal Gym® apparatus is required to perform this test.

2. Familiarize yourself with the six lifts used for this test: lateral pull-down, leg extension (quad lift), bench press, sit-up, leg curl, and arm curl. Graphic illustrations for each lift are given at the end of this chapter. For the leg curl exercise, the knees should be flexed to 90°. For the sit-up exercise, use a horizontal plane, hold the weight behind the neck, have a partner hold your feet, and keep the knees at a 100° angle. For the lateral pull-down exercise, use a sitting position and have your partner hold you down by the waist. On the leg extension lift, maintain the trunk in an upright position.

3. Determine your body weight in pounds.

4. Determine the amount of resistance to be used on each lift. To obtain this number, multiply your body weight by the percent given below for each lift.

Lift	Percent of Body Weight	
	Men	Women
Lateral Pull-Down	.70	.45
Leg Extension (Quad Lift)	.65	.50
Bench Press	.75	.45
Sit-Up	.16	.10
Leg Curl	.32	.25
Arm Curl	.35	.18

5. Perform the maximum continuous number of repetitions possible.

6. Based on the number of repetitions performed, look up the percentile rank for each lift in the far left column of Table 3.1.

7. An overall strength fitness category can be obtained by determining an average percentile score for all six lifts (see Figure 3.4). Determine your overall muscular endurance fitness category according to the following ratings:

Average Score	Endurance Classification
80+	Excellent
60-79	Good
40-59	Average
20-39	Fair
<19	Poor

Test developed by Hoeger, W. W. K., and D. R. Hopkins. "A Six-Item Muscular Strength Test Based on Selected Percentages of Body Weight." Copyright 1986.

Figure 3.4. *Data form for the Muscular Strength and Endurance Test*

Name: _____ Sex: _____ Date: _____

Body Weight: _____ lbs.

Lift	% Body Weight		Resistance	Repetitions	% Rank
	Men	Women			
Lateral Pull-Down	.70	.45			
Leg Extension	.65	.50			
Bench Press	.75	.45			
Sit-Up	.16	.10			
Leg Curl	.32	.25			
Arm Curl	.35	.18			

Total: _____

Average Percentile Rank (divide total by 6): _____

Overall Strength Category: _____

are not familiar with the different lifts, graphic illustrations are provided at the end of this chapter.

A strength/endurance rating is determined according to the maximum number of repetitions that you are able to perform on each lift. A sixteen-station, fixed resistance, Universal Gym® apparatus is necessary to administer the test. For individuals who perform a low number of repetitions, the test will primarily measure absolute strength. For those who are able to perform a large number of repetitions, the test will be an indicator of muscular endurance. A percentile rank for each lift is given based on the number of repetitions performed (see Table 3.1), and an overall muscular strength/endurance rating can be determined by taking an average of the percentile ranks obtained for each lift. A form for recording these data is provided in Figure 3.4.

2. **Muscular Endurance Test.** Three exercises were selected for this test to assess the endurance of the upper body, lower body, and

abdominal muscle groups (see Figure 3.5). The advantage of this test is that no strength-training equipment is required. You will need only a stopwatch, a metronome, a bench or gymnasium bleacher 16¼ inches high, three chairs (males only), and a partner to perform the test. As with the Muscular Strength and Endurance Test, a percentile rank is given for each exercise according to the number of repetitions performed (see Table 3.2). An overall endurance rating can be obtained through the average percentile rank for the three exercises. The data recording form is given in Figure 3.6

3. **Strength-to-Body Weight Ratio Test.** This is an absolute strength test that will require you to determine your 1 RM on six different lifts (see Figure 3.7). Each 1 RM is expressed as a percentage of your body weight (1 RM divided by body weight) and points are awarded based on the ratio obtained for each lift (see Table 3.3). The final strength score is obtained by totaling the points received for each lift

Table 3.1.
Muscular Strength and Endurance Scoring Table

MEN

Percentile Rank	Lateral Pull-Down	Leg Extension	Bench Press	Sit-Up	Leg Curl	Arm Curl
99	30	25	26	30	24	25
95	25	20	21	26	20	21
90	19	19	19	23	19	19
80	16	15	16	17	15	15
70	13	14	13	14	13	12
60	11	13	11	12	11	10
50	10	12	10	10	10	9
40	9	10	7	8	8	8
30	7	9	5	5	6	7
20	6	7	3	3	4	5
10	4	5	1	2	3	3
5	3	3	0	1	1	2

WOMEN

Percentile Rank	Lateral Pull-Down	Leg Extension	Bench Press	Sit-Up	Leg Curl	Arm Curl
99	30	25	27	32	20	25
95	25	20	21	27	17	21
90	21	18	20	22	12	20
80	16	13	16	14	10	16
70	13	11	13	11	9	14
60	11	10	11	6	7	12
50	10	9	10	5	6	10
40	9	8	5	4	5	8
30	7	7	3	2	4	7
20	6	5	1	1	3	6
10	3	3	0	0	1	3
5	2	1	0	0	0	2

Figure 3.5. *Procedure for the Muscular Endurance Test*

1. Three exercises are conducted on this test: bench-jumps, chair-dips (men) or modified push-ups (women), and bent-leg curl-ups. All exercises should be conducted with the aid of a partner. The correct procedures for performing each exercise are as follows:

Bench-jumps. Using a bench or gymnasium bleacher 16¼ inches high, attempt to jump up and down the bench as many times as possible in a one-minute period. If you cannot jump the full minute, you may step up and down. A repetition is counted each time both feet return to the floor.

Chair-dips. This upper-body exercise is performed by men only. Using three sturdy chairs, place one hand each on a chair, with the fingers pointing forward. Place the feet on a third chair in front of you. The hips should be bent at approximately 90°. Lower your body by flexing the elbows until you reach a 90° angle at this joint, then return to the starting position (*see* Exercise 6 at the end of this chapter). The repetition does not count if you fail to reach 90°. The repetitions are performed to a two-step cadence (down-up), regulated with a metronome set at fifty-six beats per minute. Perform as many continuous repetitions as possible. You can no longer count the repetitions if you fail to follow the metronome cadence.

Modified push-ups. Women will perform the modified push-up exercise instead of the chair-dip exercise. Lie down on the floor (face down), bend the knees (feet up in the air), and place the hands on the floor by the shoulders with the fingers pointing forward. The lower body will be supported at the knees (as opposed to the feet) throughout the test (*see* Exercise 3 at the end of this chapter). The chest must touch the floor on each repetition. As with the chair-dip exercise, the repetitions are performed to a two-step cadence (up-down) regulated with a metronome set at fifty-six beats per minute. Perform as many continuous repetitions as possible. You cannot count any more repetitions if you fail to follow the metronome cadence.

Bent-leg curl-ups. Lie down on the floor (face up) and bend both legs at the knees at approximately 100°. The feet should be on the floor, and you must hold them in place yourself throughout the test. Cross the arms in front of the chest, each hand on the opposite shoulder. Now raise the head off the floor, placing the chin against the chest. This is the starting and finishing position for each curl-up. **The back of the head may not come in contact with the floor, the hands cannot be removed from the shoulders, nor may the feet or hips be raised off the floor at any time during the test. The test is terminated if any of these four conditions occurs.** When you curl up, the upper body must come to an upright position before going back down (*see* Exercise 4 at the end of this chapter). The repetitions are performed to a two-step cadence (up-down) regulated with the metronome set at forty beats per minute. For this exercise, you should allow a brief practice period of five to ten seconds to familiarize yourself with the cadence (the up movement is initiated with the first beat, then you must wait for the next beat to initiate the down movement — one repetition is accomplished every two beats of the metronome). Count as many repetitions as you are able to perform following the proper cadence. The test is also terminated if you fail to maintain the appropriate cadence or if you accomplish 100 repetitions. Have your partner check the angle at the knees throughout the test to make sure that the 100° angle is maintained as closely as possible.

2. According to your results, look up your percentile rank for each exercise in the far left column of Table 3.2.

3. Total the percentile scores obtained for each exercise, and divide by 3 to obtain an average score (see Figure 3.6). Determine your overall muscular endurance fitness category according to the following ratings:

Average Score	Endurance Classification
80 +	Excellent
60-79	Good
40-59	Average
20-39	Fair
< 19	Poor

From Hoeger, W. W. K. *Principles and Laboratories for Physical Fitness & Wellness*. Englewood, CO: Morton Publishing Company, 1988.

Figure 3.6. *Data form for the Muscular Endurance Test*

Name: _____ Sex: _____ Date: _____

	Exercise	Metronome Cadence	Repetitions	% Rank
Men	Bench-Jumps Chair-Dips Abdominal Curl-Ups			
Women	Bench-Jumps Modified Push-Ups Abdominal Curl-Ups			
			Total:	

Average Percentile Rank (divide total by 3): _____

Overall Endurance Category: _____

Table 3.2.
Muscular Endurance Scoring Table

MEN				WOMEN			
Percentile Rank	Bench Jumps	Chair Dips	Bent-leg Curl-ups	Percentile Rank	Bench Jumps	Modified Push-ups	Bent-leg Curl-ups
99	66	54	100	99	58	95	100+
95	63	50	81	95	54	70	100
90	62	38	65	90	52	50	97
80	58	32	51	80	48	41	77
70	57	30	44	70	44	38	57
60	56	27	31	60	42	33	45
50	54	26	28	50	39	30	37
40	51	23	25	40	38	28	28
30	48	20	22	30	36	25	22
20	47	17	17	20	32	21	17
10	40	11	10	10	28	18	9
5	34	7	3	5	26	15	4

(see Figure 3.8). Because the 1 RM is determined through trial and error, individual assessments require about twenty to thirty minutes or longer to conduct. As with the Muscular Strength and Endurance Test (first test), a sixteen-station, fixed resistance, Universal Gym® apparatus is necessary to administer the test.

After you have established your own strength fitness category, record this information in Figure 3.9 and in your fitness and wellness profile in Appendix A. If you wish to conduct periodic strength assessments, additional blanks have been provided in Figure 3.9 for you to monitor your improvements.

Figure 3.7. *Procedure for the Strength-to-Body Weight Ratio Test*

1. Familiarize yourself with the six lifts used for this test: bench press, arm curl, lateral pull-down, leg press, leg extension, and leg curl (a graphic illustration of each lift is given at the end of this chapter).

2. Determine your body weight in pounds.

3. Determine your one repetition maximum (1 RM) for each lift. This is done through trial and error. Estimate the amount of resistance (weight) that you think you will be able to lift. If the load is too light, increase the resistance by five to ten pounds; if it is too heavy, decrease by the same amount. Allow two to three minutes between trials. Continue the process until you have determined the maximal amount of resistance that you can lift in one single effort. Record this information under the 1 RM column in Figure 3.8.

4. Express each 1 RM as a percentage of your body weight. To obtain this number, divide the 1 RM for each lift by your weight. Enter this number under the ratio column in Figure 3.8. For example, the strength-to-body weight ratio for a 150-pound male who bench pressed 180 pounds would be 1.20 (180 divided by 150).

5. Using Table 3.3, look up on the far right column the number of points scored for the ratio obtained on each lift. In the case of the previous example, a ratio of 1.2 on the bench press for a male would score seven points. Record this information in the appropriate points column in Figure 3.8.

6. Total the number of points obtained on each lift, and determine your overall strength fitness category according to the following ratings:

Total Points	Strength Category
48+	Excellent
37-47	Good
25-36	Average
13-24	Fair
<12	Poor

Figure 3.8. *Data form for the Strength-to-Body Weight Ratio Test*

Name: _____ Sex: _____ Date: _____

Body Weight: _____ lbs.

Lift	1 RM	Ratio	Points
Bench Press			
Leg Press			
Arm Curl			
Lateral Pull-Down			
Leg Extension			
Leg Curl			

Overall

Strength Category

_____

Total Points: _____

Table 3.3.
Strength-to-Body Weight Ratio Scoring Table

			MEN			
BENCH PRESS	ARM CURL	LATERAL PULL-DOWN	LEG PRESS	LEG EXTENSION[a]	LEG CURL	POINTS
1.50	0.70	1.20	3.00	1.30	0.70	10
1.40	0.65	1.15	2.80	1.35	0.65	9
1.30	0.60	1.10	2.60	1.20	0.60	8
1.20	0.55	1.05	2.40	1.10	0.55	7
1.10	0.50	1.00	2.20	1.00	0.50	6
1.00	0.45	0.95	2.00	0.90	0.45	5
0.90	0.40	0.90	1.80	0.80	0.40	4
0.80	0.35	0.85	1.60	0.70	0.35	3
0.70	0.30	0.80	1.40	0.60	0.30	2
0.60	0.25	0.75	1.20	0.50	0.25	1
			WOMEN			
0.90	0.50	0.85	2.70	1.05	0.60	10
0.85	0.45	0.80	2.50	1.00	0.55	9
0.80	0.42	0.75	2.30	0.95	0.52	8
0.70	0.38	0.73	2.10	0.90	0.50	7
0.65	0.35	0.70	2.00	0.85	0.45	6
0.60	0.32	0.65	1.80	0.80	0.40	5
0.55	0.28	0.63	1.60	0.75	0.35	4
0.50	0.25	0.60	1.40	0.70	0.30	3
0.45	0.21	0.55	1.20	0.65	0.25	2
0.35	0.18	0.50	1.00	0.60	0.20	1

From Heyward, V. H. *Designs for Fitness.* Macmillan Publishing Company, New York, 1984.
[a]Leg extension ratios adapted with permission by the author. (This exercise is also referred to as Quadriceps Lift.)

Figure 3.9. *Muscular strength report*

Name: _____ Age: _____ Sex: _____

Date	Test Used	Score	Fitness Classification

PHYSIOLOGICAL FACTORS THAT AFFECT STRENGTH

Over the years it has been well documented that muscle cells will increase and decrease their capacity to exert force according to the demands placed upon the muscular system. If muscle cells are overloaded beyond their normal use, such as in strength-training programs, the cells will increase in size (hypertrophy) and strength. If the demands placed on the muscle cells decrease, such as in sedentary living or required rest resulting from illness or injury, the cells will decrease in size (atrophy) and lose strength.

There are several physiological factors related to muscle contraction and subsequent strength gains. These factors are neural stimulation, muscle fiber type, overload principle, and specificity of training. Basic knowledge of these factors is important to understand the principles involved in strength training.

Neural Stimulation

Within the neuromuscular system, single motor neurons (nerves traveling from the central nervous system to the muscle) branch and attach to multiple muscle fibers. The combination of the motor neuron and the muscle fibers that it innervates is called a motor unit. The number of fibers that a motor neuron can innervate varies from just a few to as many as 200. Stimulation of a motor neuron causes the muscle fibers to contract maximally or not at all. Variations in the number of fibers innervated and the frequency of their stimulation determine the strength of the muscle contraction. As the number of fibers innervated and frequency of stimulation increase, so does the strength of the muscular contraction.

Fiber Types

There are primarily two types of muscle fibers that determine muscle response: slow-twitch or red fibers and fast-twitch or white fibers. Slow-twitch fibers have a greater capacity for aerobic work. Fast-twitch fibers have a greater capacity for anaerobic work. The latter produce a greater overall force and are important for quick and powerful movements commonly used in strength-training activities. The proportion of slow- and fast-twitch fibers are genetically determined, and consequently vary from one person to another. Nevertheless, training will increase the functional capacity of both fiber types, and more specifically, strength training increases their ability to exert force.

During muscular contraction, slow-twitch fibers are always recruited first. As the force and speed of muscular contraction increase, the relative importance of the fast-twitch fibers also increases. An activity must be intense and powerful for activation of the fast-twitch fibers to occur.

Overload Principle

Strength gains are achieved in two ways: (1) through an increased ability of individual muscle fibers to elicit a stronger contraction, and (2) by recruiting a greater proportion of the total available fibers for each contraction. The development of these two factors can be accomplished by the use of the overload principle. This principle states that for strength improvements to occur, the demands placed on the muscle must be systematically and progressively increased over a period of time, and the resistance must be of a magnitude significant enough to cause physiologic adaptation. In simpler terms, just like all other organs and systems of the human body, muscles have to be taxed beyond their regular accustomed loads to increase in physical capacity.

Specificity of Training

Another important aspect of training is the concept of specificity of training. This principle indicates that for a muscle to increase in strength or endurance, the training program must be specific to obtain the desired effects. In like manner, to increase isometric (static) versus isotonic (dynamic) strength, an individual must use static against dynamic training procedures to achieve the appropriate results. Furthermore, if a person is trying to improve a particular movement or skill through strength increases, the selected strength-training exercises must resemble the actual movement or skill as closely as possible.

PRINCIPLES OF STRENGTH-TRAINING PRESCRIPTION

Similar to the prescription of cardiovascular exercise, several principles should be observed to improve muscular strength and endurance. These principles are mode, resistance, sets, and frequency of training.

Mode of Training

Two basic types of training methods are used to improve strength: isometric and isotonic. Isometric or static training refers to a muscular contraction producing little or no movement, such as pushing or pulling against immovable objects. Isotonic or dynamic training refers to a muscular contraction with movement, such as lifting an object over the head. Isotonic training programs can be conducted without weights or with free weights (barbells and dumbbells), fixed resistance machines, variable resistance machines, and isokinetic equipment.

When a person performs isotonic exercises without weights (e.g., pull-ups, push-ups), with free weights, or with fixed resistance machines, a constant resistance (weight) is moved through a joint's full range of motion. The greatest resistance (weight) that can be lifted equals the maximum weight that can be moved at the weakest angle of the joint. This is because of changes in muscle length and angle of pull as the joint moves through its range of motion.

As the popularity of strength training increased, new strength-training machines were developed. This new technology brought about the introduction of isokinetic and variable resistance training. These training programs require the use of special machines equipped with mechanical devices that provide a variable resistance, with the intent of overloading the muscle group maximally through the entire range of motion. A distinction of isokinetic training is that the speed of the muscular contraction is kept constant because the machine provides an accommodating resistance to match the user's force through the range of motion.

The mode of training an individual uses depends largely on the type of equipment available and the specific objective that the training program is attempting to accomplish. Isometric training does not require much equipment and was commonly used several years ago, but its popularity has significantly decreased in recent years. Because strength gains with isometric training are specific to the angle at which the contraction is being performed, this type of training is beneficial in a sport such as gymnastics, in which static contractions are used regularly during routines.

Isotonic training is the most popular mode used in strength training. The primary advantage is that strength gains occur through the full range of motion. Most daily activities are isotonic in nature. We are constantly lifting, pushing, and pulling objects, where strength is needed through a complete range of motion. Another advantage is that improvements are easily measured by the amount lifted.

The benefits of isokinetic and variable resistance training are similar to the other isotonic training methods. Theoretically, strength gains should be better because maximum resistance is applied at all angles. Research, however, has not shown this type of training to be more effective than other modes of isotonic training. A possible advantage is that specific speeds used in various sport skills can be more closely duplicated with isokinetic strength training, which may enhance performance (specificity of training). A disadvantage is that the equipment is not readily available to many people.

Resistance

Resistance in strength training is the equivalent of intensity in cardiovascular exercise prescription. The amount of resistance used, or weight lifted, depends on whether the individual is trying to develop muscular strength or muscular endurance.

To stimulate strength development, a resistance of approximately 80 percent of the maximum capacity (1 RM) is recommended. For example, a person who can press 150 pounds should work with at least 120 pounds (150 × .80). Using less than 80 percent will help increase muscular endurance rather than strength. Because of the time factor involved in constantly determining the 1 RM on each lift to ensure that the person is indeed working above 80 percent, a rule of thumb widely accepted by many authors and coaches is that individuals should perform between three and ten repetitions maximum for adequate strength gains. For instance, if a person is training with a resistance of 120 pounds and cannot lift it more than ten times, training stimuli are adequate for strength development. Once the weight can be lifted more than ten times, the resistance should be increased by five to ten pounds and the person should again build up to ten repetitions. If training is conducted with more than ten repetitions, primarily muscular endurance will be developed.

Strength research indicates that the closer a person trains to the 1 RM, the greater will be the strength gains. A disadvantage of constantly working at or near the 1 RM is that it increases the risk of injury. Three to six repetitions maximum are frequently used by highly trained athletes who seek maximum strength development. From a health/fitness point of view, six to ten repetitions maximum are ideal for adequate development. We live in an "isotonic world" in which muscular strength and endurance are both required to lead an enjoyable life; therefore, working near the ten-repetition threshold seems best to improve overall performance.

Sets

A set in strength training has been defined as the number of repetitions performed for a given exercise. For example, a person lifting 120 pounds eight times has performed one set of eight repetitions. The number of sets recommended for optimum development is anywhere from three to five sets, with about ninety seconds of recovery time between each set. Because of the physiology of muscle fiber, there is a limit to the number of sets that can be done. As the number of sets increases, so does the amount of muscular fatigue and subsequent recovery time; therefore, strength gains may be lessened if too many sets are performed. A recommended program for beginners in their first year of training is three heavy sets (up to the maximum number of repetitions) preceded by one or two light warm-up sets using about 50 percent of the 1 RM.

To make the exercise program more time-effective, two or three exercises that require different muscle groups may be alternated. In this manner, an individual will not have to wait the full ninety seconds before proceeding to the next set. For example, bench press, leg extensions, and sit-ups exercises may be combined so that the person can go almost directly from one set to the next.

Additionally, to avoid muscle soreness and stiffness, new participants ought to build up gradually to the three sets of maximal repetitions. This can be accomplished by doing only one set of each exercise with a lighter resistance on the first day. On the second session, two sets of each exercise can be performed — one light and the second with the regular resistance. On the third session, three sets could be performed — one light and two heavy ones. Thereafter, a person should be able to do all three heavy sets.

Frequency of Training

Strength training should be done either with a total body workout three times per week, or more frequently if a split-body routine (upper body one day and lower body the next) is used. Following a maximum workout, it is necessary to rest the muscles for about forty-eight hours to allow adequate recovery. If complete recovery has not occurred in two or three days, the person is most likely overtraining and therefore not reaping the full benefits of the program. In such a case, a decrease in the total number of sets and/or exercises performed on the previous workout is recommended.

To achieve significant strength gains, a minimum of eight weeks of consecutive training is needed. Once an ideal level of strength is achieved, one training session per week will be sufficient to maintain the new strength level.

STRENGTH TRAINING PROGRAMS

Three strength-training programs are illustrated at the end of this chapter. These programs have been developed to provide a complete body workout. Only a minimum of equipment is required for the first program, "Strength-Training Exercises Without Weights" (exercises 1 through 10). This program can be conducted within the walls of your own home. Your body weight is used as the primary resistance for most exercises. In a few instances, a friend's help or some basic implements from around your home are used to provide greater resistance.

The second program, "Universal Gym® Equipment Strength-Training Exercises" (exercises 11 through 27), requires the use of gym machines such as those shown in the various photographs. Some of these machines use fixed resistance; others use variable resistance. Many of these exercises also can be performed with free weights. The first eight exercises (11 to 18) and exercise 27 are recommended to get a complete workout. The rest are optional. If one of the optional exercises involves the same body parts, however, the person may substitute the latter for one of the basic nine (exercise 21 for 11, 19 or 20 for 12, 26 for 13, 23 or 24 for 14, 22 for 16, and 25 for 18).

The third program, "Nautilus® Strength-Training Exercises" (exercises 28 through 39) also require the use of machines, as illustrated in the various photos. All of these machines use variable resistance. In this last program, exercises 28 through 38 are recommended for a complete body workout, and exercise 39 may be substituted for exercise 31.

Setting Up Your Own Strength-Training Program

Depending on the facilities available to you, choose one of the three training programs illustrated at the end of this chapter. The resistance and the number of repetitions that you use should be based on whether you want to increase muscular strength or muscular endurance. Up to ten repetitions maximum should be used for strength gains and more than ten for muscular endurance. As pointed out previously, three training sessions per week conducted on nonconsecutive days is an ideal program for proper development, and because both strength and endurance are required in daily activities, three to five sets of about ten repetitions maximum for each exercise are sufficient. In this manner you will obtain good strength gains and yet be close to the endurance threshold.

Perhaps the only exercises in which more than ten repetitions are recommended are the abdominal exercises. The abdominal muscles are considered primarily antigravity or postural muscles; hence, a little more endurance may be required. Most people perform about twenty repetitions when doing abdominal work. Once you initiate your strength-training program, you may use the form provided in Figure 3.10 to keep a record of your training sessions. Figure 3.11 graphically points out the major muscles of the human body referred to in the exercises.

Bibliography

Allsen, P. E. *Strength Training: Beginners, Bodybuilders, and Athletes.* Glenview, IL: Scott, Foresman, 1987.

Fox, E. L., and D. K. Mathews. *The Physiological Basis of Physical Education and Athletics.* Philadelphia: Saunders College Publishing, 1981.

Heyward, V. H. *Designs for Fitness: A Guide to Physical Fitness Appraisal and Exercise Prescription.* Minneapolis: Burgess Publishing, 1984.

Hoeger, W. W. K. *Principles and Laboratories for Physical Fitness & Wellness.* Englewood, CO: Morton Publishing, 1988.

Hoeger, W. W. K., S. L. Barette, D. F. Hale, and D. R. Hopkins. "Relationship Between Repetitions and Selected Percentages of One Repetition Maximum." *Journal of Applied Sports Science* 1(1):11-13, 1987.

McArdle, W. D., F. I. Katch, and V. L. Katch. *Exercise Physiology: Energy, Nutrition and Human Performance.* Philadelphia: Lea and Febiger, 1986.

O'Shea, J. P. *Scientific Principles and Methods of Strength Fitness.* Reading, MA: Addison-Wesley, 1976.

Figure 3.10. *Strength training record form*

Name _____

Date										
Exercise	**St/Reps/Res***	**St/Reps/Res**	**St/Reps/Res**	**St/Reps/Res**	**St/Reps/Res**	**St/Reps/Res**	**St/Reps/Res**	**St/Reps/Res**	**St/Reps/Res**	**St/Reps/Res**

*St/Reps/Res = Sets, Repetitions, and Resistance (e.g., 1/6/125 = 1 set of 6 repetitions with 125 pounds).

Figure 3.10. *Strength training record form (Continued)*

Name _____

Date	St/Reps/Res*	St/Reps/Res	St/Reps/Res	St/Reps/Res	St/Reps/Res	St/Reps/Res	St/Reps/Res	St/Reps/Res	St/Reps/Res
Exercise									

*St/Reps/Res = Sets, Repetitions, and Resistance (e.g., 1/6/125 = 1 set of 6 repetitions with 125 pounds).

Figure 3.11. *Major muscles of the human body*

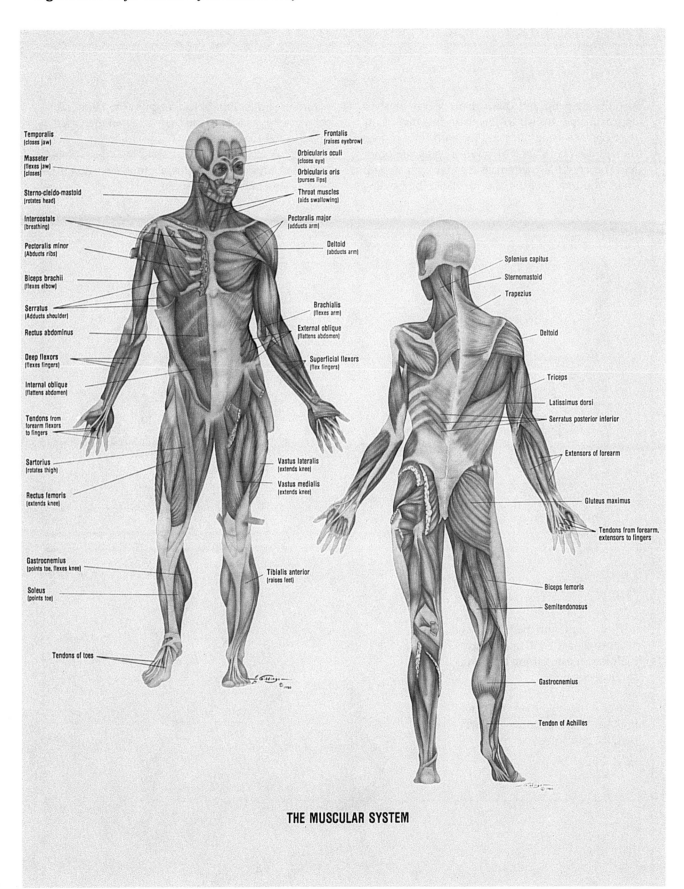

THE MUSCULAR SYSTEM

Strength-Training Exercises Without Weights

Exercise 1:   STEP-UP

Action: Step up and down using a box or chair approximately twelve to fifteen inches high. Conduct one set using the same leg each time you go up and then conduct a second set using the other leg. You could also alternate legs on each step-up cycle. You may increase the resistance by holding a child or some other object in your arms (hold the child or object close to the body to avoid increased strain in the lower back).

Muscles Developed: Gluteal muscles, quadriceps, gastrocnemius, and soleus.

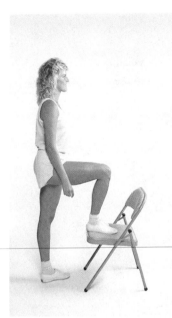
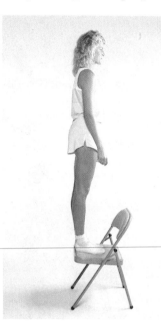
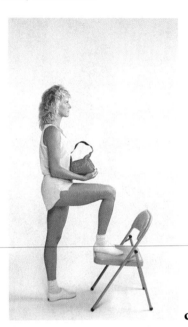

a

b

c

Exercise 2: HIGH JUMPER

Action: Start with the knees bent at approximately 150° and jump as high as you can, raising both arms simultaneously.

Muscles Developed: Gluteal muscles, quadriceps, gastrocnemius, and soleus.

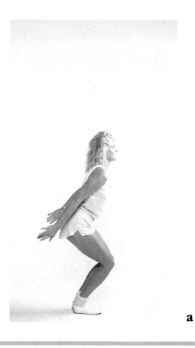
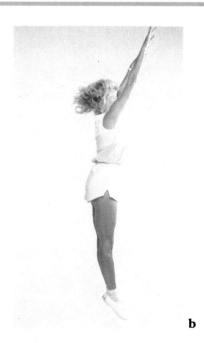

a

b

Exercise 3: PUSH-UP

Action: Maintaining your body as straight as possible, flex the elbows, lowering the body until you almost touch the floor, then raise yourself back up to the starting position. If you are unable to perform the push-up as indicated, you can decrease the resistance by supporting the lower body with the knees rather than the feet (see illustration c) or using an incline plane and supporting your

hands at a higher point than the floor (see illustration d). If you wish to increase the resistance, have someone else add resistance to your shoulders as you are coming back up (see illustration e).

Muscles Developed: Triceps, deltoid, pectoralis major, erector spinae, and abdominals.

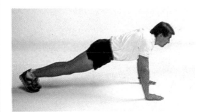
a

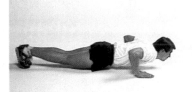
b

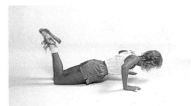
c

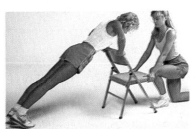
d

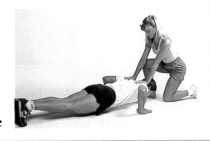
e

Exercise 4: SIT-UP

Action: Start with your head and shoulders off the floor, arms crossed on your chest, and knees slightly bent (the greater the flexion of the knee, the more difficult the sit-up). Now curl all the way up, then return to the starting position without letting the head or shoulders touch the floor, or allowing the hips to come off the floor. If you allow the hips to raise off the floor and the head and shoulders to touch the floor (see illustration c), you will most likely "swing up" on the next sit-up, which minimizes the work of the abdominal muscles. If you cannot curl up with the arms on the chest, place the hands by the side of the hips or even help yourself up by holding on to your thighs (illustrations d and e). Do not perform the sit-up exercise with your legs completely extended, as this will cause strain on the lower back.

Muscles Developed: Abdominal muscles and hip flexors.

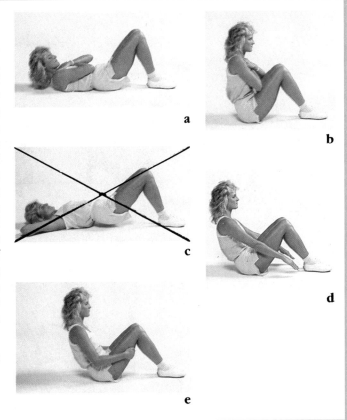
a
b
c
d
e

Exercise 5: LEG CURL

Action: Lie on the floor face down. Cross the right ankle over the left heel. Apply resistance with your right foot, while you bring the left foot up to 90° at the knee joint. (Apply enough resistance so that the left foot can only be brought up slowly). Repeat the exercise, crossing the left ankle over the right heel.

Muscles Developed: Hamstrings (and quadriceps).

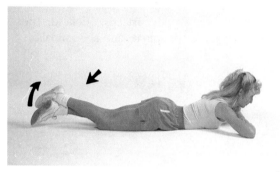

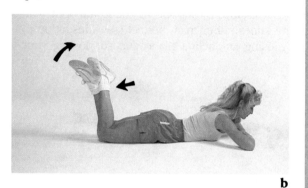

a

b

Exercise 6: MODIFIED DIP

Action: Place your hands and feet on opposite chairs with knees slightly bent (make sure that the chairs are well stabilized). Dip down at least to a 90° angle at the elbow joint, then return to the initial position. To increase the resistance, have someone else hold you down by the shoulders on the way up (see illustration c).

Muscles Developed: Triceps, deltoid, and pectoralis major.

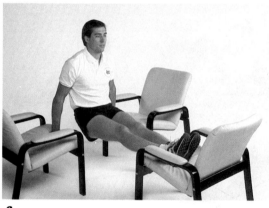

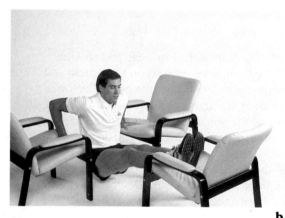

a

b

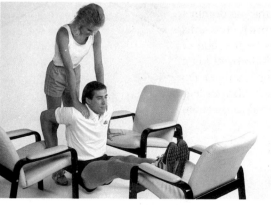

c

Exercise 7: PULL-UP

Action: Suspend yourself from a bar with a pronated grip (thumbs in). Pull your body up until your chin is above the bar, then lower the body slowly to the starting position. If you are unable to perform the pull-up as described, either have a partner hold your feet to push off and facilitate the movement upward (illustrations c and d) or use a lower bar and support your feet on the floor (illustration e).

Muscles Developed: Biceps, brachioradialis, brachialis, trapezius, and latissimus dorsi.

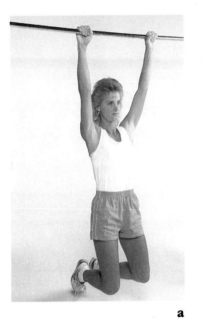

a

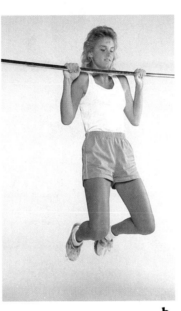

b

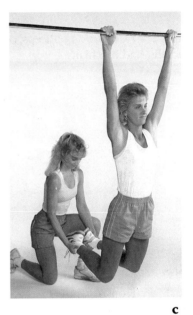

c

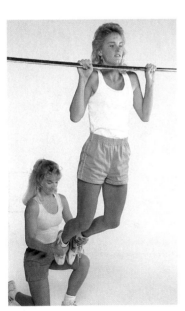

d

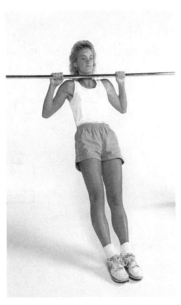

e

Exercise 8: ARM CURL

Action: Using a palms-up grip, start with the arm completely extended, and with the aid of a sandbag or bucket filled (as needed) with sand or rocks, curl up as far as possible, then return to the initial position. Repeat the exercise with the other arm.

Muscles Developed: Biceps, brachio-radialis, and brachialis.

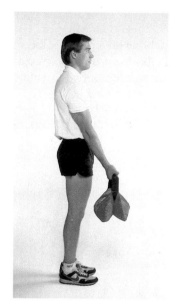 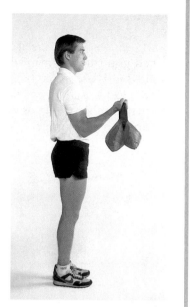

a   **b**

Exercise 9: HEEL RAISE

Action: From a standing position with feet flat on the floor, raise and lower your body weight by moving at the ankle joint only (for added resistance, have someone else hold your shoulders down as you perform the exercise).

Muscles Developed: Gastrocnemius and soleus.

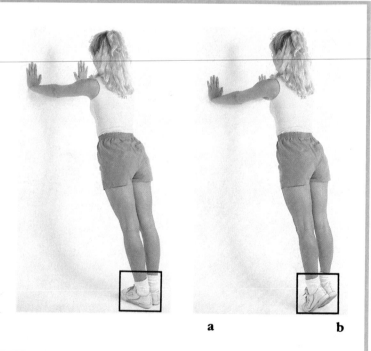

a   **b**

Exercise 10: LEG ABDUCTION AND ADDUCTION

Action: Both participants sit on the floor. The subject on the left places the feet on the inside of the other participant's feet. Simultaneously, the subject on the left presses the legs laterally (to the outside — abduction), while the subject on the right presses the legs medially (adduction). Hold the contraction for five to ten seconds. Repeat the exercise at all three angles, and then reverse the pressing sequence. The subject on the left places the feet on the outside and presses inward, while the subject on the right presses outward.

Muscles Developed: Hip abductors and adductors.

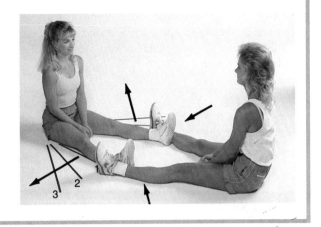

Universal Gym® Equipment Strength-Training Exercises*

Exercise 11: ARM CURL

Action: Use a supinated or palms-up grip, and start with the arms almost completely extended. Now curl up as far as possible, then return to the starting position.

Muscles Developed: Biceps, brachioradialis, and brachialis.

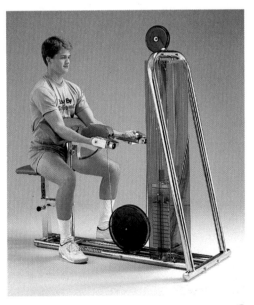

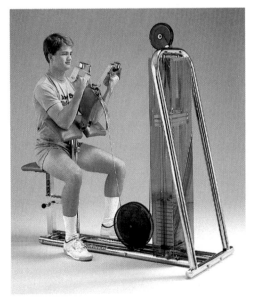

a   b

*Photographs courtesy of Universal Gym® Equipment, Inc., 930 27th Avenue, S.W., Cedar Rapids, IA 52406.

Exercise 12: LEG PRESS

Action: From a sitting position with the knees flexed at about 90° and both feet on the footrest, fully extend the legs, then return slowly to the starting position.

Muscles Developed: Quadriceps and gluteal muscles.

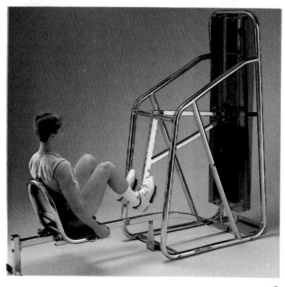
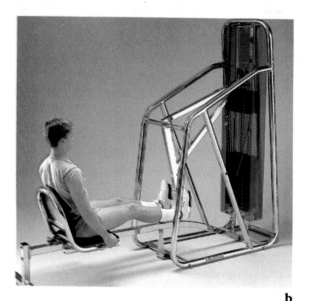

a

b

Exercise 13: SIT-UP

Action: Using either a horizontal or an inclined board, stabilize your feet and flex the knees to about 100 to 120 degrees. Start with the head and shoulders off the board, curl all the way up, then return to the starting position without letting the head and shoulders touch the board (do not swing up, but rather curl up). You may curl straight up or use a twisting motion (twisting as you first start to come up), alternating on each sit-up.

Muscles Developed: Abdominals and hip flexors.

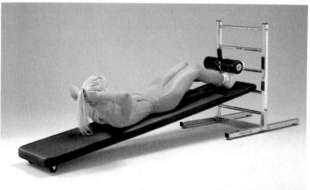

a

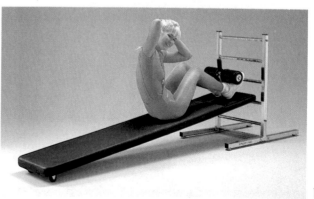

b

Exercise 14:   BENCH PRESS

Action: Lie down on the bench with the head toward the weight stack, feet flat on the floor, and the bench press bar above the chest. Press upward until the arms are completely extended, then return to the starting position. Do not arch the back during the exercise.

Muscles Developed: Pectoralis   major, triceps, and deltoid.

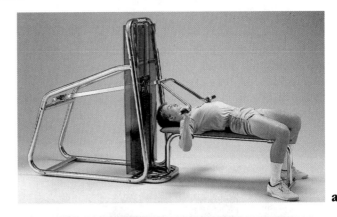
a

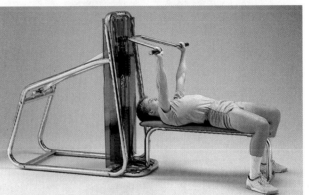
b

Exercise 15:   LEG CURL

Action: Lie with the face down on the bench and legs straight with the back of the feet against the bar. Curl up to at least 90°, then return to the original position.

Muscles Developed: Hamstrings.

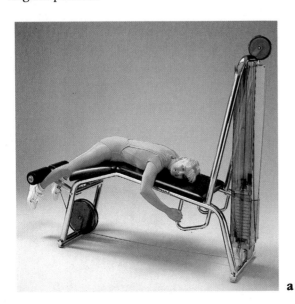
a

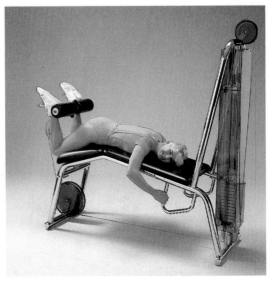
b

Exercise 16:   LATERAL PULL-DOWN

Action: Start from a sitting position, and hold the exercise bar with a wide grip. Pull the bar down until it touches the base of the neck, then return to the starting position (if a heavy resistance is used, stabilization of the body may be required by either using equipment as shown or by having someone else hold you down by the waist or shoulders).

Muscles Developed: Latissimus dorsi, pectoralis major, and biceps.

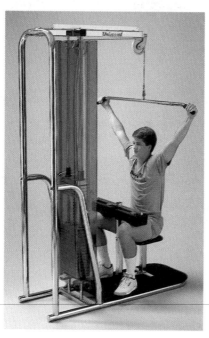

a

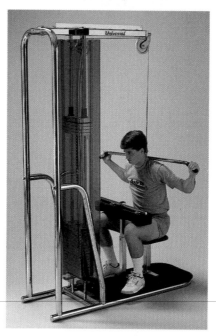

b

Exercise 17:   HEEL RAISE

Action: Start with your feet either flat on the floor or the front of the feet on an elevated block, then raise and lower yourself by moving at the ankle joint only. If additional resistance is needed, you can use the squat machine, illustrated in Exercise 19.

Muscles Developed: Gastrocnemius and soleus.

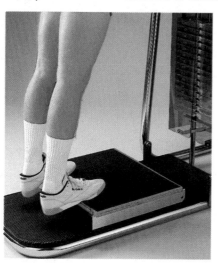

a

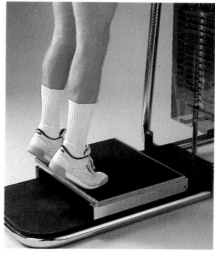

b

Exercise 18: TRICEPS EXTENSION

Action: Using a palms-down grip, grasp the bar slightly closer than shoulder width, and start with the elbows almost completely bent. Fully extend the arms, then return to starting position.

Muscle Developed: Triceps.

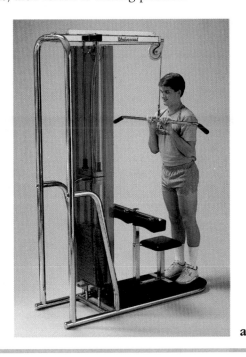

a

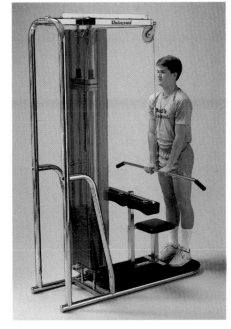

b

Exercise 19: SQUAT

Action: Start with the knees bent at about 120° and shoulders under the padded bars. Completely extend the legs, then return to the original position.

Muscles Developed: Quadriceps, gluteal muscles, hamstrings, gastrocnemius, soleus, and erector spinae.

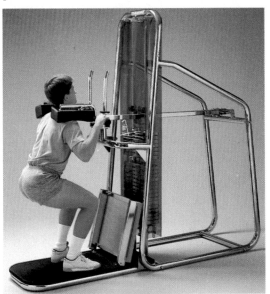

a

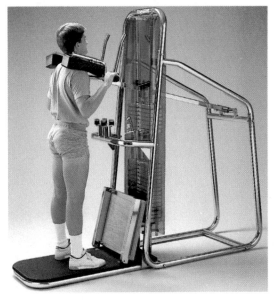

b

Exercise 20: LEG EXTENSION

Action: Sit in an upright position with feet under the padded bar. Extend the legs until they are completely straight, then return to the starting position.

Muscles Developed: Quadriceps.

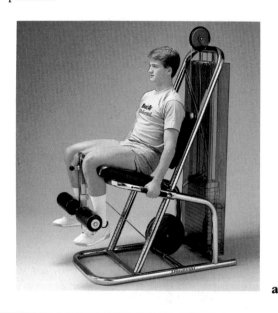

a

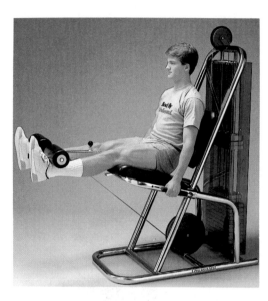

b

Exercise 21: UPRIGHT ROWING

Action: Start with the arms extended and grip the handles with the palms down. Pull all the way up to the chin, then return to the starting position.

Muscles Developed: Biceps, brachioradialis, brachialis, deltoid, and trapezius.

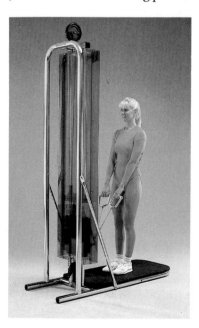

a

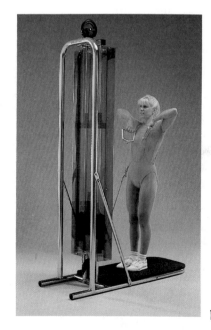

b

Exercise 22:   BENT-ARM PULLOVER

Action: Sit back into the chair and grasp the bar behind your head. Pull the bar over your head all the way down to your abdomen and slowly return to the original position.

Muscles Developed: Latissimus dorsi, pectoral muscles, deltoid, and serratus anterior.

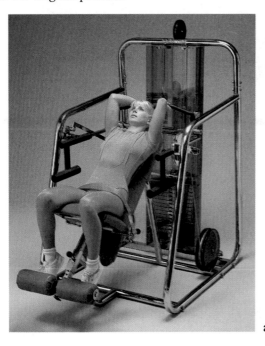   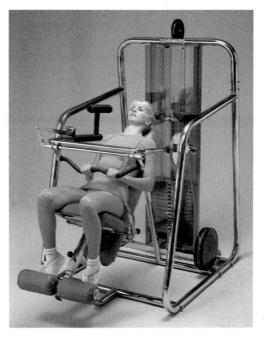

a   b

Exercise 23:   CHEST PRESS

Action: Start with the arms to the side and elbows bent at 90°. Press your arms forward until the padded bars touch in front of your chest, then return to the starting position.

Muscles Developed:
Pectoralis major and deltoid.

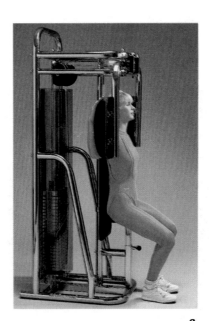   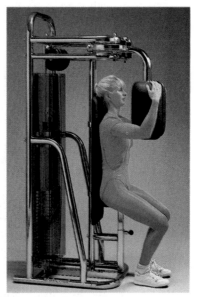

a   b

Exercise 24: SHOULDER PRESS

Action: Sit in an upright position and grasp the bar wider than the shoulder width. Press the bar all the way up until the arms are fully extended, then return to the initial position.

Muscles Developed: Triceps, deltoid, and pectoralis major.

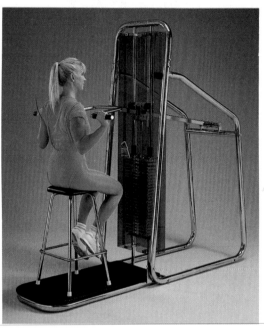

a

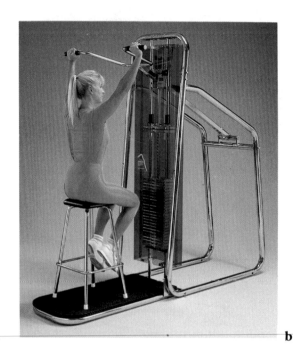

b

Exercise 25: DIP

Action: Start with the elbows flexed, then fully extend the arms, and slowly return to the initial position.

Muscles Developed: Triceps, deltoid, and pectoralis major.

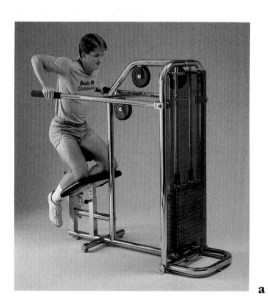

a

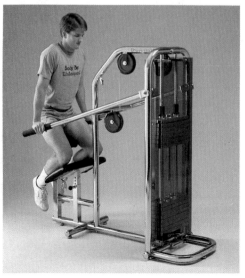

b

Exercise 26:   ABDOMINAL CRUNCH

Action: Sit back into the machine and place the hands inside the straps. Slowly crunch forward to a seated upright position, then return to the starting position.

Muscles Developed: Abdominals.

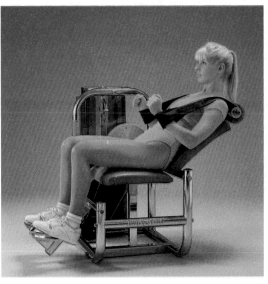

a

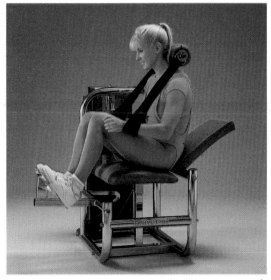

b

Exercise 27:   SEATED BACK

Action: Sit in the machine with your trunk flexed and the upper back against the shoulder pad. Place the feet under the padded bar and hold on with your hands to the bars on the sides. Start the exercise by pressing backward, simultaneously extending the trunk and hip joints. Slowly return to the original position.

Muscles Developed: Erector spinae and gluteus maximus.

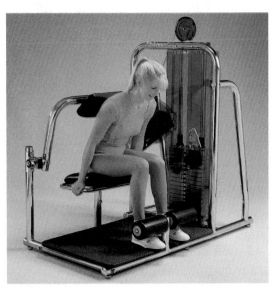

a

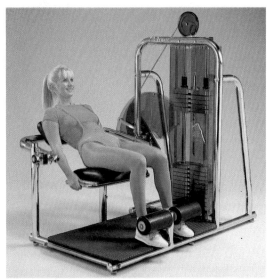

b

Nautilus® Strength-Training Exercises*

Exercise 28:   MULTI-BICEPS (Arm Curl)

Action: Sit into the machine and grasp the bar with the arms completely extended using a supinated or palms up grip. Curl up as far as possible, and then return to the starting position.

Muscles Developed: Biceps, brachioradialis, and brachialis.

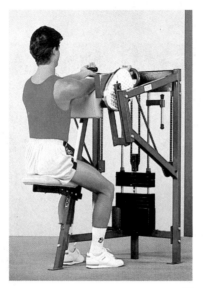
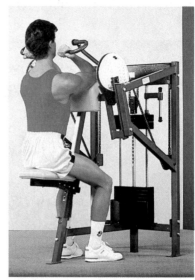

a

b

Exercise 29:   ABDOMINAL CRUNCH

Action: Sit in an upright position with the chest against the padded bar. Place the hands on the abdomen and crunch forward, bringing the chest toward the knees. Slowly return to the original position.

Muscles Developed: Abdominals.

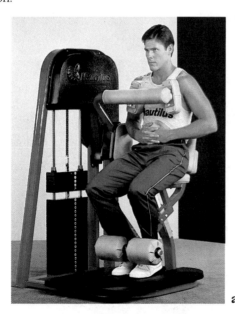
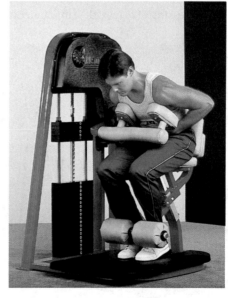

a

b

*Photographs used by permission from Nautilus®, a registered trademark of Nautilus® Sports/Medical Industries, Inc., P.O. Box 809014, Dallas, TX 75380-9014.

Exercise 30:   LEG EXTENSION

Action: Sit in an upright position with the feet under the padded bar and grasp the handles at the sides. Extend the legs until they are completely straight, then return to the starting position.

Muscles Developed: Quadriceps.

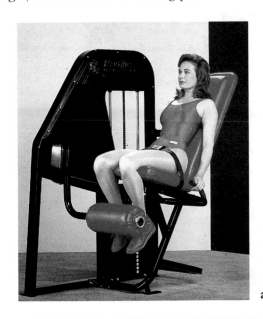

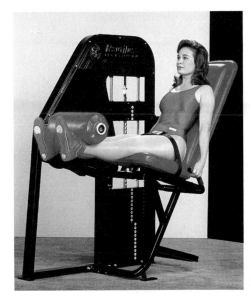

a

b

Exercise 31:   BENCH PRESS

Action: Lie down on the bench with the head by the weight stack, the bench press bar above the chest, and keep the feet on the floor. Grasp the bar handles and press upward until the arms are completely extended, then return to the original position. Do not arch the back during this exercise.

Muscles Developed: Pectoralis major, triceps, and deltoid.

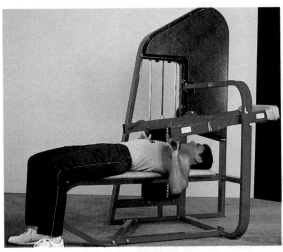

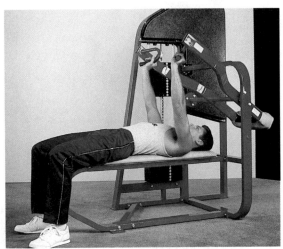

a

b

Exercise 32: LEG CURL

Action: Lie with the face down on the bench, legs straight, and place the back of the feet under the padded bar. Curl up to at least 90°, and return to the original position.

Muscles Developed: Hamstrings.

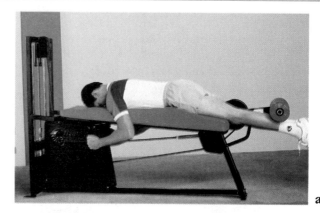

a

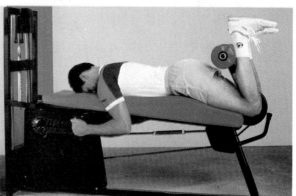

b

Exercise 33: LOWER BACK

Action: Place yourself in the machine so that the front of the thigh and the upper back rest against the padded bars. Slowly press backward against the padded bar until the back is fully extended. Slowly return to the original position.

Muscles Developed: Erector spine and gluteus maximus.

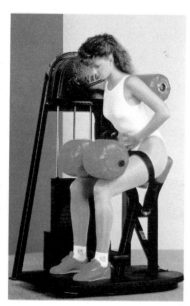

a

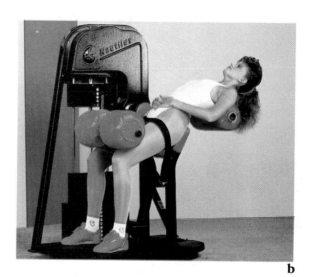

b

Exercise 34: ROWING TORSO

Action: Sit in the machine with your arms in front of you, elbows bent and resting against the padded bars. Press back as far as possible, drawing the shoulder blades together. Return to the original position.

Muscles Developed: Posterior deltoid, rhomboids, and trapezius.

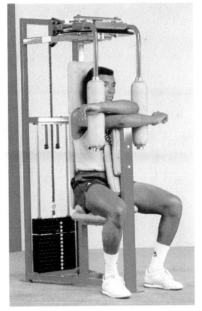 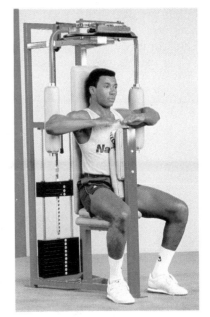

a b

Exercise 35: DUO HIP AND BACK

Action: Lie face up on the bench, grasp handles at sides, and place the back of the knees against the padded bars. Alternately press the legs downward until fully extended. Return to the original position. Repeat with the other leg.

Muscle Developed: Gluteus maximus.

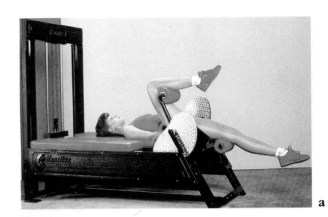

a

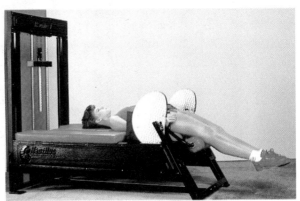

b

Exercise 36: PULLOVER

Action: Sit back into the chair, arms bent. Place the elbows against the padded end of the movement arm, and grasp the bar behind your head. Press forward and downward with your arms, pulling the bar over your head all the way down to your abdomen. Slowly return to the starting position.

Muscles Developed: Latissimus dorsi, pectoral muscles, deltoid, and serratus anterior.

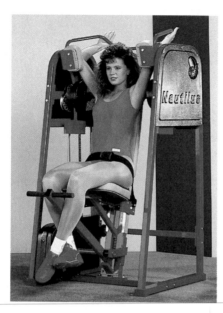 a

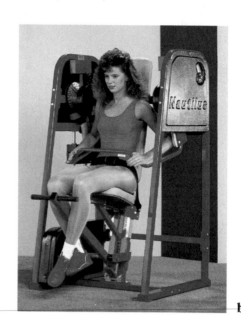 b

Exercise 37: ROTARY TORSO

Action: Sit upright into the machine and place the elbows behind the padded bars. Rotate the torso as far as possible to one side and then slowly return to the starting position. Repeat the exercise to the opposite side.

Muscles Developed: Internal and external oblique (abdominal muscles).

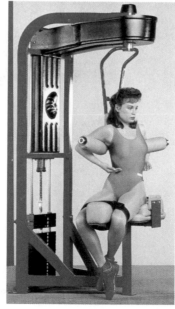 a

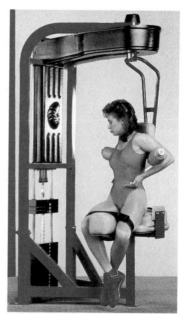 b

Exercise 38: MULTI-TRICEPS (Triceps Extension)

Action: Sit in an upright position, arms up, elbows bent, and place the little finger side of the hands and wrists against the pads, palms of the hands facing each other. Fully extend the arms, and then return to the original position.

Muscle Developed: Triceps.

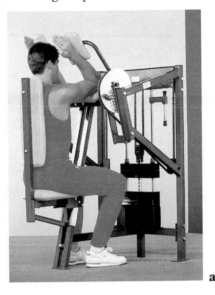 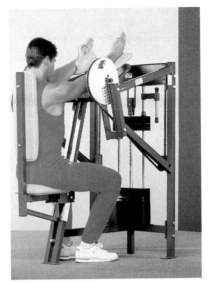

a   b

Exercise 39: CHEST PRESS

Action: Start with the arms up to the side, hands resting against the handle bars, and elbows bent at 90°. Press the movement arms forward as far as possible, leading with the elbows. Slowly return to the starting position.

Muscles Developed: Pectoralis major and deltoid.

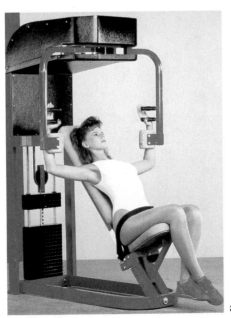 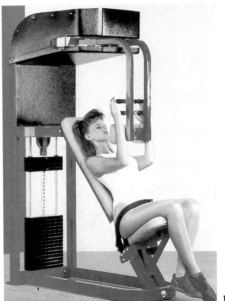

a   b

Muscular Flexibility Assessment And Prescription

Flexibility is defined as the ability of a joint to move freely through its full range of motion. The contribution of good muscular flexibility to overall fitness and preventive health care has been generally underestimated and overlooked by health care professionals, practitioners, and even coaches and athletes.

Total range of motion about a joint is highly specific and varies significantly from one joint to the other (hip, trunk, shoulder), as well as from one individual to the next. The amount of muscular flexibility individuals possess is primarily related to genetic factors and an index of physical activity. Because of the specificity of flexibility, it is difficult to precisely indicate what constitutes an ideal level of flexibility. Nevertheless, the development and maintenance of some level of flexibility are important components of everyone's health enhancement program, and even more so during the aging process.

THE VALUE OF MUSCULAR FLEXIBILITY

Sports medicine specialists have indicated that many muscular/skeletal problems and injuries, especially among adults, are related to a lack of flexibility. Improving and maintaining good joint range of motion is important to enhance the quality of life. Approximately 80 percent of all low back problems in the United States results from improper alignment of the vertebral column and pelvic girdle — a direct result of inflexible and weak muscles. This backache syndrome costs American industry in excess of $1 billion each year in lost productivity and services alone and an extra $225 million in Workmen's Compensation.

Additionally, in daily life we often are required to make rapid or strenuous movements that we are not accustomed to make, leading to potential injury. Physical therapists also have indicated that improper body mechanics are often the result of inadequate flexibility levels.

Most experts agree that participating in a regular flexibility program will help a person maintain good joint mobility, increase resistance to muscle injury and soreness, prevent low back and other spinal column problems, improve and maintain good postural alignment, enhance proper and graceful body movement, improve personal appearance and self-image, and facilitate the development and maintenance of motor skills throughout life. Flexibility exercises also have been used successfully in the treatment of patients suffering from dysmenorrhea and general neuromuscular tension.

Furthermore, stretching exercises in conjunction with calisthenics are helpful in warm-up routines to prepare the human body for more vigorous aerobic or strength-training exercises. They are also used in cool-down routines to help the body return to the normal resting state.

FACTORS AFFECTING FLEXIBILITY

Flexibility seems to be determined by heredity and exercise. Joint range of motion is limited by factors such as joint structure, ligaments, tendons, muscles, skin, tissue injury, adipose tissue, body temperature, age, gender, and index of physical activity.

The range of motion about a given joint depends largely on the structure of that particular joint. Fortunately, greater range of motion is attainable and can be accomplished through "plastic" or "elastic" elongation. Plastic elongation refers to a permanent lengthening of soft tissue. Even though joint capsules, ligaments, and tendons are primarily nonelastic in nature, they can undergo plastic elongation. This permanent lengthening leads to increases in joint range of motion and is best attained using slow, sustained stretching exercises. Muscle tissue, on the other hand, has elastic properties and will respond to stretching exercises by undergoing elastic or temporary lengthening. This form of elongation increases the extensibility of the muscles.

Changes in muscle temperature can increase or decrease flexibility by as much as 20 percent. Properly warmed-up individuals exhibit better flexibility levels than non-warmed-up subjects. Cool temperatures have the opposite effect, decreasing joint range of motion. Because of the effects of temperature on muscular flexibility, many people prefer to conduct their stretching exercises following the aerobic phase of their workout. Aerobic activities raise the temperature of connective tissue, facilitating plastic elongation.

Another factor that influences flexibility is the amount of adipose tissue in and around joints and muscle tissue. Large amounts of adipose tissue not only increase resistance to movement, but the additional bulk restricts joint mobility because of the premature contact between contiguous body surfaces.

On the average, women enjoy higher flexibility levels than men and seem to retain this advantage throughout life. Aging decreases the extensibility of soft tissue, resulting in decreased flexibility. The most significant contributors to decrements in flexibility, however, are sedentary living and lack of physical activity. As physical activity decreases, muscles lose elasticity, and tendons and ligaments tighten and shorten. In addition, inactivity frequently leads to an increase in adipose tissue, which further decreases joint range of motion. Finally, injury to muscle tissue and tight skin resulting in excessive scar tissue, has a negative effect on joint range of motion.

FLEXIBILITY ASSESSMENT TECHNIQUES

Many flexibility tests can be found in the literature, but most of them are specific to certain

sports and are not practical for use with the general population. Consequently, their application in health and fitness programs is very limited. For example, the Back Hyperextension Test, the Front-to-Rear Splits Test, and the Bridge-Up Test (see Figure 4.1) all may have applications in sports such as gymnastics and several track and field events, but they are not indicative of actions

Figure 4.1. *Back Hyperextension Test (a), Front-to-Rear Splits Test (b), and Bridge-Up Test (c). These tests are not practical for use with the general population because they are not indicative of actions most people encounter in daily life.*

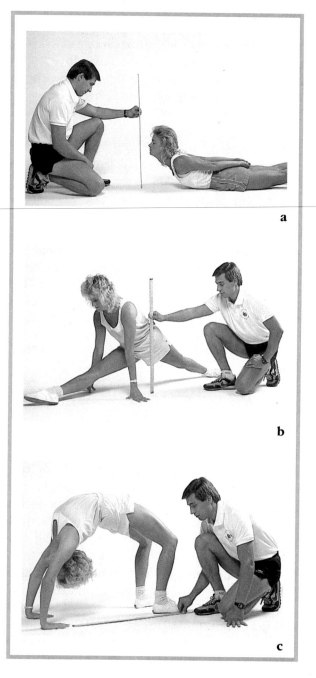

people encounter in daily life. Because of the lack of practical flexibility tests, most health/fitness centers have relied strictly on the Sit-and-Reach Test (see Figure 4.2) as an indicator of overall flexibility. This test, however, measures only the flexibility of the lower back and the hamstring muscles (back of the thigh).

Because flexibility is joint-specific and a high degree of flexibility in one joint does not necessarily indicate a high degree in other joints, two

additional tests that are indicative of everyday movements such as reaching, bending, and turning, have been included to determine your flexibility profile. These tests are the Total Body Rotation Test (previously referred to as Trunk Rotation Test) and the Shoulder Rotation Test.

The Sit-and-Reach Test also has been modified from the traditional test in that arm/leg length discrepancies are taken into consideration to determine the flexibility score (see test procedure in Figure 4.3). The procedures and norms for the battery of flexibility tests are described in Figures 4.3 through 4.5 and Tables 4.1 through 4.3.* For the flexibility profile, instead of a choice of tests, you will need to take all three tests.

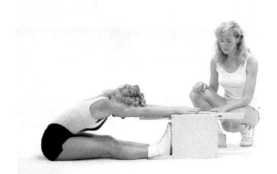

Figure 4.2. *Sit-and-Reach Test*

---

* The norms for the Modified Sit-and-Reach Test, Total Body Rotation Test (previously referred to as Trunk Rotation Test), and Shoulder Rotation Test contained in this chapter are reproduced with permission from Hoeger, W. W. K. *The Complete Guide for the Development and Implementation of Health Promotion Programs.* Englewood, CO: Morton Publishing Company, 1987.

Figure 4.3. *Procedure for the Modified Sit-and-Reach Test[a]*

1. To perform this test you will need the Acu-flex I Sit-and-Reach Flexibility Tester[b], or you may simply place a yardstick on top of a box approximately twelve inches high.

2. Be sure to properly warm up prior to the first trial.

3. Remove your shoes. Sit on the floor with the back and head against a wall, legs fully extended, and the bottom of the feet against the Acuflex I or sit-and-reach box.

4. Place the hands one on top of the other, and reach forward as far as possible without letting the head and back come off the wall. (The shoulders may be rounded as much as possible, but neither the head nor back should come off the wall at this time.) The technician can then slide the reach indicator on the Acuflex I (or yardstick) along the top of the box until the end of the indicator touches the participant's fingers (see Figure 4.3a). The indicator then must be held firmly in place throughout the rest of the test.

5. The head and back can now come off the wall. Gradually reach forward three times, the third time stretching forward as far as possible on the indicator (or yardstick) and holding the final position for at least two seconds (see Figure 4.2). Be sure that during the test the back of the knees are kept flat against the floor. Record the final number of inches reached to the nearest one-half inch.

6. You are allowed two trials, and an average of the two scores is used as the final test score. The respective percentile ranks and fitness categories for this test are given in Tables 4.1 and 4.4.

---

[a] Unlike the traditional Sit-and-Reach Test, the modified protocol varies in that the arm and leg lengths are taken into consideration to determine the score. In the original test procedure, the fifteen-inch mark of the yardstick is always set at the edge of the box where the feet are placed. This procedure does not differentiate between an individual with long arms and/or short legs and someone with short arms and/or long legs. All other factors being equal, an individual with longer arms and/or shorter legs would receive a better rating because of the structural advantage.

[b] The Acuflex I Flexibility Tester for the Modified Sit-and-Reach Test can be obtained from Novel Products Figure Finder Collection, 80 Fairbanks, Unit 12, Addison, IL 60101, (312) 628-1787.

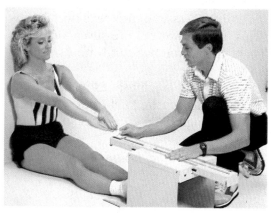

Figure 4.3a. *Determining the starting position for the Sit-and-Reach Test.*

Table 4.1.
Percentile Ranks for the
Modified Sit-and-Reach Test

	Percentile Rank	Age Category		
		<35	36–49	50>
Men	99	24.7	18.9	16.2
	95	19.5	18.2	15.8
	90	17.9	16.1	15.0
	80	17.0	14.6	13.3
	70	15.8	13.9	12.3
	60	15.0	13.4	11.5
	50	14.4	12.6	10.2
	40	13.5	11.6	9.7
	30	13.0	10.8	9.3
	20	11.6	9.9	8.8
	10	9.2	8.3	7.8
	05	7.9	7.0	7.2
	01	7.0	5.1	4.0
Women	99	19.8	19.8	17.2
	95	18.7	19.2	15.7
	90	17.9	17.4	15.0
	80	16.7	16.2	14.2
	70	16.2	15.2	13.6
	60	15.8	14.5	12.3
	50	14.8	13.5	11.1
	40	14.5	12.8	10.1
	30	13.7	12.2	9.2
	20	12.6	11.0	8.3
	10	10.1	9.7	7.5
	05	8.1	8.5	3.7
	01	2.6	2.0	1.5

Figure 4.4. *Procedure for the Total Body Rotation Test*

1. To perform this test you will need an Acuflex II Total Body Rotation Flexibility Tester[a] or a measuring scale with a sliding panel. Place the Acuflex II or scale on the wall at shoulder height. It should be adjustable to accommodate individual differences in height. If you need to build your own scale, use two measuring tapes and glue them above and below the sliding panel — centered at the fifteen-inch mark. Each tape should be at least thirty inches long. If no sliding panel is available, simply tape the measuring tapes onto a wall. A line that is centered with the fifteen-inch mark must also be drawn on the floor (*see* Figures 4.4a, 4.4b, 4.4c, and 4.4d).

2. Be sure to properly warm up prior to initiating this test.

3. Stand sideways, an arm's length away from the wall, with the feet straight ahead, slightly separated, and the toes right up to the corresponding line drawn on the floor. Hold the arm opposite the wall horizontally from the body, making a fist with the hand. The Acuflex II, measuring scale, or tapes should be shoulder height at this time.

4. Rotate the trunk, the extended arm going backward (always maintaining a horizontal plane) and making contact with the panel, gradually sliding it forward as far as possible (*see* Figure 4.4d). If no panel is available, slide the fist alongside the tapes as far as possible. Hold the final position for at least two seconds. Position the hand with the little finger side forward during the entire sliding movement (Figure 4.4e). **It is crucial that the proper hand position be used. Many people will attempt to either open the hand, push with extended fingers, or slide the panel with the knuckles, none of which are acceptable test procedures.** During the test, the knees can be slightly bent, but **the feet cannot be moved. They must always point straight forward.** The body must be kept as straight (vertical) as possible.

5. The test can be conducted on either the right or left side of the body. You are allowed two trials. Record the farthest point reached, measured to the nearest one-half inch, and held for at least two seconds. The average of the two trials is used as the final test score. Using Tables 4.2 and 4.4, determine the percentile rank and flexibility fitness classification.

[a] The Acuflex II Flexibility Tester for total body rotation can be obtained from Novel Products Figure Finder Collection, 80 Fairbanks, Unit 12, Addison, IL 60101, (312) 628-1787.

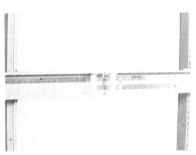

Figure 4.4a. *Acuflex II measuring device for the Total Body Rotation Test*

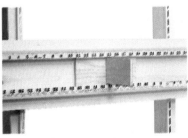

Figure 4.4b. *Homemade measuring device for the Total Body Rotation Test*

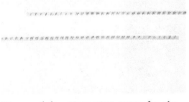

Figure 4.4c. *Measuring tapes for the Total Body Rotation Test*

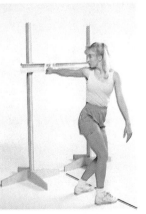

Figure 4.4d. *Total Body Rotation Test*

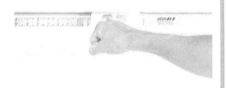

Figure 4.4e. *Proper hand position for the Total Body Rotation Test*

Table 4.2.
Percentile Ranks for the Total Body Rotation Test

	Percentile Rank	Age:	Right Rotation			Left Rotation		
			<35	36–49	50>	<35	36–49	50>
Men	99		27.8	25.2	22.2	28.0	26.6	21.0
	95		25.6	23.8	20.7	24.8	24.5	20.0
	90		24.1	22.5	19.3	23.6	23.0	17.7
	80		22.3	21.0	16.3	22.0	21.2	15.5
	70		20.7	18.7	15.7	20.3	20.4	14.7
	60		19.0	17.3	14.7	19.3	18.7	13.9
	50		17.2	16.3	12.3	18.0	16.7	12.7
	40		16.3	14.7	11.5	16.8	15.3	11.7
	30		15.0	13.3	10.7	15.0	14.8	10.3
	20		13.3	11.2	8.7	13.3	13.7	9.5
	10		11.3	8.0	2.7	10.5	10.8	4.3
	05		8.3	5.5	0.3	8.9	8.8	0.3
	01		2.9	2.0	0.0	1.7	5.1	0.0
Women	99		29.4	27.1	21.7	28.6	27.1	23.0
	95		25.3	25.9	19.7	24.8	25.3	21.4
	90		23.0	21.3	19.0	23.0	23.4	20.5
	80		20.8	19.6	17.9	21.5	20.2	19.1
	70		19.3	17.3	16.8	20.5	18.6	17.3
	60		18.0	16.5	15.6	19.3	17.7	16.0
	50		17.3	14.6	14.0	18.0	16.4	14.8
	40		16.0	13.1	12.8	17.2	14.8	13.7
	30		15.2	11.7	8.5	15.7	13.6	10.0
	20		14.0	9.8	3.9	15.2	11.6	6.3
	10		11.1	6.1	2.2	13.6	8.5	3.0
	05		8.8	4.0	1.1	7.3	6.8	0.7
	01		3.2	2.8	0.0	5.3	4.3	0.0

Figure 4.5. *Procedure for the Shoulder Rotation Test*

1. Perform this test using the Acuflex III Flexibility Tester[a], which consists of a shoulder caliper and a measuring device for shoulder rotation. If it is unavailable, you can quite easily construct your own device. The caliper can be built with three regular yardsticks. Nail and glue two of the yardsticks at one end at a 90° angle, and use the third one as the sliding end of the caliper. Construct the rotation device by placing a sixty-inch measuring tape on an aluminum or wood stick, starting at about six or seven inches from the end of the stick.

2. Be sure to properly warm up prior to the test.

3. Using the shoulder caliper, measure the biacromial width to the nearest one-fourth inch (use the red scale on the Acuflex III). Biacromial width is measured between the lateral edges of the acromion processes of the shoulders, as shown in Figure 4.4a.

[a] The Acuflex III Flexibility Tester for the Shoulder Rotation Test can be obtained from Novel Products Figure Finder Collection, 80 Fairbanks, Unit 12, Addison, IL 60101, (312) 628-1787.

4. Place the Acuflex III or homemade device behind your back and use a reverse (thumbs out) grip to hold on to the device (Figure 4.5b). Place the right hand next to the zero point of the scale (blue scale on the Acuflex III) or tape and hold firmly in place throughout the test. Place the left hand on the other end of the measuring device, as wide as needed.

5. Standing straight up and extending both arms to full length, **with elbows locked,** slowly bring the measuring device over the head until it reaches forehead level (Figure 4.5c). For succeeding trials, depending on the resistance encountered when rotating the shoulders, move the left grip in one-half to one inch at a time. Repeat the task until you can no longer rotate the shoulders without undue strain or you start bending the elbows to do so. Always keep the righthand grip against the zero point of the scale. Measure the last successful trial to the nearest one-half inch. Take this measurement at the very inner edge of the left hand — on the side of the little finger.

6. Determine the final score for this test by subtracting the biacromial width from the best score (shortest distance) between both hands on the rotation test. For example, if the best score is thirty-five inches and the biacromial width is fifteen inches, the final score would be twenty inches (35 − 15 = 20). Using Tables 4.3 and 4.4, determine the percentile rank and flexibility fitness classification for this test.

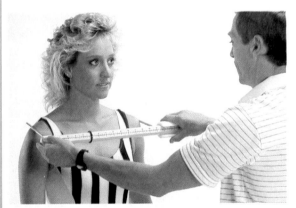

Figure 4.5a. *Measuring Biacromial Width*

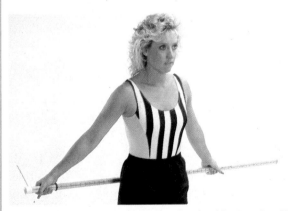

Figure 4.5.b. *Starting position for the Shoulder Rotation Test (note the reverse grip used for this test)*

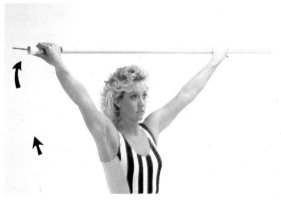

Figure 4.5.c. *Shoulder Rotation Test*

Table 4.3.
Percentile Ranks for the Shoulder Rotation Test

	Percentile Rank	Age Category		
		<35	36-49	50>
Men	99	−1.0	18.1	21.5
	95	10.4	20.4	27.0
	90	15.5	20.8	27.9
	80	18.4	23.3	28.5
	70	20.5	24.7	29.4
	60	22.9	26.6	29.9
	50	24.4	28.0	30.5
	40	25.7	30.0	31.0
	30	27.3	31.9	31.7
	20	30.1	33.3	33.1
	10	31.8	36.1	37.2
	05	33.5	37.8	38.7
	01	42.6	43.0	44.1
Women	99	−2.4	11.5	13.1
	95	6.2	15.4	16.5
	90	9.7	16.8	20.9
	80	14.5	19.2	22.5
	70	17.2	21.5	24.3
	60	18.7	23.1	25.1
	50	20.0	23.5	26.2
	40	21.4	24.4	28.1
	30	24.0	25.9	29.9
	20	25.9	29.8	31.5
	10	29.1	31.1	33.1
	05	31.3	33.4	34.1
	01	37.1	34.9	35.4

INTERPRETATION OF THE FLEXIBILITY TESTS

After obtaining your score and percentile rank for each test, you can determine the fitness category for each flexibility test using the guidelines given in Table 4.4. The overall flexibility fitness classification (see Figure 4.6) is obtained by computing an average percentile rank from all three tests and using the same guidelines given in Table 4.4.

Table 4.4.
Flexibility Fitness Categories

Percentile Rank	Fitness Category
80+	Excellent
60-79	Good
40-59	Average
20-39	Fair
<19	Poor

PRINCIPLES OF MUSCULAR FLEXIBILITY PRESCRIPTION

The overload and specificity of training principles discussed in conjunction with strength development in Chapter 3 also apply to the development of muscular flexibility. To increase the total range of motion of a given joint, the specific muscles that surround that particular joint have to be progressively stretched beyond their normal accustomed length. Principles of mode,

Figure 4.6. *Muscular flexibility report*

Name: _____ Age: _____ Sex: _____

Date: _____

Test	Score	% Rank	Classification
Modified Sit-and-Reach			
Total Body Rotation ___ Right ___ Left			
Shoulder Rotation			

Total:

Average Percentile Rank (divide total by 3): _____

Overall Flexibility Classification: _____

Date: _____

Test	Score	% Rank	Classification
Modified Sit-and-Reach			
Total Body Rotation ___ Right ___ Left			
Shoulder Rotation			

Total:

Average Percentile Rank (divide total by 3): _____

Overall Flexibility Classification: _____

intensity, repetitions, and frequency of exercise can also be used for the prescription of flexibility programs.

Mode of Exercise

Three modes of stretching exercises can be used to increase flexibility: (a) ballistic stretching, (b) slow-sustained stretching, and (c) proprioceptive neuromuscular facilitation stretching. Although research has indicated that all three types of stretching are effective in developing better flexibility, there are certain advantages to each technique.

Ballistic or dynamic stretching exercises are performed using jerky, rapid, and bouncy movements that provide the necessary force to lengthen the muscles. Even though studies have indicated that this type of stretching helps to develop flexibility, the ballistic actions may lead to increased muscle soreness and injury because of small tears to the soft tissue. In addition, proper precautions must be taken to not overstretch ligaments, because they will undergo plastic or permanent elongation. If the magnitude of the stretching force cannot be adequately controlled in the fast, jerky movements, ligaments can be easily overstretched. This, in turn, leads to excessively loose joints, increasing the risk for injuries, including joint dislocation and subluxation (partial dislocation). Consequently, most authorities do not recommend ballistic exercises for flexibility development.

With the slow-sustained stretching technique, muscles are gradually lengthened through a joint's complete range of motion, and the final position is held for a few seconds. Using a slow-sustained stretch causes the muscles to relax; hence, greater length can be achieved. This type of stretch causes relatively little pain and has a very low risk of injury. Slow-sustained stretching exercises are the most frequently used and recommended for flexibility development programs.

Proprioceptive neuromuscular facilitation (PNF) stretching (see Figure 4.7) has become more popular in the last few years. This technique is based on a "contract and relax" method and requires the assistance of another person. The procedure used is as follows:

1. The person assisting with the exercise provides an initial force by slowly pushing in the direction of the desired stretch. The initial stretch does not cover the entire range of motion.

2. The person being stretched then applies force in the opposite direction of the stretch, against the assistant, who will try to hold the initial degree of stretch as closely as possible. An isometric contraction is being performed at that angle.

3. After four or five seconds of isometric contraction, the muscles being stretched are completely relaxed. The assistant then slowly increases the degree of stretch to a greater angle.

4. The isometric contraction is then repeated for another four or five seconds, after which the muscles are relaxed again. The assistant can then slowly increase the degree of stretch one more time. This procedure is repeated from two to five times, until mild discomfort occurs. On the last trial, the final stretched position should be held for several seconds.

Theoretically, with the PNF technique, the isometric contraction aids in the relaxation of the muscles being stretched, which results in greater muscle length. Although some researchers have indicated that PNF is more effective than slow-sustained stretching, the disadvantages are that the degree of pain incurred with PNF is greater, a second person is required to perform the exercises, and a greater period of time is needed to conduct each session.

Intensity of Exercise

Before starting any flexibility exercises, the muscles should be adequately warmed up with some calisthenic exercises. A good time to do flexibility exercises is following aerobic workouts. Increased body temperature can significantly increase joint range of motion. Failing to conduct a proper warm-up increases the risk for muscle pulls and tears.

The intensity or degree of stretch when doing flexibility exercises should be only to a point of mild discomfort. Pain does not have to be a part of the stretching routine. Excessive pain is an indication that the load is too high and may lead to injury. Stretching should be done to slightly below the pain threshold. As you reach this point, you should try to relax the muscles being stretched as much as possible. After completing the stretch, bring the body part gradually back to the original starting point.

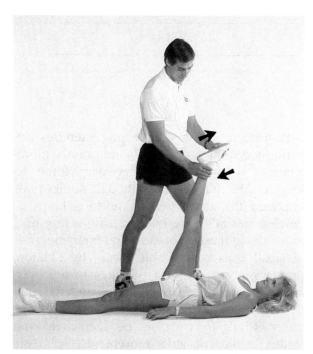

Figure 4.7. *Proprioceptive neuromuscular facilitation stretching technique*

Repetitions

The duration of an exercise session for flexibility development is based on the repetitions performed for each exercise and the length of time that each repetition (final stretched position) is held. The general recommendations are that each exercise be done four or five times, and each time the final position should be held for five to ten seconds. As the flexibility levels increase, the subject can progressively increase the time that each repetition is held, to a maximum of one minute.

Frequency of Exercise

Flexibility exercises should be conducted five to six times per week in the initial stages of the program. After a minimum of six to eight weeks of almost daily stretching, flexibility levels can be maintained with only two or three sessions per week, using about three repetitions of ten to fifteen seconds each.

FLEXIBILITY EXERCISES

To improve body flexibility, at least one stretching exercise should be used for each major muscle group. A complete set of exercises for the development of muscular flexibility is given at the end of this chapter. For some of these exercises (e.g., lateral head tilts and arm circles) you may not be able to hold a final stretched position, but you should still perform the exercise through the joint's full range of motion. Depending on the number and the length of the repetitions performed, a complete workout will last between fifteen and thirty minutes.

PREVENTION AND REHABILITATION OF LOW BACK PAIN

Very few people make it through life without suffering from low back pain at some point. Current estimates indicate that 75 million Americans suffer from chronic low back pain each year. Approximately 80 percent of the time, backache syndrome is preventable and is caused by: (a) physical inactivity, (b) poor postural habits and body mechanics, and (c) excessive body weight.

Lack of physical activity is the most common cause contributing to chronic low back pain. The deterioration or weakening of the abdominal and gluteal muscles, along with a tightening of the lower back (erector spinae) muscles, brings about an unnatural forward tilt of the pelvis (see Figure 4.8). This tilt puts extra pressure on the spinal vertebrae, causing pain in the lower back. In addition, excessive accumulation of fat around the midsection of the body contributes to the forward tilt of the pelvis, which further aggravates the condition.

Low back pain is also frequently associated with faulty posture and improper body mechanics in all of life's daily activities — sleeping, sitting, standing, walking, driving, working, and exercising. Incorrect posture and poor mechanics, as explained in Figure 4.9, lead to increased strain not only on the lower back, but on many other bones, joints, muscles, and ligaments as well.

The incidence and frequency of low back pain can be greatly reduced by including some specific stretching and strengthening exercises in your regular fitness program. When suffering from backache, in most cases pain is present only with movement and physical activity. If the pain is severe and persists even at rest, the initial step

Figure 4.8. *A comparison of incorrect (left) and correct (right) pelvic alignment*

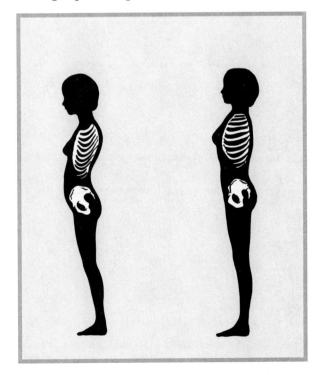

is to consult a physician. If disc damage is ruled out, correct bed rest will most likely be prescribed, using several pillows under the knees for adequate leg support (see Figure 4.9). This position helps relieve muscle spasms by stretching the muscles involved. A physician may additionally prescribe a muscle relaxant or anti-inflammatory medication (or both) and some type of physical therapy.

Once the individual is pain-free in the resting state, he/she needs to start correcting the muscular imbalance by stretching the tight muscles and strengthening weak ones (stretching exercises are always performed first). Because of the significance of these exercises in prevention and rehabilitation of the backache syndrome, they are included at the end of this chapter. You should conduct these exercises twice or more daily when suffering from backache. Under normal conditions, three to four times per week is sufficient to prevent the syndrome.

Bibliography

Billing, H., and E. Loewendahl. *Mobilization of the Human Body.* Palo Alto, CA: Stanford University Press, 1949.

Chapman, E. A., H. A. deVries, and R. Swezey. "Joint Stiffness: Effects of Exercise on Young and Old Men." *Journal of Gerontology* 27:218-221, 1972.

Dickerson, R. V. "The Specificity of Flexibility." *Research Quarterly* 33:222-229, 1962.

Fleishman, E. A. *Examiners Manual for Basic Fitness Tests.* Englewood Cliffs, NJ: Prentice-Hall, 1964.

Fox, E. L., and D. K. Mathews. *The Physiological Basis of Physical Education and Athletics.* Philadelphia: Saunders College Publishing, 1988.

Heyward, V. H. *Designs for Fitness: A Guide to Physical Fitness Appraisal and Exercise Prescription.* Minneapolis: Burgess Publishing, 1984.

Hoeger, W. W. K. *The Complete Guide for the Development & Implementation of Health Promotion Programs.* Englewood, CO: Morton Publishing, 1987.

Hoeger, W. W. K., D. R. Hopkins, and L. C. Johnson. *Assessment of Muscular Flexibility: Test Protocols for the Modified Sit-and-Reach Test, Total Body Rotation Test, and Shoulder Rotation Test.* Addison, IL: Novel Products Figure Finder Collection, 1988.

Holt, L. E., T. M. Travis, and T. Okita. "Comparative Study of Three Stretching Techniques." *Perceptual and Motor Skills* 31:611-616, 1970.

Johnson, B. L., and J. K. Nelson. *Practical Measurements for Evaluation in Physical Education.* Minneapolis: Burgess Publishing, 1979.

Johnson, L. C. "Trunk Rotation Flexibility Test." Unpublished test protocol. Lake Geneva, WI: Fitness Monitoring Preventive Medicine Clinic, 1979.

Sapega, A. A., T. C. Quedenfeld, R. A. Moyer, and R. A. Butler, "Biophysical Factors in Range-of-Motion Exercise." *Physician and Sportsmedicine* 9:57-65, 1981.

Wright, V., and R. J. Johns. "Physical Factors Concerned with Stiffness of Normal and Diseased Joints." *Bulletin of Johns Hopkins Hospital* 106:215-231, 1960.

Your Back and How to Care For It. Kenilworth, NJ: Schering Corp., 1965.

Figure 4.9. *Your back and how to care for it*

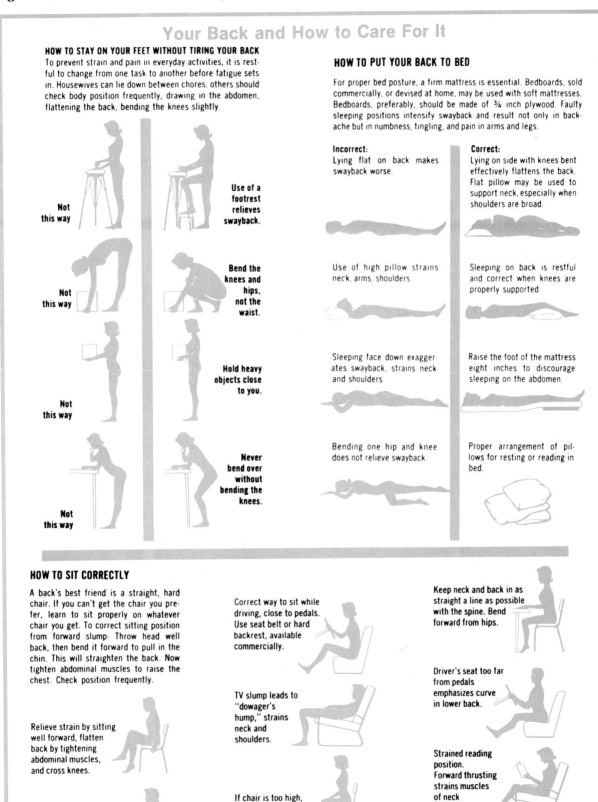

Your Back and How to Care For It

HOW TO STAY ON YOUR FEET WITHOUT TIRING YOUR BACK

To prevent strain and pain in everyday activities, it is restful to change from one task to another before fatigue sets in. Housewives can lie down between chores; others should check body position frequently, drawing in the abdomen, flattening the back, bending the knees slightly.

Not this way

Use of a footrest relieves swayback.

Not this way

Bend the knees and hips, not the waist.

Not this way

Hold heavy objects close to you.

Not this way

Never bend over without bending the knees.

HOW TO PUT YOUR BACK TO BED

For proper bed posture, a firm mattress is essential. Bedboards, sold commercially, or devised at home, may be used with soft mattresses. Bedboards, preferably, should be made of ¾ inch plywood. Faulty sleeping positions intensify swayback and result not only in backache but in numbness, tingling, and pain in arms and legs.

Incorrect:
Lying flat on back makes swayback worse.

Correct:
Lying on side with knees bent effectively flattens the back. Flat pillow may be used to support neck, especially when shoulders are broad.

Use of high pillow strains neck, arms, shoulders.

Sleeping on back is restful and correct when knees are properly supported.

Sleeping face down exaggerates swayback, strains neck and shoulders.

Raise the foot of the mattress eight inches to discourage sleeping on the abdomen.

Bending one hip and knee does not relieve swayback.

Proper arrangement of pillows for resting or reading in bed.

HOW TO SIT CORRECTLY

A back's best friend is a straight, hard chair. If you can't get the chair you prefer, learn to sit properly on whatever chair you get. To correct sitting position from forward slump: Throw head well back, then bend it forward to pull in the chin. This will straighten the back. Now tighten abdominal muscles to raise the chest. Check position frequently.

Relieve strain by sitting well forward, flatten back by tightening abdominal muscles, and cross knees.

Use of footrest relieves swayback. Aim is to have knees higher than hips.

Correct way to sit while driving, close to pedals. Use seat belt or hard backrest, available commercially.

TV slump leads to "dowager's hump," strains neck and shoulders.

If chair is too high, swayback is increased.

Keep neck and back in as straight a line as possible with the spine. Bend forward from hips.

Driver's seat too far from pedals emphasizes curve in lower back.

Strained reading position. Forward thrusting strains muscles of neck and head.

Flexibility Exercises

Exercise 1: LATERAL HEAD TILT

Action: Slowly and gently tilt the head laterally. Repeat several times to each side.

Areas Stretched: Neck flexors and extensors and ligaments of the cervical spine.

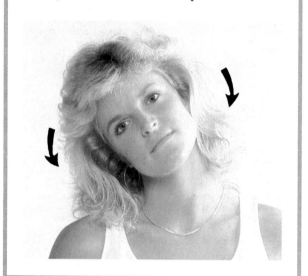

Exercise 2:   ARM CIRCLES

Action: Gently circle your arms all the way around. Conduct the exercise in both directions.

Areas Stretched: Shoulder muscles and ligaments.

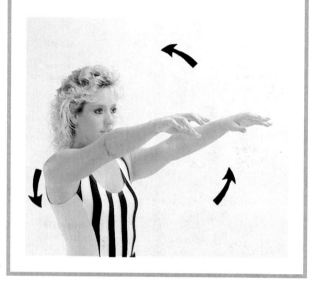

Exercise 3:   SIDE STRETCH

Action: Stand straight up, feet separated to shoulder width, and place your hands on your waist. Now move the upper body to one side and hold the final stretch for a few seconds. Repeat on the other side.

Areas Stretched: Muscles and ligaments in the pelvic region.

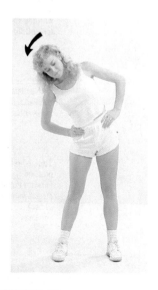

Exercise 4: BODY ROTATION

Action: Place your arms slightly away from your body and rotate the trunk as far as possible, holding the final position for several seconds. Conduct the exercise for both the right and left sides of the body. You can also perform this exercise by standing about two feet away from the wall (back toward the wall), and then rotate the trunk, placing the hands against the wall.

Areas Stretched: Hip, abdominal, chest, back, neck, and shoulder muscles; hip and spinal ligaments.

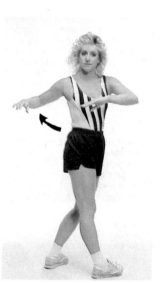

Exercise 5: CHEST STRETCH

Action: Kneel down behind a chair and place both hands on the back of the chair. Gradually push your chest downward and hold for a few seconds.

Areas Stretched: Chest (pectoral) muscles and shoulder ligaments.

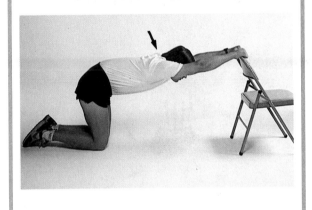

Exercise 6: SHOULDER HYPEREXTENSION STRETCH

Action: Have a partner grasp your arms from behind by the wrists and slowly push them upward. Hold the final position for a few seconds.

Areas Stretched: Deltoid and pectoral muscles, and ligaments of the shoulder joint.

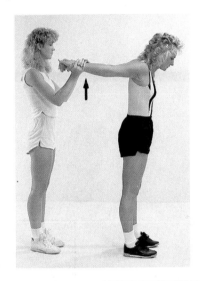

Exercise 7: SHOULDER ROTATION STRETCH

Action: With the aid of an aluminum or wood stick or surgical tubing, place the stick or tubing behind your back and grasp the two ends using a reverse (thumbs-out) grip. Slowly bring the stick over your head, keeping the elbows straight. Repeat several times (bring the hands closer together for additional stretch).

Areas Stretched: Deltoid, latissimus dorsi, and pectoral muscles; shoulder ligaments.

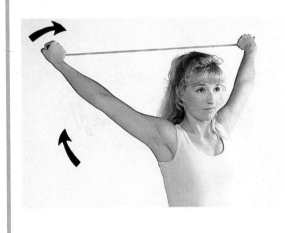

Exercise 8: QUAD STRETCH

Action: Stand straight up and bring up one foot, flexing the knee. Grasp the front of the ankle and pull the ankle toward the gluteal region. Hold for several seconds. Repeat with the other leg.

Areas Stretched: Quadriceps muscle, and knee and ankle ligaments.

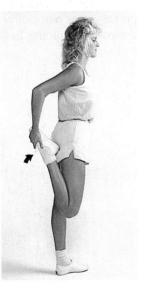

Exercise 9:
HEEL CORD STRETCH

Action: Stand against the wall or at the edge of a step and stretch the heel downward, alternating legs. Hold the stretched position for a few seconds.

Areas Stretched: Heel cord (Achilles tendon), gastrocnemius, and soleus muscles.

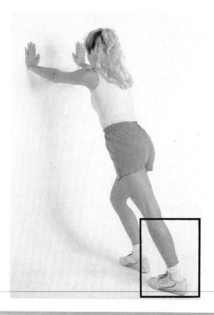

Exercise 10:
ADDUCTOR STRETCH

Action: Stand with your feet about twice shoulder width and place your hands slightly above the knee. Flex one knee and slowly go down as far as possible, holding the final position for a few seconds. Repeat with the other leg.

Areas Stretched: Hip adductor muscles.

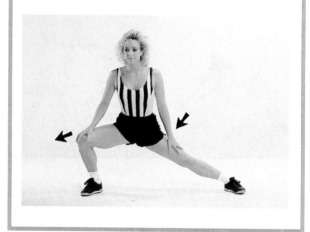

Exercise 11:
SITTING ADDUCTOR STRETCH

Action: Sit on the floor and bring your feet in close to you, allowing the soles of the feet to touch each other. Now place your forearms (or elbows) on the inner part of the thigh and push the legs downward, holding the final stretch for several seconds.

Areas Stretched: Hip adductor muscles.

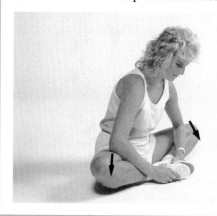

Exercise 12:
SIT-AND-REACH STRETCH

Action: Sit on the floor with legs together and gradually reach forward as far as possible. Hold the final position for a few seconds. This exercise may also be performed with the legs separated, reaching to each side as well as to the middle.

Areas Stretched: Hamstrings and lower back muscles, and lumbar spine ligaments.

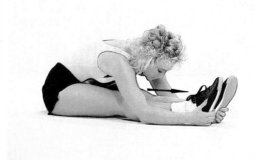

Exercises for the Prevention and Rehabilitation of Low Back Pain

---

Exercise 13:   SINGLE-KNEE TO CHEST STRETCH

Action: Lie down flat on the floor. Bend one leg at approximately 100° and gradually pull the opposite leg toward your chest. Hold the final stretch for a few seconds. Switch legs and repeat the exercise.

Areas Stretched: Lower back and hamstring muscles, and lumbar spine ligaments.

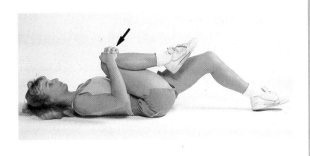

Exercise 14:   DOUBLE-KNEE TO CHEST STRETCH

Action: Lie flat on the floor and then slowly curl up into a fetal position. Hold for a few seconds.

Areas Stretched: Upper and lower back and hamstring muscles; spinal ligaments.

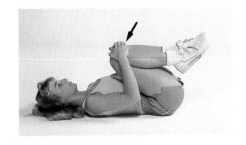

Exercise 15:   UPPER AND LOWER BACK STRETCH

Action: Sit in a chair with feet separated greater than shoulder width. Place your arms to the inside of the thighs and bring your chest down toward the floor. At the same time, attempt to reach back as far as you can with your arms.

Areas Stretched: Upper and lower back muscles and ligaments.

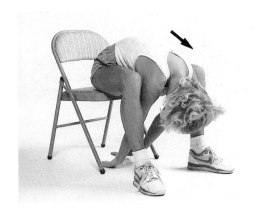

Exercise 16:   SIT-AND-REACH STRETCH
(see Exercise 12 in this chapter)

Exercise 17: TRUNK ROTATION AND LOWER BACK STRETCH

Action: Sit on the floor and bend the left leg, placing the left foot on the outside of the right knee. Place the right elbow on the left knee and push against it. At the same time, try to rotate the trunk to the left (counterclockwise). Hold the final position for a few seconds. Repeat the exercise with the other side.

Areas Stretched: Lateral side of the hip and thigh; trunk, and lower back.

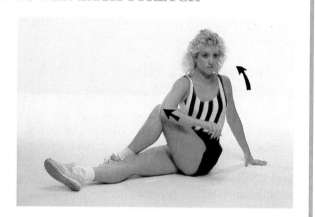

Exercise 18: PELVIC TILT

Action: Lie flat on the floor with the knees bent at about a 70° angle. Tilt the pelvis by tightening the abdominal muscles, flattening your back against the floor, and raising the lower gluteal area ever so slightly off the floor (see illustration b). Hold the final position for several seconds. The exercise can also be performed against a wall (as shown in illustration c).

Areas Stretched:
Low back muscles and ligaments.

Areas Strengthened:
Abdominal and gluteal muscles.

Note: This is perhaps the most important exercise for the care of the lower back. It should be included as a part of your daily exercise routine and should be performed several times throughout the day when pain in the lower back is present as a result of muscle imbalance.

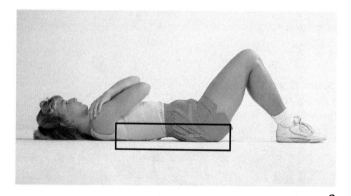

a

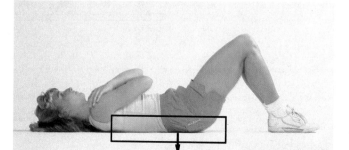

b

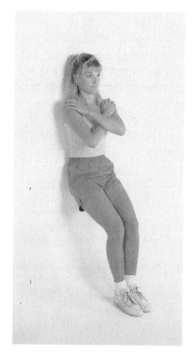

c

Exercise 19:   ABDOMINAL CURL-UP (see Exercise 4 in Chapter 3)

It is important that you do not stabilize your feet when performing this exercise, because doing so decreases the work of the abdominal muscles. Also, remember not to "swing up" but rather to curl up as you perform the exercise.

Body Composition Assessment

Obesity has become a health hazard of epidemic proportions in most developed countries around the world. Current statistical estimates indicate that 35 percent of the adult population in developed countries is obese, and approximately half of all adults in the U.S. have a weight problem. The evidence further shows that the prevalence is still increasing. Consider the following two facts: The average weight of American adults increased by about fifteen pounds in just the last decade. When Yankee Stadium in New York was renovated several years ago, total seating capacity had to be reduced to accommodate the wider bodies of our adult population!

Obesity by itself has been associated with several serious health problems, accounting for 15 to 20 percent of the annual U.S. mortality rate. Obesity has long been recognized as a major risk factor for diseases of the cardiovascular system, including coronary heart disease, hypertension, congestive heart failure, elevated blood lipids, atherosclerosis, strokes, thromboembolitic disease, varicose veins, and intermittent claudication.

New evidence points toward a possible link between obesity and cancer of the colon, rectum, prostate, gallbladder, breast, uterus, and ovaries. It is interesting to note that if all deaths from cancer could be eliminated, the average life span would increase by approximately two years. If obesity were eliminated, the life span could increase by as many as seven years. In addition, obesity has been associated with diabetes, osteoarthritis, ruptured intervertebral discs, gallstones, gout, respiratory insufficiency, and complications during pregnancy and delivery. Furthermore, it can lead to psychologic maladjustment and increased accidental death rate. Life insurance companies are also quick to point out that the mortality rate among overweight males is 150 percent greater than the average mortality rate.

There is little disagreement regarding a greater mortality rate among obese people, but scientific evidence also points to the reality that the same is true for underweight people. Although a slight change has been seen in recent years, the social pressure to achieve model-like thinness is still with us and continues to cause a gradual increase in the number of people who develop eating disorders (anorexia nervosa and bulimia). Extreme weight loss can lead to medical conditions such as heart damage, gastrointestinal problems, shrinkage of internal organs, immune system abnormalities, disorders of the reproductive system, loss of muscle tissue, damage to the nervous system, and even death. Additional information on eating disorders is given in Chapter 6.

WHAT DOES "BODY COMPOSITION" MEAN?

The term "body composition" is used in reference to the fat and nonfat components of the human body. The fat component is usually referred to as fat mass or percent body fat. The nonfat component is termed lean body mass. Although for many years people have relied on height/weight charts to determine ideal body weight, we now know that these tables can be highly inaccurate for many people. The proper way of determining ideal weight is through body composition — by finding out what percent of total body weight is fat and what amount is lean tissue. Once the fat percentage is known, ideal body weight can be calculated from ideal body fat, the recommended amount at which there is no detriment to human health.

In spite of the fact that various techniques to determine percent body fat were developed several years ago, many people are still unaware of these procedures and continue to depend on height/weight charts to find out what their "ideal" body weight should be. These standard height/weight tables, first published in 1912, were based on average weights (including shoes and clothing) for men and women who obtained life insurance policies between 1888 and 1905. The ideal weight in the tables is obtained according to gender, height, and frame size. Because no scientific guidelines are given to determine frame size, most people choose their size based on the column containing their body weight!

To determine whether people are truly obese or "falsely" at ideal body weight, body composition must be established. Obesity is related to excessive body fat accumulation. If body weight is used as the only criteria, an individual can easily be overweight according to height/weight charts, yet not be obese. This is commonly seen among football players, body builders, weight lifters, and other athletes with large muscle size. Some of these athletes in reality have very little body fat but appear to be twenty or thirty pounds overweight.

The inaccuracy of the height/weight charts in predicting ideal weight for many people was clearly illustrated when a young man who weighed about 225 pounds applied to join a city police force but was turned down without having been granted an interview. The reason: He was "too fat" according to the height/weight charts. When this young man's body composition was later assessed at a preventive medicine clinic, he was shocked to find out that only 5 percent of his total body weight was in the form of fat (considerably lower than the ideal standard). In the words of the technical director of the clinic: "The only way that this fellow could come down to the chart's target weight would have been through surgical removal of a large amount of his muscle tissue."

On the other end of the spectrum, some people who weigh very little and are viewed by many as "skinny" or underweight can actually be classified as obese because of their high body fat content. Not at all uncommon are cases of people weighing as little as 100 pounds who are over 30 percent fat (about one-third of their total body weight). Such cases are more readily observed among sedentary people and those who are constantly dieting. Both physical inactivity and constant negative caloric balance lead to a loss in lean body mass. It is clear from these examples that body weight alone does not always tell the true story.

ESSENTIAL AND STORAGE FAT

Total fat in the human body is classified into two types, essential fat and storage fat. The essential fat is needed for normal physiological functions, and without it, human health begins to deteriorate. This essential fat constitutes about 3 percent of the total fat in men and 10 to 12 percent in women. The percentage is higher in women because it includes gender-specific fat, such as that found in the breast tissue, the uterus, and other gender-related fat deposits. The amount varies from 10 to 12 percent in women because of morphological (body build) differences from one woman to another.

Storage fat constitutes the fat that is stored in adipose tissue, mostly beneath the skin (subcutaneous fat) and around major organs in the body. This fat serves three basic functions: (a) as an insulator to retain body heat, (b) as energy substrate for metabolism, and (c) as padding against physical trauma to the body. The amount of storage fat does not differ between men and women, except that men tend to store fat around the waist, and women more so around the hips and thighs.

TECHNIQUES FOR ASSESSING BODY COMPOSITION

Several different procedures can be used to determine body composition. The most common techniques are: (a) hydrostatic or underwater weighing, (b) electrical impedance, (c) skinfold thickness, and (d) girth measurements.

Hydrostatic weighing is the most accurate technique available to assess body composition, but it also requires a considerable amount of

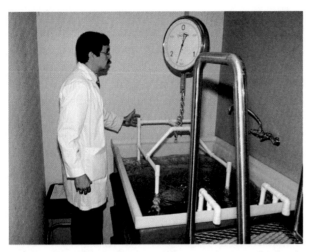

Figure 5.1. *Hydrostatic weighing technique for body composition assessment*

time, skill, space, equipment, and complex procedures. The person's residual lung volume (the amount of air left in the lungs following complete forceful exhalation) must also be measured while the person is in the water. If the residual volume cannot be measured, as is the case in many health/fitness centers, the volume is estimated using predicting equations, which may sacrifice the accuracy of hydrostatic weighing. The psychological factor of being weighed while submerged underwater also makes hydrostatic weighing difficult to administer to the aquaphobic.

The electrical impedance technique is much simpler to administer but does require costly equipment. This technique requires the subject to be hooked up to a machine, and a weak electrical current (totally painless) is run through the body to analyze body composition (body fat, lean body mass, and body water). There is still disagreement, nevertheless, regarding the accuracy of the current equations used in estimating percent body fat according to electrical impedance.

Because of cost, time, and complexity of test procedures, most health and fitness programs prefer the use of anthropometric measurement techniques that correlate quite well with hydrostatic weighing. These techniques, primarily skinfold thickness and girth measurements, provide a quick, simple, and inexpensive estimate of body composition.

Skinfold Thickness Technique

The assessment of body composition using skinfold thickness is based on the principle that approximately 50 percent of the fatty tissue in the body is deposited directly beneath the skin. If this tissue is estimated validly and reliably, a good indication of percent body fat can be obtained. This test is regularly performed with the aid of pressure calipers (see Figure 5.2); several sites must be measured to reflect the total percentage of fat. The protocols used in this book require the measurement of triceps, suprailium, and thigh skinfolds for women; and chest, abdomen, and thigh for men. All measurements should be taken on the right side of the body.

Even with the skinfold technique, a minimum amount of training is necessary to achieve accurate measurements. Also, small variations in measurements on the same subject may be found when these are taken by different observers. Therefore, it is recommended that pre- and post-measurements be conducted by the same technician. Furthermore, measurements should be taken at the same time of the day, preferably in the morning, because water hydration changes as a result of activity and exercise can increase skinfold girth up to 15 percent. The procedure for assessing percent body fat using skinfold

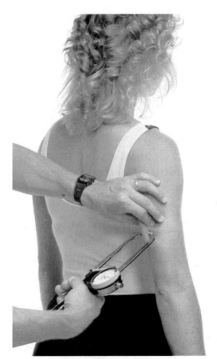

Figure 5.2. *Skinfold thickness technique for body composition assessment*

thickness is outlined in Figure 5.3. If skinfold calipers* are available to you, you may proceed to assess your percent body fat with the help of your instructor or an experienced technician.

Girth Measurements Technique

A simpler method to determine body fat is by measuring circumferences at various body sites. All this technique requires is the use of a standard measuring tape, and with little practice good accuracy can be achieved. The limitation of this procedure is that it may not be valid for athletic individuals (men or women) who actively participate in strenuous physical activity, or subjects who visually can be classified as thin or obese. The required procedure for this technique is given in Figure 5.4. The girth measurements for women are the upper arm, hip, and wrist; for men, the waist and wrist are used.

LEAN BODY MASS AND IDEAL BODY WEIGHT DETERMINATION

After finding out your percent body fat, you can determine your current body composition classification according to Table 5.6. In this same table you can find the healthy or ideal amount of fat that you should have under the "Ideal" column. For example, the ideal fat percentage for a twenty-year-old female is 18 percent. Ideal percent body fat is established at the point at which there is no detriment to your health. The ideal percentage does not mean that you cannot be somewhat below this number. Many highly trained male athletes are as low as 3 percent fat, and some female distance runners have been assessed around 8 percent body fat.

Although there is little disagreement regarding a greater mortality rate among obese people, some evidence seems to indicate that the same is true for underweight people. Being underweight and thin does not necessary mean the same thing. A healthy, thin person has total body fat around the ideal percentage, while an underweight person has extremely low body fat, even to the point of compromising the essential fat.

The 3 percent essential fat for men and 10 to 12 percent for women are the lower limits for most people to maintain good health. Below these percentages, normal physiologic functions can be seriously impaired. In addition, some experts point out that a little storage fat (over the essential fat) is better than none at all. As a result, the standards for ideal percent fat in Table 5.6 are set higher than the minimum essential fat requirements, at a point that is conducive to good health. Additionally, because lean tissue decreases with age, one extra percentage point is allowed for every additional decade of life.

This discussion on ideal percent body fat is important, because ideal body weight is computed based on the ideal fat percentage for your respective age and gender. To compute ideal body weight, take the following steps:

1. Determine the pounds of body weight in fat (FW). Multiply body weight (BW) by the current percent fat (%F) expressed in decimal form (FW = BW × %F).

2. Determine lean body mass (LBM) by subtracting the weight in fat from the total body weight (LBM = BW − FW). Remember that anything which is not fat must be part of the lean component.

3. Look up the ideal body fat percentage (IFP) in Table 5.6.

4. Compute ideal body weight (IBW) according to the following formula: IBW = LBM/(1.0 − IFP).

An example of these computations may be helpful. A nineteen-year-old female who weighs 136 pounds and is 25 percent fat would like to know what her ideal body weight should be.

Gender: female
Age: 19
BW: 136 lbs.
%F: 25% (.25 in decimal form)

1. FW = BW x %F
   FW = 136 × .25 = 34 lbs.

2. LBM = BW − FW
   LBM = 136 − 34 = 102 lbs.

3. IFP: 17% (.17 in decimal form)

4. IBW = LBM/(1.0 − IFP)
   IBW = 102/(1.0 − .17)
   IBW = 102/(.83) = 122.9 lbs.

---

* This instrument is available at most colleges and universities around the country. If unavailable, you can purchase an inexpensive, yet reliable Adipometer Skinfold Caliper from Ross Laboratories, Department #441, 625 Cleveland Avenue, Columbus, OH 43216.

Figure 5.3. *Procedure for body fat assessment according to skinfold thickness technique*

1. Select the proper anatomical sites. For men, chest, abdomen, and thigh skinfolds are used. For women, use triceps, suprailium, and thigh skinfolds. All measurements should be taken on the right side of the body with the subject standing. The correct anatomical landmarks for skinfolds are:

   Chest: a diagonal fold halfway between the shoulder crease and the nipple.

   Abdomen: a vertical fold about one inch to the right of the umbilicus.

   Triceps: a vertical fold on the back of the upper arm, halfway between the shoulder and the elbow.

   Thigh: a vertical fold on the front of the thigh, midway between the knee and hip.

   Suprailium: a diagonal fold above the crest of the ilium (on the side of the hip).

2. Measure each site by grasping a double thickness of skin firmly with the thumb and forefinger, pulling the fold slightly away from the muscular tissue. Hold the calipers perpendicular to the fold, and take the measurement one-half inch below the finger hold. Measure each site three times and read the values to the nearest .1 to .5 mm. Record the average of the two closest readings as the final value. Take the readings without delay to avoid excessive compression of the skinfold. Releasing and refolding the skinfold is required between readings.

3. When doing pre- and post-assessments, conduct the measurement at the same time of day. The best time is early in the morning to avoid water hydration changes resulting from activity or exercise.

4. Obtain percent fat by adding together all three skinfold measurements and looking up the respective values on Tables 5.1 for women, 5.2 for men under forty, and 5.3 for men over forty.

   For example, if the skinfold measurements for an eighteen-year-old female are: (a) triceps = 16, (b) suprailium = 4, and (c) thigh = 30 (total = 50), the percent body fat would be 20.6 percent.

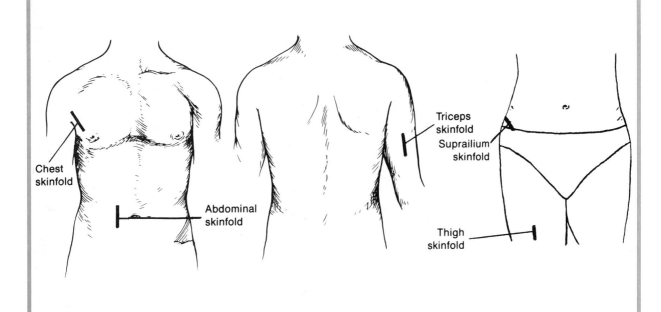

Anatomical landmarks for skinfolds

Table 5.1.
Percent Fat Estimates for Women Calculated from Triceps, Suprailium, and Thigh Skinfold Thickness

Sum of 3 Skinfolds	Under 22	23 to 27	28 to 32	33 to 37	38 to 42	43 to 47	48 to 52	53 to 57	Over 58
23- 25	9.7	9.9	10.2	10.4	10.7	10.9	11.2	11.4	11.7
26- 28	11.0	11.2	11.5	11.7	12.0	12.3	12.5	12.7	13.0
29- 31	12.3	12.5	12.8	13.0	13.3	13.5	13.8	14.0	14.3
32- 34	13.6	13.8	14.0	14.3	14.5	14.8	15.0	15.3	15.5
35- 37	14.8	15.0	15.3	15.5	15.8	16.0	16.3	16.5	16.8
38- 40	16.0	16.3	16.5	16.7	17.0	17.2	17.5	17.7	18.0
41- 43	17.2	17.4	17.7	17.9	18.2	18.4	18.7	18.9	19.2
44- 46	18.3	18.6	18.8	19.1	19.3	19.6	19.8	20.1	20.3
47- 49	19.5	19.7	20.0	20.2	20.5	20.7	21.0	21.2	21.5
50- 52	20.6	20.8	21.1	21.3	21.6	21.8	22.1	22.3	22.6
53- 55	21.7	21.9	22.1	22.4	22.6	22.9	23.1	23.4	23.6
56- 58	22.7	23.0	23.2	23.4	23.7	23.9	24.2	24.4	24.7
59- 61	23.7	24.0	24.2	24.5	24.7	25.0	25.2	25.5	25.7
62- 64	24.7	25.0	25.2	25.5	25.7	26.0	26.2	26.4	26.7
65- 67	25.7	25.9	26.2	26.4	26.7	26.9	27.2	27.4	27.7
68- 70	26.6	26.9	27.1	27.4	27.6	27.9	28.1	28.4	28.6
71- 73	27.5	27.8	28.0	28.3	28.5	28.8	29.0	29.3	29.5
74- 76	28.4	28.7	28.9	29.2	29.4	29.7	29.9	30.2	30.4
77- 79	29.3	29.5	29.8	30.0	30.3	30.5	30.8	31.0	31.3
80- 82	30.1	30.4	30.6	30.9	31.1	31.4	31.6	31.9	32.1
83- 85	30.9	31.2	31.4	31.7	31.9	32.2	32.4	32.7	32.9
86- 88	31.7	32.0	32.2	32.5	32.7	32.9	33.2	33.4	33.7
89- 91	32.5	32.7	33.0	33.2	33.5	33.7	33.9	34.2	34.4
92- 94	33.2	33.4	33.7	33.9	34.2	34.4	34.7	34.9	35.2
95- 97	33.9	34.1	34.4	34.6	34.9	35.1	35.4	35.6	35.9
98-100	34.6	34.8	35.1	35.3	35.5	35.8	36.0	36.3	36.5
101-103	35.2	35.4	35.7	35.9	36.2	36.4	36.7	36.9	37.2
104-106	35.8	36.1	36.3	36.6	36.8	37.1	37.3	37.5	37.8
107-109	36.4	36.7	36.9	37.1	37.4	37.6	37.9	38.1	38.4
110-112	37.0	37.2	37.5	37.7	38.0	38.2	38.5	38.7	38.9
113-115	37.5	37.8	38.0	38.2	38.5	38.7	39.0	39.2	39.5
116-118	38.0	38.3	38.5	38.8	39.0	39.3	39.5	39.7	40.0
119-121	38.5	38.7	39.0	39.2	39.5	39.7	40.0	40.2	40.5
122-124	39.0	39.2	39.4	39.7	39.9	40.2	40.4	40.7	40.9
125-127	39.4	39.6	39.9	40.1	40.4	40.6	40.9	41.1	41.4
128-130	39.8	40.0	40.3	40.5	40.8	41.0	41.3	41.5	41.8

Body density calculated based on the generalized equation for predicting body density of men developed by Jackson, A. S., and M. L. Pollock. *British Journal of Nutrition* 40:497-504, 1978. Percent body fat determined from the calculated body density using the Siri formula (W. E. Siri, *Body Composition from Fluid Spaces and Density*, Berkeley, CA: University of California, Donner Laboratory of Medical Physics, 1956).

Table 5.2.
Percent Fat Estimates for Men Under 40 Calculated from Chest, Abdomen, and Thigh Skinfold Thickness

Sum of 3 Skinfolds	Under 19	20 to 22	23 to 25	26 to 28	29 to 31	32 to 34	35 to 37	38 to 40
8- 10	.9	1.3	1.6	2.0	2.3	2.7	3.0	3.3
11- 13	1.9	2.3	2.6	3.0	3.3	3.7	4.0	4.3
14- 16	2.9	3.3	3.6	3.9	4.3	4.6	5.0	5.3
17- 19	3.9	4.2	4.6	4.9	5.3	5.6	6.0	6.3
20- 22	4.8	5.2	5.5	5.9	6.2	6.6	6.9	7.3
23- 25	5.8	6.2	6.5	6.8	7.2	7.5	7.9	8.2
26- 28	6.8	7.1	7.5	7.8	8.1	8.5	8.8	9.2
29- 31	7.7	8.0	8.4	8.7	9.1	9.4	9.8	10.1
32- 34	8.6	9.0	9.3	9.7	10.0	10.4	10.7	11.1
35- 37	9.5	9.9	10.2	10.6	10.9	11.3	11.6	12.0
38- 40	10.5	10.8	11.2	11.5	11.8	12.2	12.5	12.9
41- 43	11.4	11.7	12.1	12.4	12.7	13.1	13.4	13.8
44- 46	12.2	12.6	12.9	13.3	13.6	14.0	14.3	14.7
47- 49	13.1	13.5	13.8	14.2	14.5	14.9	15.2	15.5
50- 52	14.0	14.3	14.7	15.0	15.4	15.7	16.1	16.4
53- 55	14.8	15.2	15.5	15.9	16.2	16.6	16.9	17.3
56- 58	15.7	16.0	16.4	16.7	17.1	17.4	17.8	18.1
59- 61	16.5	16.9	17.2	17.6	17.9	18.3	18.6	19.0
62- 64	17.4	17.7	18.1	18.4	18.8	19.1	19.4	19.8
65- 67	18.2	18.5	18.9	19.2	19.6	19.9	20.3	20.6
68- 70	19.0	19.3	19.7	20.0	20.4	20.7	21.1	21.4
71- 73	19.8	20.1	20.5	20.8	21.2	21.5	21.9	22.2
74- 76	20.6	20.9	21.3	21.6	22.0	22.2	22.7	23.0
77- 79	21.4	21.7	22.1	22.4	22.8	23.1	23.4	23.8
80- 82	22.1	22.5	22.8	23.2	23.5	23.9	24.2	24.6
83- 85	22.9	23.2	23.6	23.9	24.3	24.6	25.0	25.3
86- 88	23.6	24.0	24.3	24.7	25.0	25.4	25.7	26.1
89- 91	24.4	24.7	25.1	25.4	25.8	26.1	26.5	26.8
92- 94	25.1	25.5	25.8	26.2	26.5	26.9	27.2	27.5
95- 97	25.8	26.2	26.5	26.9	27.2	27.6	27.9	28.3
98-100	26.6	26.9	27.3	27.6	27.9	28.3	28.6	29.0
101-103	27.3	27.6	28.0	28.3	28.6	29.0	29.3	29.7
104-106	27.9	28.3	28.6	29.0	29.3	29.7	30.0	30.4
107-109	28.6	29.0	29.3	29.7	30.0	30.4	30.7	31.1
110-112	29.3	29.6	30.0	30.3	30.7	31.0	31.4	31.7
113-115	30.0	30.3	30.7	31.0	31.3	31.7	32.0	32.4
116-118	30.6	31.0	31.3	31.6	32.0	32.3	32.7	33.0
119-121	31.3	31.6	32.0	32.3	32.6	33.0	33.3	33.7
122-124	31.9	32.2	32.6	32.9	33.3	33.6	34.0	34.3
125-127	32.5	32.9	33.2	33.5	33.9	34.2	34.6	34.9
128-130	33.1	33.5	33.8	34.2	34.5	34.9	35.2	35.5

Body density calculated based on the generalized equation for predicting body density of men developed by Jackson, A. S., and M. L. Pollock. *British Journal of Nutrition* 40:497-504, 1978. Percent body fat determined from the calculated body density using the Siri formula (W. E. Siri, *Body Composition from Fluid Spaces and Density*, Berkeley, CA: University of California, Donner Laboratory of Medical Physics, 1956).

Table 5.3.
Percent Fat Estimates for Men Over 40 Calculated from Chest, Abdomen, and Thigh Skinfold Thickness

Sum of 3 Skinfolds	Age to the Last Year							
	41 to 43	44 to 46	47 to 49	50 to 52	53 to 55	56 to 58	59 to 61	Over 62
8- 10	3.7	4.0	4.4	4.7	5.1	5.4	5.8	6.1
11- 13	4.7	5.0	5.4	5.7	6.1	6.4	6.8	7.1
14- 16	5.7	6.0	6.4	6.7	7.1	7.4	7.8	8.1
17- 19	6.7	7.0	7.4	7.7	8.1	8.4	8.7	9.1
20- 22	7.6	8.0	8.3	8.7	9.0	9.4	9.7	10.1
23- 25	8.6	8.9	9.3	9.6	10.0	10.3	10.7	11.0
26- 28	9.5	9.9	10.2	10.6	10.9	11.3	11.6	12.0
29- 31	10.5	10.8	11.2	11.5	11.9	12.2	12.6	12.9
32- 34	11.4	11.8	12.1	12.4	12.8	13.1	13.5	13.8
35- 37	12.3	12.7	13.0	13.4	13.7	14.1	14.4	14.8
38- 40	13.2	13.6	13.9	14.3	14.6	15.0	15.3	15.7
41- 43	14.1	14.5	14.8	15.2	15.5	15.9	16.2	16.6
44- 46	15.0	15.4	15.7	16.1	16.4	16.8	17.1	17.5
47- 49	15.9	16.2	16.6	16.9	17.3	17.6	18.0	18.3
50- 52	16.8	17.1	17.5	17.8	18.2	18.5	18.8	19.2
53- 55	17.6	18.0	18.3	18.7	19.0	19.4	19.7	20.1
56- 58	18.5	18.8	19.2	19.5	19.9	20.2	20.6	20.9
59- 61	19.3	19.7	20.0	20.4	20.7	21.0	21.4	21.7
62- 64	20.1	20.5	20.8	21.2	21.5	21.9	22.2	22.6
65- 67	21.0	21.3	21.7	22.0	22.4	22.7	23.0	23.4
68- 70	21.8	22.1	22.5	22.8	23.2	23.5	23.9	24.2
71- 73	22.6	22.9	23.3	23.6	24.0	24.3	24.7	25.0
74- 76	23.4	23.7	24.1	24.4	24.8	25.1	25.4	25.8
77- 79	24.1	24.5	24.8	25.2	25.5	25.9	26.2	26.6
80- 82	24.9	25.3	25.6	26.0	26.3	26.6	27.0	27.3
83- 85	25.7	26.0	26.4	26.7	27.1	27.4	27.8	28.1
86- 88	26.4	26.8	27.1	27.5	27.8	28.2	28.5	28.9
89- 91	27.2	27.5	27.9	38.2	28.6	28.9	29.2	29.6
92- 94	27.9	28.2	28.6	28.9	29.3	29.6	30.0	30.3
95- 97	28.6	29.0	29.3	29.7	30.0	30.4	30.7	31.1
98-100	29.3	29.7	30.0	30.4	30.7	31.1	31.4	31.8
101-103	30.0	30.4	30.7	31.1	31.4	31.8	32.1	32.5
104-106	30.7	31.1	31.4	31.8	32.1	32.5	32.8	33.2
107-109	31.4	31.8	32.1	32.4	32.8	33.1	33.5	33.8
110-112	32.1	32.4	32.8	33.1	33.5	33.8	34.2	34.5
113-115	32.7	33.1	33.4	33.8	34.1	34.5	34.8	35.2
116-118	33.4	33.7	34.1	34.4	34.8	35.1	35.5	35.8
119-121	34.0	34.4	34.7	35.1	35.4	35.8	36.1	36.5
122-124	34.7	35.0	35.4	35.7	36.1	36.4	36.7	37.1
125-127	35.3	35.6	36.0	36.3	36.7	37.0	37.4	37.7
128-130	35.9	36.2	36.6	36.9	37.3	37.6	38.0	38.35

Body density calculated based on the generalized equation for predicting body density of men developed by Jackson, A. S., and M. L. Pollock. *British Journal of Nutrition* 40:497-504, 1978. Percent body fat determined from the calculated body density using the Siri formula (W. E. Siri, *Body Composition from Fluid Spaces and Density*, Berkeley, CA: University of California, Donner Laboratory of Medical Physics, 1956).

Figure 5.4. *Procedure for body fat assessment according to girth measurements*

Girth Measurements for Women*

1. Using a regular tape measure, determine the following girth measurements in centimeters (cm):

   Upper Arm: measure halfway between the shoulder and the elbow.
   Hip: measure at the point of largest circumference.
   Wrist: measure the girth in front of the bones where the wrist bends.

2. Use the correct age.

3. Referring to Table 5.4, find the girth measurement for each site and age in the lefthand columns. Look up the constant values in the righthand columns. These values will allow you to derive body density (BD) by substituting the constants in the following formula:

   BD = A − B − C + D

4. Using the derived body density, calculate percent body fat (%F) according to the following equation:**

   %F = (495 ÷ BD) − 450

5. Example: Jane is twenty years old, with the following girth measurements: upper arm = 27 cm, hip = 99.5 cm, wrist = 15.4 cm.

Data	Constant	
Upper Arm = 27 cm	A = 1.0813	
Age = 20	B = .0102	BD = A − B − C + D
Hip = 99.5 cm	C = .1206	%F = (495 ÷ BD) − 450
Wrist = 15.4 cm	D = .0971	

   BD = 1.0813 − .0102 − .1206 + .0971 = 1.0476

   %F = (495 ÷ 1.0476) − 450 = 22.5

Girth Measurements for Men

1. Using a regular tape measure, determine the following girth measurements in inches (the men's measurements are taken in inches as opposed to centimeters for women):

   Waist: measure at the umbilicus (belly button)

   Wrist: measure in front of the bones where the wrist bends.

2. Subtract the wrist from the waist measurement.

3. Obtain the weight of the subject in pounds.

4. Look up the percent body fat (%F) in Table 5.5*** by using the difference obtained in number 2 above and the subject's body weight.

5. Example. John weighs 160 pounds, and his waist and wrist girth measurements are 36.5 and 7.5 inches, respectively.

   Waist girth = 36.5 inches

   Wrist girth = 7.5 inches

   Difference = 29.0 inches

   Body weight = 160.0 lbs.

   %F = 22

*Reproduced with permission from Lambson, R. B. "Generalized Body Density Prediction Equations for Women Using Simple Anthropometric Measurements." Unpublished doctoral dissertation, Brigham Young University, August 1987.

**From Siri, W. E. *Body Composition From Fluid Spaces and Density.* Berkeley, CA: University of California, Donner Laboratory of Medical Physics, 1956.

***Table 5.5 reproduced by permission from Fisher, A. G., and P. E. Allsen. *Jogging.* Dubuque, IA: Wm. C. Brown, 1987. This table was developed according to the generalized body composition equation for men using simple measurement techniques by Penrouse, K. W., A. G. Nelson, and A. G. Fisher. *Medicine and Science in Sports and Exercise* 17(2):189, 1985, © American College of Sports Medicine.

Table 5.4.
Conversion Constants from Girth Measurements (centimeters) to Calculate Body Density for Women

Upper Arm (cm)	Constant A	Age	Constant B	Hip (cm)	Constant C	Hip (cm)	Constant C	Wrist (cm)	Constant D
20.5	1.0966	17	.0086	79	.0957	114.5	.1388	13.0	.0819
21	1.0954	18	.0091	79.5	.0963	115	.1394	13.2	.0832
21.5	1.0942	19	.0096	80	.0970	115.5	.1400	13.4	.0845
22	1.0930	20	.0102	80.5	.0976	116	.1406	13.6	.0857
22.5	1.0919	21	.0107	81	.0982	116.5	.1412	13.8	.0870
23	1.0907	22	.0112	81.5	.0988	117	.1418	14.0	.0882
23.5	1.0895	23	.0117	82	.0994	117.5	.1424	14.2	.0895
24	1.0883	24	.0122	82.5	.1000	118	.1430	14.4	.0908
24.5	1.0871	25	.0127	83	.1006	118.5	.1436	14.6	.0920
25	1.0860	26	.0132	83.5	.1012	119	.1442	14.8	.0933
25.5	1.0848	27	.0137	84	.1018	119.5	.1448	15.0	.0946
26	1.0836	28	.0142	84.5	.1024	120	.1454	15.2	.0958
26.5	1.0824	29	.0147	85	.1030	120.5	.1460	15.4	.0971
27	1.0813	30	.0152	85.5	.1036	121	.1466	15.6	.0983
27.5	1.0801	31	.0157	86	.1042	121.5	.1472	15.8	.0996
28	1.0789	32	.0162	86.5	.1048	122	.1479	16.0	.1009
28.5	1.0777	33	.0168	87	.1054	122.5	.1485	16.2	.1021
29	1.0775	34	.0173	87.5	.1060	123	.1491	16.4	.1034
29.5	1.0754	35	.0178	88	.1066	123.5	.1497	16.6	.1046
30	1.0742	36	.0183	88.5	.1072	124	.1503	16.8	.1059
30.5	1.0730	37	.0188	89	.1079	124.5	.1509	17.0	.1072
31	1.0718	38	.0193	89.5	.1085	125	.1515	17.2	.1084
31.5	1.0707	39	.0198	90	.1091	125.5	.1521	17.4	.1097
32	1.0695	40	.0203	90.5	.1097	126	.1527	17.6	.1109
32.5	1.0683	41	.0208	91	.1103	126.5	.1533	17.8	.1122
33	1.0671	42	.0213	91.5	.1109	127	.1539	18.0	.1135
33.5	1.0666	43	.0218	92	.1115	127.5	.1545	18.2	.1147
34	1.0648	44	.0223	92.5	.1121	128	.1551	18.4	.1160
34.5	1.0636	45	.0228	93	.1127	128.5	.1558	18.6	.1172
35	1.0624	46	.0234	93.5	.1133	129	.1563		
35.5	1.0612	47	.0239	94	.1139	129.5	.1569		
36	1.0601	48	.0244	94.5	.1145	130	.1575		
36.5	1.0589	49	.0249	95	.1151	130.5	.1581		
37	1.0577	50	.0254	95.5	.1157	131	.1587		
37.5	1.0565	51	.0259	96	.1163	131.5	.1593		
38	1.0554	52	.0264	96.5	.1169	132	.1600		
38.5	1.0542	53	.0269	97	.1176	132.5	.1606		
39	1.0530	54	.0274	97.5	.1182	133	.1612		
39.5	1.0518	55	.0279	98	.1188	133.5	.1618		
40	1.0506	56	.0284	98.5	.1194	134	.1624		
40.5	1.0495	57	.0289	99	.1200	134.5	.1630		
41	1.0483	58	.0294	99.5	.1206	135	.1636		
41.5	1.0471	59	.0300	100	.1212	135.5	.1642		
42	1.0459	60	.0305	100.5	.1218	136	.1648		
42.5	1.0448	61	.0310	101	.1224	136.5	.1654		
43	1.0434	62	.0315	101.5	.1230	137	.1660		
43.5	1.0424	63	.0320	102	.1236	137.5	.1666		
44	1.0412	64	.0325	102.5	.1242	138	.1672		
		65	.0330	103	.1248	138.5	.1678		
		66	.0335	103.5	.1254	139	.1685		
		67	.0340	104	.1260	139.5	.1691		
		68	.0345	104.5	.1266	140	.1697		

(continued)

Table 5.4.
Conversion Constants from Girth Measurements (centimeters) to Calculate Body Density for Women
(continued)

Upper Arm (cm)	Constant A	Age	Constant B	Hip (cm)	Constant C	Hip (cm)	Constant C	Wrist (cm)	Constant D
		69	.0350	105	.1272	140.5	.1703		
		70	.0355	105.5	.1278	141	.1709		
		71	.0360	106	.1285	141.5	.1715		
		72	.0366	106.5	.1291	142	.1721		
		73	.0371	107	.1297	142.5	.1728		
		74	.0376	107.5	.1303	143	.1733		
		75	.0381	108	.1309	143.5	.1739		
				108.5	.1315	144	.1745		
				109	.1321	144.5	.1751		
				109.5	.1327	145	.1757		
				110	.1333	145.5	.1763		
				110.5	.1339	146	.1769		
				111	.1345	146.5	.1775		
				111.5	.1351	147	.1781		
				112	.1357	147.5	.1787		
				112.5	.1363	148	.1794		
				113	.1369	148.5	.1800		
				113.5	.1375	149	.1806		
				114	.1382	149.5	.1812		
						150	.1818		

Table 5.5.

Estimated Percent Body Fat for Men Obtained from Waist Minus Wrist Girth Measurements (Inches) and Body Weight

Body Weight (lbs)	22	22.5	23	23.5	24	24.5	25	25.5	26	26.5	27	27.5	28	28.5	29	29.5	30	30.5	31	31.5	32	32.5	33	33.5	34	34.5	35	35.5	36	36.5	37	37.5	38	38.5	39	39.5	40	40.5	41	41.5	42	42.5	43	43.5	44	44.5	45	45.5	46	46.5	47	47.5	48	48.5	49	49.5	50
120	4	6	8	10	12	14	16	18	20	21	23	25	27	29	31	33	35	37	39	41	43	45	47	49	50	52	54	56	58																												
125	4	6	7	9	11	13	15	17	19	20	22	24	26	28	30	32	33	35	37	39	41	43	45	46	48	50	52	54	56	58																										
130	3	5	7	9	11	12	14	16	18	20	21	23	25	27	28	30	32	34	36	37	39	41	43	44	46	48	50	52	53	55	57																								
135	3	5	7	8	10	12	14	15	17	19	20	22	24	26	27	29	31	32	34	36	38	39	41	43	44	46	48	50	51	53	54	56																							
140	3	5	6	8	10	11	13	15	16	18	20	21	23	24	26	28	29	31	33	34	36	38	39	41	43	44	46	48	49	51	53	54	56																					
145	3	4	6	7	9	11	12	14	15	17	19	20	22	23	25	27	28	30	31	33	35	36	38	39	41	43	44	46	47	49	51	52	54	55																				
150	2	4	6	7	9	10	12	14	15	17	18	20	21	23	25	26	28	29	31	33	34	36	38	39	41	43	44	46	47	49	50	52	53	55																				
155	2	4	5	7	9	10	12	13	15	16	18	20	21	23	24	26	28	29	31	32	34	35	37	38	40	41	43	44	46	48	49	50	52	53	55																			
160	2	4	5	6	8	9	11	12	14	15	17	18	20	22	23	25	26	28	30	31	33	34	36	37	39	40	41	43	44	46	47	48	50	51	53	54																		
165	2	3	5	6	8	9	10	12	13	15	16	18	19	21	22	24	26	27	29	30	31	33	34	36	37	38	40	41	43	44	45	47	48	50	51	52	54																
170	2	3	4	6	7	9	10	11	13	14	16	17	19	20	22	24	25	26	28	29	30	32	33	35	36	37	39	40	41	43	44	45	47	48	49	51	52	54															
175	2	3	4	6	7	8	10	11	12	14	15	17	18	20	21	23	24	25	27	28	29	31	32	34	35	36	38	39	40	41	43	44	45	47	48	49	51	52	53														
180		3	4	5	7	8	9	11	12	13	15	16	17	19	20	21	23	24	25	27	28	29	31	32	33	35	36	37	39	40	41	43	44	45	47	48	49	50	52	53													
185		3	4	5	6	8	9	10	11	13	14	15	17	18	19	21	22	23	25	26	27	28	30	31	32	34	35	36	38	39	40	41	43	44	45	46	48	49	50	51	53												
190		2	4	5	6	7	9	10	11	12	14	15	16	18	19	20	22	23	24	26	27	28	29	31	32	33	35	36	37	38	40	41	43	44	45	46	48	49	50	51	52												
195		2	3	5	6	7	8	10	11	12	13	15	16	17	19	20	21	22	24	25	26	28	29	30	31	33	34	35	37	38	39	40	41	43	44	45	46	47	49	50	51	52											
200		2	3	4	6	7	8	9	11	12	13	14	16	17	18	20	21	22	23	25	26	27	28	30	31	32	33	35	36	37	38	40	41	42	43	44	46	47	48	49	50	51	52										
205		2	3	4	5	6	8	9	10	11	13	14	15	16	18	19	20	21	23	24	25	26	28	29	30	31	32	34	35	36	37	38	40	41	42	43	44	45	46	47	48	49	51	52								
210		2	3	4	5	6	7	8	10	11	12	13	15	16	17	18	20	21	22	23	25	26	27	28	29	31	32	33	34	35	37	38	39	40	41	42	43	44	45	46	47	48	50	51	52							
215		2	3	4	5	6	7	8	9	11	12	13	14	15	17	18	19	20	21	23	24	25	26	27	28	30	31	32	33	34	36	37	38	39	40	41	42	43	44	45	46	47	48	49	50	51						
220			2	3	4	5	6	7	8	9	10	11	13	14	15	16	17	19	20	21	22	23	24	26	27	28	29	30	31	32	34	35	36	37	38	39	40	42	43	44	45	46	47	48	49	50	51					
225			2	3	4	5	6	7	8	9	10	11	12	14	15	16	17	18	19	21	22	23	24	25	26	27	28	30	31	32	33	34	35	36	37	38	40	41	42	43	44	45	46	47	48	49	50	51				
230			2	3	4	5	6	7	8	9	10	11	12	13	14	16	17	18	19	20	21	22	24	25	26	27	28	29	30	31	32	33	35	36	37	38	39	40	41	42	43	44	45	46	47	48	49	50	51			
235			2	3	4	5	6	7	8	9	10	11	12	13	14	15	16	18	19	20	21	22	23	24	25	26	28	29	30	31	32	33	34	35	36	37	38	39	41	42	43	44	45	46	47	48	49	50	51			
240			2	3	4	5	6	7	8	9	10	11	12	13	15	16	17	18	19	20	21	22	23	24	25	26	27	28	30	31	32	33	34	35	36	37	38	39	40	41	42	44	45	46	47	48	49	50				
245			2	3	4	5	6	7	8	9	10	11	12	13	14	15	16	17	18	20	21	22	23	24	25	26	27	28	29	30	31	32	33	34	35	36	37	38	39	40	41	42	43	44	45	46	47	48	49	50		
250			2	3	4	4	5	6	7	8	9	10	11	12	13	14	15	16	17	18	19	20	21	22	23	24	25	26	27	28	29	30	31	32	33	34	35	36	37	38	39	40	41	42	43	44	45	46	47	48	49	
255			2	3	4	4	5	6	7	8	9	10	11	11	12	13	14	15	16	17	18	19	20	21	22	23	24	25	26	27	28	29	30	31	32	33	34	35	36	37	38	39	40	41	42	43	44	45	46	47	48	49
260			2	2	3	4	5	6	7	7	8	9	10	11	12	13	14	15	16	17	18	19	20	21	22	23	24	25	26	27	28	29	30	31	32	33	34	35	36	37	38	39	40	41	42	43	44	45	46	47	48	49
265			2	2	3	4	5	6	6	7	8	9	10	11	12	13	14	15	16	17	18	19	20	21	22	23	24	25	26	27	28	29	30	31	32	33	34	35	36	37	38	39	40	41	42	43	44	45	46	47	48	49
270			2	2	3	4	4	5	6	7	8	8	9	10	11	12	13	14	15	16	17	18	19	20	21	22	23	24	25	26	27	28	29	30	31	32	33	34	35	36	37	38	39	40	41	42	43	44	45	46	47	48
275			2	2	3	4	4	5	6	7	8	8	9	10	11	12	13	14	15	16	17	17	18	19	20	21	22	23	24	25	26	27	28	29	30	31	32	33	34	35	36	37	38	39	40	41	42	43	44	45	46	48
280			2	2	3	3	4	5	6	6	7	8	9	10	10	11	12	13	14	15	16	17	18	19	20	21	22	23	24	25	26	27	28	29	30	31	32	33	34	35	36	37	38	38	39	40	41	42	43	44	45	47
285			2	2	3	3	4	5	5	6	7	8	8	9	10	11	12	13	14	15	16	17	18	19	20	21	22	23	24	25	26	27	28	29	30	31	32	33	34	35	36	37	38	38	39	40	41	42	43	44	45	46
290			2	2	3	3	4	5	5	6	7	8	8	9	10	11	11	12	13	14	15	16	17	18	19	20	21	22	23	24	25	26	27	28	29	30	30	31	32	33	34	35	36	37	38	39	40	41	42	43	44	45
295			2	2	2	3	4	4	5	6	6	7	8	9	10	10	11	12	13	14	14	15	16	17	18	18	19	20	21	22	23	24	24	25	26	27	28	29	30	31	32	33	34	34	35	36	37	38	39	40	41	42	43
300			2	2	2	3	4	4	5	6	6	7	8	9	9	10	11	12	13	13	14	15	16	17	17	18	19	20	21	22	22	23	24	25	26	27	28	29	29	30	31	32	33	34	35	36	37	38	39	39	40	41	42	43

Body Weight (pounds)

Table 5.6.
Body Composition Classification According to Percent Body Fat

			MEN		
Age	Ideal	Good	Moderate	Fat	Obese
<19	12	12.5-17.0	17.5-22.0	22.5-27.0	27.5+
20-29	13	13.5-18.0	18.5-23.0	23.5-28.0	28.5+
30-39	14	14.5-19.0	19.5-24.0	24.5-29.0	29.5+
40-49	15	15.5-20.0	20.5-25.0	25.5-30.0	30.5+
50+	16	16.5-21.5	21.5-26.0	26.5-31.0	31.5+
			WOMEN		
<19	17	17.5-22.0	22.5-27.0	27.5-32.0	32.5+
20-29	18	18.5-23.0	23.5-28.0	28.5-33.0	33.5+
30-39	19	19.5-24.0	24.5-29.0	29.5-34.0	34.5+
40-49	20	20.5-25.0	25.5-30.0	30.5-35.0	35.5+
50+	21	21.5-26.5	26.5-31.0	31.5-36.0	36.5+

Now it is your turn. Figure 5.5 provides a form for recording measurements for the skinfold thickness technique and/or the girth measurements technique. After determining your percent body fat, calculate your own ideal body weight using the form provided in Figure 5.6. If skinfold calipers are available, use the skinfold thickness technique to assess percent body fat. If calipers are unavailable, estimate the percent fat according to the girth measurements technique (you may wish to use both techniques and compare the results).

If you are on a diet/exercise program, it is recommended that you repeat the computations about once a month to monitor changes in body composition. This is important because lean body mass is affected by weight reduction programs as well as by physical activity. A negative caloric balance does lead to a decrease in lean body mass (these effects will be explained in more detail in Chapter 6). As lean body mass changes, so will your ideal body weight. Also, when you conduct post-assessments, always use the same technique (skinfold or girth measurements) to make valid comparisons.

An example of the changes in body composition resulting from a weight control/exercise program was seen in a coed aerobic dance course taught at The University of Texas of the Permian Basin in Odessa, Texas. The class was taught during a six-week summer term, and students participated in aerobic dance routines four times per week for sixty minutes each time. The first and last days of classes were used to assess several physiological parameters, including body composition. Students were also given information on diet and nutrition and basically followed their own weight control program. At the end of the six weeks, the average weight loss for the entire class was only three pounds. Because body composition was assessed, however, members of the class were surprised to find out that in reality the average fat loss was six pounds, accompanied by a three-pound increase in lean body mass.

Figure 5.5. *Data form for body composition assessment*

I. Percent Body Fat According to Skinfold Thickness

Men	Women
Chest (mm): _____	Triceps (mm): _____
Abdomen (mm): _____	Suprailium (mm): _____
Thigh (mm): _____	Thigh (mm): _____
Total (mm): _____	Total (mm): _____
Percent Fat: _____	Percent Fat: _____

II. Percent Fat According to Girth Measurements

Men

Waist (inches): _____

Wrist (inches): _____

Difference: _____

Body Weight: _____

Percent Fat: _____

Women

Upper Arm (cm): _____   Constant A = _____

Age: _____   Constant B = _____

Hip (cm): _____   Constant C = _____

Wrist (cm): _____   Constant D = _____

BD* = A−B−C+D = _____ − _____ − _____ + _____ =

Percent Fat = (495/BD) − 450 = (495/_____) − 450 =

*Body density

Figure 5.6. *Computation form for ideal body weight*

A.   Body Weight (BW):   _____

B.   Current Percent Fat (%F)*:   _____

C.   Fat Weight (FW) = BW $\times$ %F = _____ $\times$ _____ =

D.   Lean Body Mass (LBM) = BW $-$ FW = _____ $-$ _____ =

E.   Age: _____

F.   Ideal Fat Percent (IFP — *see* Table 6.6):   _____

G.   Ideal Body Weight (IBW) = LBM $\div$ (1.0 $-$ IFP*)

  IBW = _____ $\div$ (1.0 $-$ _____) =

*Express percentages in decimal form (e.g., 25% = .25)

Bibliography

Fisher, A. G., and P. E. Allsen. *Jogging.* Dubuque, IA: Wm. C. Brown, 1987.

Hoeger, W. W. K. *Principles and Laboratories for Physical Fitness & Wellness.* Englewood, CO: Morton Publishing, 1988.

Jackson, A. S., and M. L. Pollock. "Generalized Equations for Predicting Body Density of Men." *British Journal of Nutrition* 40:497-504, 1978.

Jackson, A. S., M. L. Pollock, and A. Ward. "Generalized Equations for Predicting Body Density of Women." *Medicine and Science in Sports and Exercise* 3:175-182, 1980.

Lambson, R. B. *Generalized Body Density Prediction Equations for Women Using Simple Anthropometric Measurements.* Unpublished doctoral dissertation, Brigham Young University, August 1987.

Penrouse, K. W., A. G. Nelson, and A. G. Fisher. "Generalized Body Composition Equation for Men Using Simple Measurement Techniques." *Medicine and Science in Sports and Exercise* 17(2): 189, 1985.

Siri, W. E. *Body Composition from Fluid Spaces and Density.* Berkeley, CA: Donner Laboratory of Medical Physics, University of California, 19 March 1956.

Nutrition For Weight Control And Wellness

The science of nutrition studies the relationship of foods to optimal health and performance. Ample scientific evidence has long linked good nutrition to overall health and well-being. Proper nutrition signifies that a person's diet is supplying all of the essential nutrients to carry out normal tissue growth, repair, and maintenance. It also implies that the diet will provide sufficient substrates to obtain the energy necessary for work, physical activity, and relaxation.

Unfortunately, the typical American diet is too high in calories, sugars, fats, sodium, and alcohol, and too low in complex carbohydrates and fiber — none of which are conducive to good health. Over-consumption is now a major concern for many Americans. In fact, according to a 1988 report on nutrition and health issued by the United States Surgeon General, the first ever of its kind, diseases of dietary excess and imbalance are among the leading causes of death in the country. Of the total 2.1 million deaths in 1987, an estimated 1.5 million people died of diseases associated with faulty nutrition. Coronary heart disease, stroke, atherosclerosis, diabetes, and cancer, all related to poor nutritional habits, account for more than two-thirds of all deaths in the United States. In this report, based on more than 2,000 scientific studies, the Surgeon General indicates that dietary changes "can bring a substantial measure of better health to all Americans."

NUTRIENTS

The essential nutrients required by the human body are carbohydrates, fats, protein, vitamins, minerals, and water. The first three have been referred to as fuel nutrients because they are the only substances used to supply the energy (commonly measured in calories) necessary for work and normal body functions. Vitamins, minerals, and water have no caloric value but are still essential for normal body functions and maintenance of good health. In addition, many nutritionists like to add to this list a seventh nutrient that has received a great deal of attention recently — dietary fiber.

Carbohydrates, fats, protein, and water are called *macronutrients* because large amounts are needed on a daily basis. Vitamins and minerals are necessary only in very small amounts; therefore, nutritionists commonly refer to them as *micronutrients*.

Depending on the amount of nutrients and calories, foods can be categorized into high nutrient density and low nutrient density. High nutrient density is used in reference to foods that contain a low or moderate amount of calories but are packed with nutrients. Foods that are high in calories but contain few nutrients are of low nutrient density. The latter frequently are referred to as "junk food."

The term *calorie* is used as a unit of measure to indicate the energy value of food and cost of physical activity. Technically, a kilocalorie (kcal) or large calorie is the amount of heat necessary to raise the temperature of one kilogram of water from 14.5 to 15.5 degrees Centigrade, but for the purpose of simplicity, people refer to it as a calorie rather than kcal. For example, if the caloric value of a given food is 100 calories (kcal), the energy contained in this food could raise the temperature of 100 kilograms of water by one degree Centigrade.

Carbohydrates

Carbohydrates are the major source of calories used by the body to provide energy for work, cell maintenance, and heat. They also play a crucial role in the digestion and regulation of fat and protein metabolism. Each gram of carbohydrates provides the human body with approximately four calories. Carbohydrates are classified into simple and complex carbohydrates. The major sources of carbohydrates are breads, cereals, fruits, vegetables, and milk and other dairy products.

Simple carbohydrates, frequently denoted as sugars, are formed by simple or double sugar units with little nutritive value (e.g., candy, ice cream, pop, cakes). Simple carbohydrates are divided into monosaccharides and disaccharides; they can be easily recognized because of their -ose endings. Eating too many simple carbohydrates often takes the place of more nutritive foods in the diet.

Monosaccharides are the simplest sugars, formed by five- or six-carbon skeletons. The three most common monosaccharides are glucose, fructose, and galactose. *Glucose* is a natural sugar found in food, but it is also produced in the body from other simple and complex carbohydrates. *Fructose*, or fruit sugar, occurs naturally in fruits and honey. *Galactose* is produced from milk sugar in the mammary glands of lactating animals. Both fructose and galactose are readily converted to glucose in the body.

Disaccharides are formed when two monosaccharide units, one of which is glucose, are linked together. The major disaccharides are *sucrose*, or table sugar (glucose + fructose), *lactose* (glucose + galactose), and maltose (glucose + glucose).

Complex carbohydrates are formed when three or more simple sugar molecules link together. Therefore, they also are referred to as *polysaccharides*. Anywhere from about ten to thousands of monosaccharide molecules can unite to form a single polysaccharide. Two examples of complex carbohydrates are starches and dextrins. *Starches* are commonly found in seeds, corn, nuts, grains, roots, potatoes, and legumes. *Dextrins* are formed from the breakdown of large starch molecules exposed to dry heat, such as when bread is baked or cold cereals are produced. Complex carbohydrates provide many valuable nutrients to the body and can be an excellent source of fiber or roughage. Fiber, also considered a complex carbohydrate, is discussed later in this chapter. Figure 6.1 summarizes all these types of carbohydrates.

Fats

Fats, or *lipids*, are also used as a source of energy in the human body. They are the most concentrated source of energy. Each gram of fat supplies nine calories to the body. Fats are also a

Figure 6.1. *Major types of carbohydrates*

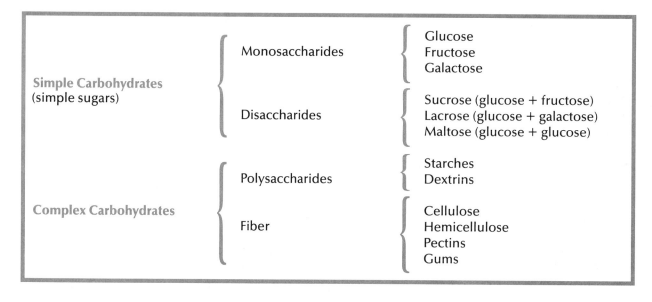

Simple Carbohydrates (simple sugars)	Monosaccharides	Glucose Fructose Galactose
	Disaccharides	Sucrose (glucose + fructose) Lacrose (glucose + galactose) Maltose (glucose + glucose)
Complex Carbohydrates	Polysaccharides	Starches Dextrins
	Fiber	Cellulose Hemicellulose Pectins Gums

part of the cell structure. They are used as stored energy and as an insulator for body heat preservation. They provide shock absorption, supply essential fatty acids, and carry the fat-soluble vitamins A, D, E, and K. Fats can be classified into three main groups: simple, compound, and derived. The basic sources of fat are milk and other dairy products, and meats and alternates.

Simple fats consist of a glyceride molecule linked to one, two, or three units of fatty acids. According to the number of fatty acids attached, simple fats are divided into *monoglycerides* (one fatty acid), *diglycerides* (two fatty acids), and *triglycerides* (three fatty acids). More than 90 percent of the weight of fat in foods and over 95 percent of the stored fat in the human body are in the form of triglycerides.

Fatty acids vary in the length of the carbon atom chain and in the degree of hydrogen saturation. Based on the degree of saturation, fatty acids are said to be saturated or unsaturated. Unsaturated fatty acids can be further classified as monounsaturated and polyunsaturated. Saturated fatty acids are primarily of animal origin; unsaturated fats are generally found in plant products.

In *saturated* fatty acids the carbon atoms are fully saturated with hydrogens; therefore only single bonds link the carbon atoms on the chain

(see Figure 6.2). These saturated fatty acids, frequently referred to as saturated fats, are contained in meats, cheese, and butter, as examples. If the carbon atoms are not completely saturated with hydrogen, double bonds are formed between the unsaturated carbons, and the fatty acid unit is said to be *unsaturated* (an unsaturated fat). In *monounsaturated* fatty acids (MUFA) only one double bond is found along the chain. Olive oil and avocado are two examples of triglycerides high in monounsaturated fatty acids. *Polyunsaturated* fatty acids (PUFA) contain two or more double bonds between unsaturated carbon atoms along the chain. Corn and cottonseed oils are high in polyunsaturated fatty acids.

Saturated fats do not melt at room temperature, whereas unsaturated fats are usually liquid at room temperature (coconut and palm oils are exceptions because they are high in saturated fats). Shorter fatty acid chains also tend to be liquid at room temperature. In general, saturated fats increase the blood cholesterol level, and polyunsaturated fats tend to decrease cholesterol. The role of cholesterol in health and disease is discussed in Chapter 7.

Compound fats are a combination of simple fats and other chemicals. Examples of compound fats are phospholipids, glucolipids, and

Figure 6.2. *Chemical structure of saturated and unsaturated fats*

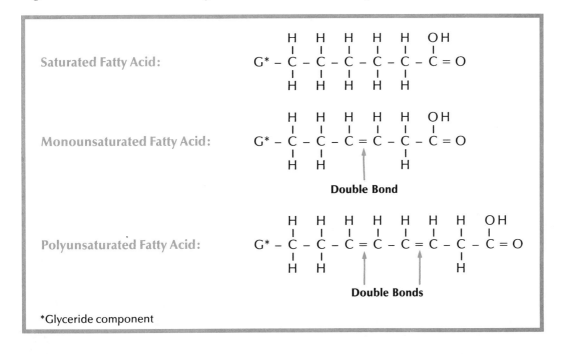

lipoproteins. *Phospholipids* are similar to triglycerides, except that phosphoric acid takes the place of one of the fatty acid units. *Glucolipids* are formed by a combination of carbohydrates, fatty acids, and nitrogen. *Lipoproteins* are water-soluble aggregates of protein with either triglycerides, phospholipids, or cholesterol. Lipoproteins transport fats (cholesterol and triglycerides) in the blood and have a significant role in the development and prevention of heart disease (see total cholesterol/HDL-cholesterol ratio and triglycerides in Chapter 7).

Derived fats are a combination of simple and compound fats. *Sterols* are an example of derived fats. Although sterols contain no fatty acids, they are viewed as fats because they are insoluble in water. The most often mentioned sterol is *cholesterol,* which is found in many foods or can be manufactured from saturated fats in the body. Figure 6.3 gives a breakdown of the types of fats.

Proteins

Proteins are the main substances used to build and repair tissues such as muscles, blood, internal organs, skin, hair, nails, and bones. They are a part of hormones, enzymes, and antibodies and help maintain normal body fluid balance. Proteins also can be used as a source of energy but only if there are not enough carbohydrates and fats available. Each gram of protein yields four calories of energy. The primary sources are meats and alternates, milk and other dairy products, and some breads and cereals.

The human body uses approximately twenty *amino acids* or basic building blocks to build different types of protein. Amino acids contain nitrogen, carbon, hydrogen, and oxygen. Nine of the twenty amino acids are referred to as essential amino acids because they cannot be produced in the body. The other eleven can be manufactured by the body if sufficient nitrogen is provided from food proteins in the diet.

Proteins that contain all of the essential amino acids are known as *complete* or higher-quality protein. These types of proteins are usually of animal source. If one or more of the essential amino acids are missing, the proteins are referred to as *incomplete* or lower-quality protein.

The only concern in regard to protein intake is that individuals get enough protein in the diet to ensure nitrogen for adequate amino acid production, as well as to get enough high-quality protein to obtain the essential amino acids. Protein deficiency is not a significant problem in the American diet.

Vitamins

Vitamins are organic substances essential for normal metabolism, growth, and development of the body. They are classified into two types based on their solubility: *fat-soluble vitamins* (A, D, E, and K), and *water-soluble vitamins* (B complex and C). Vitamins cannot be manufactured by the body; they can be obtained only through a well-balanced diet. A description of the functions of each vitamin is presented in Figure 6.4.

Figure 6.3. *Major types of fats (lipids)*

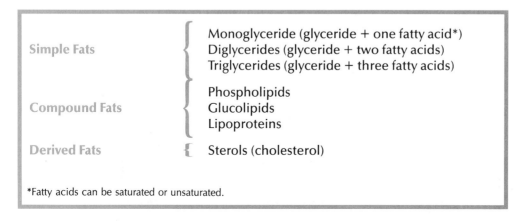

Simple Fats	{	Monoglyceride (glyceride + one fatty acid*)
		Diglycerides (glyceride + two fatty acids)
		Triglycerides (glyceride + three fatty acids)
Compound Fats	{	Phospholipids
		Glucolipids
		Lipoproteins
Derived Fats	{	Sterols (cholesterol)

*Fatty acids can be saturated or unsaturated.

Figure 6.4. *Major functions of vitamins*

NUTRIENT	GOOD SOURCES	MAJOR FUNCTIONS	DEFICIENCY SYMPTOMS
Vitamin A	Milk, cheese, eggs, liver, and yellow/dark green fruits and vegetables	Required for healthy bones, teeth, skin, gums, and hair; maintenance of inner mucous membranes, thus increasing resistance to infection; adequate vision in dim light	Night blindness, decreased growth, decreased resistance to infection, rough-dry skin
Vitamin D	Fortified milk, cod liver oil, salmon, tuna, egg yolk	Necessary for bones and teeth; needed for calcium and phosphorus absorption	Rickets (bone softening), fractures, and muscle spasms
Vitamin E	Vegetable oils, yellow and green leafy vegetables, margarine, wheat germ, whole grain breads and cereals	Related to oxydation and normal muscle and red blood cell chemistry	Leg cramps, red blood cell breakdown
Vitamin K	Green leafy vegetables, cauliflower, cabbage, eggs, peas, and potatoes	Essential for normal blood clotting	Hemorrhaging
Vitamin B_1 (Thiamine)	Whole grain or enriched bread, lean meats and poultry, organ fish, liver, pork, poultry, organ meats, legumes, nuts, and dried yeast	Assists in proper use of carbohydrates; normal functioning of nervous system; maintenance of good appetite	Loss of appetite, nausea, confusion, cardiac abnormalities, muscle spasms
Vitamin B_2 (Riboflavin)	Eggs, milk, leafy green vegetables, whole grains, lean meats, dried beans and peas	Contributes to energy release from carbohydrates, fats, and proteins; needed for normal growth and development, good vision, and healthy skin	Cracking of the corners of the mouth, inflammation of the skin, impaired vision
Vitamin B_6 (Pyridoxine)	Vegetables, meats, whole grain cereals, soybeans, peanuts, and potatoes	Necessary for protein and fatty acids metabolism, and normal red blood cell formation	Depression, irritability, muscle spasms, nausea
Vitamin B_{12}	Meat, poultry, fish, liver, organ meats, eggs, shellfish, milk, and cheese	Required for normal growth, red blood cell formation, nervous system and digestive tract functioning	Impaired balance, weakness, drop in red blood cell count
Niacin	Liver and organ meats, meat, fish, poultry, whole grains, enriched breads, nuts, green leafy vegetables, and dried beans and peas	Contributes to energy release from carbohydrates, fats, and proteins; normal growth and development, and formation of hormones and nerve-regulating substances	Confusion, depression, weakness, weight loss
Biotin	Liver, kidney, eggs, yeast, legumes, milk, nuts, dark green vegetables	Essential for carbohydrate metabolism and fatty acid synthesis	Inflamed skin, muscle pain, depression, weight loss
Folic Acid	Leafy green vegetables, organ meats, whole grains and cereals, and dried beans	Needed for cell growth and reproduction and red blood cell formation	Decreased resistance to infection
Pantothenic Acid	All natural foods, especially liver, kidney, eggs, nuts, yeast, milk, dried peas and beans, and green leafy vegetables	Related to carbohydrate and fat metabolism	Depression, low blood sugar, leg cramps, nausea, headaches
Vitamin C (Ascorbic Acid)	Fruits and vegetables	Helps protect against infection; formation of collagenous tissue; normal blood vessels, teeth, and bones	Slow healing wounds, loose teeth, hemorrhaging, rough-scaly skin, irritability

Minerals

Minerals are inorganic elements found in the body and in food. They serve several important functions. Minerals are constituents of all cells, especially those found in hard parts of the body (bones, nails, teeth). They are crucial in the maintenance of water balance and the acid-base balance. They are essential components of respiratory pigments, enzymes, and enzyme systems, and they regulate muscular and nervous tissue excitability. The specific functions of some of the most important minerals are contained in Figure 6.5.

Water

Approximately 70 percent of total body weight is water. The most important nutrient, it is involved in almost every vital body process. Water is used in digestion and absorption of food, in the circulatory process, in removing waste products, in building and rebuilding cells, and in the transport of other nutrients. Water is contained in almost all foods but primarily in liquid foods, fruits, and vegetables. Besides the natural content in foods, it is recommended that every person drink at least eight to ten glasses of fluids a day.

Fiber

Dietary fiber is a type of complex carbohydrate made up of plant material that cannot be digested by the human body. It is present mainly in leaves, skins, roots, and seeds. Processing and refining foods removes almost all of the natural fiber. In our daily diets, the main sources of dietary fiber are whole-grain cereals and breads, fruits, and vegetables. The most common types of fiber are *cellulose* and *hemicellulose*, found in plant cell

Figure 6.5. *Major functions of minerals*

NUTRIENT	GOOD SOURCES	MAJOR FUNCTIONS	DEFICIENCY SYMPTOMS
Calcium	Milk, yogurt, cheese, green leafy vegetables, dried beans, sardines, and salmon	Required for strong teeth and bone formation; maintenance of good muscle tone, heart beat, and nerve function	Bone pain and fractures, periodontal disease, muscle cramps
Iron	Organ meats, lean meats, seafoods, eggs, dried peas and beans, nuts, whole and enriched grains, and green leafy vegetables	Major component of hemoglobin; aids in energy utilization	Nutritional anemia, and overall weakness
Phosphorus	Meats, fish, milk, eggs, dried beans and peas, whole grains, and processed foods	Required for bone and teeth formation; energy release regulation	Bone pain and fracture, weight loss, and weakness
Zinc	Milk, meat, seafood, whole grains, nuts, eggs, and dried beans	Essential component of hormones, insulin, and enzymes; used in normal growth and development	Loss of appetite, slow healing wounds, and skin problems
Magnesium	Green leafy vegetables, whole grains, nuts, soybeans, seafood, and legumes	Needed for bone growth and maintenance; carbohydrate and protein utilization; nerve function; temperature regulation	Irregular heartbeat, weakness, muscle spasms, and sleeplessness
Sodium	Table salt, processed foods, and meat	Body fluid regulation; transmission of nerve impulse; heart action	Rarely seen
Potassium	Legumes, whole grains, bananas, orange juice, dried fruits, and potatoes	Heart action; bone formation and maintenance; regulation of energy release; acid-base regulation	Irregular heartbeat, nausea, weakness

walls; *pectins*, found in fruits; and *gums*, also found in small quantities in foods of plant origin.

Fiber is important in the diet because it binds water, yielding a softer stool, which decreases transit time of food residues in the intestinal tract. Many researchers believe that speeding up the passage of food residues through the intestines decreases the risk for colon cancer, primarily because of the decreased time that cancer-causing agents remain in contact with the intestinal wall. The increased water content of the stool may also dilute the cancer-causing agents, decreasing the potency of these substances.

The risk for coronary heart disease also decreases with increased fiber intake. This decreased risk can be attributed to two factors. First, all too often fats take the place of dietary fiber in the diet, thereby increasing cholesterol formation and absorption. Second, some specific water-soluble fibers, such as pectin and guar gum found in beans, oats, corn, and fruits, seem to bind cholesterol in the intestines, thereby preventing its absorption. In addition, several other health disorders have been linked to low fiber intake. These include constipation, diverticulitis, hemorrhoids, ulcerative colitis, gallbladder disease, appendicitis, and obesity.

Determining the amount of fiber in your diet can be confusing at times because it can be measured either as crude fiber or dietary fiber. *Crude fiber* is the smaller portion of the dietary fiber that actually remains after chemical extraction in the digestive tract. The recommended amount of *dietary fiber* is about twenty-five grams per day, which is the equivalent of seven grams of crude fiber.

Because most nutrition labels list the fiber content in terms of dietary fiber, you should be careful to use the twenty-five gram guideline (see Table 6.1). Also, be aware that too much fiber consumption can be detrimental to health, because excessive amounts can lead to increased loss of calcium, phosphorus, and iron, not to mention increased gastrointestinal discomfort. It is also important to increase fluid intake when fiber consumption is increased, as too little fluid can lead to dehydration or constipation.

THE BALANCED DIET

Most people would like to live life to its fullest, maintain good health, and lead a productive life.

Table 6.1.
Dietary Fiber Content of Selected Foods

Food	Serving Size	Dietary Fiber (gm)
Almonds	1 oz.	3.0
Apple	1 medium	4.3
Banana	1 medium	3.3
Beans — red, kidney	.5 cup	10.2
Blackberries	.5 cup	4.9
Beets (cooked)	.5 cup	2.0
Brazil nuts	1 oz.	2.5
Broccoli (cooked)	.5 cup	3.3
Brown rice (cooked)	.5 cup	2.0
Carrots (cooked)	.5 cup	2.9
Cauliflower (cooked)	.5 cup	1.7
Cereal		
All Bran	1 oz.	8.5
Cheerios	1 oz.	1.1
Cornflakes	1 oz.	0.5
Fruit and Fibre	1 oz.	4.0
Fruit Wheats	1 oz.	2.0
Just Right	1 oz.	2.0
Wheaties	1 oz.	2.0
Corn (cooked)	.5 cup	3.9
Eggplant (cooked)	.5 cup	3.0
Lettuce (chopped)	.5 cup	0.4
Orange	1 medium	3.0
Parsnips (cooked)	.5 cup	2.1
Pear	1 medium	5.0
Peas (cooked)	.5 cup	3.7
Popcorn (plain)	1 cup	1.5
Potato (baked)	1 medium	3.9
Strawberries	.5 cup	1.6
Summer squash (cooked)	.5 cup	1.6
Watermelon	1 cup	0.8

One of the fundamental ways to accomplish this goal is by eating a well-balanced diet. Generally, daily caloric intake should be distributed so that 50 to 60 percent of the total calories come from carbohydrates (48 percent complex carbohydrates and 10 percent sugar) and less than 30 percent of the total calories from fat. Protein intake should be about .8 grams per kilogram (2.2 pounds) of body weight, or about 15 to 20 percent of the total calories. Saturated fats should constitute less than 10 percent of the total daily caloric intake. In addition, all of the vitamins, minerals, and water must be provided. To accurately rate a diet is rather difficult without conducting a complete nutrient analysis.

Achieving and maintaining a balanced diet is not as hard as most people think. The difficult part is retraining yourself to eat the right type of foods and to avoid those that have little or no nutritive value. Proper nutrition is one of the most significant factors in the development and maintenance of good health. Both cardiovascular disease and cancer are related to poor nutritional habits. A diet high in saturated fat and cholesterol increases the risk for atherosclerosis and coronary heart disease (see Chapter 7). High sodium intake has been linked to elevated blood pressure. Equally, some researchers believe that close to 50 percent of all cancer is diet-related (see Chapter 8).

In spite of the ample scientific evidence linking poor dietary habits to early disease and mortality rates, most people are not willing to change their eating patterns. Even when faced with conditions such as obesity, elevated blood lipids, and hypertension, people do not change. The motivating factor seems to be when a major health breakdown (e.g., a heart attack, a stroke, cancer) actually occurs. By this time the damage already has been done. In many cases it is irreversible and, for some, fatal.

Nutrient Analysis

The initial step to evaluate your diet is achieved by conducting your own nutrient analysis. This analysis can be quite an educational experience because most people do not realize how detrimental and non-nutritious many common foods are. To analyze your diet, keep a three-day record of everything you eat, using the forms given in Appendix B, Figure B.1. At the end of each day, look up the nutrient content for the foods you ate, in the "Nutritive Value of Selected Foods" list, also given in Appendix B. Record this information in the respective spaces provided in your three-day listing of foods in Figure B.1. If you do not find a particular food in the provided list, look for the information on the food container itself, or refer to the references provided at the end of the list. After recording the nutritive values for each day, add up each column and record the totals at the bottom of the chart.

After the third day, compute an average for the three days, using Figure B.2. To rate your diet, compare the results of the analysis to the Recommended Dietary Allowances (RDA) given at the end of Figure B.2. The results of your analysis will give a good indication of areas of strength and deficiency in your current diet.

The process of analyzing your diet by hand is quite time consuming. It can be simplified by using the computer software for this analysis (also available through Morton Publishing Company, Englewood, Colorado). If you use this software, you will only have to record the foods by code and by the number of servings based on the standard amounts given in the list of selected foods at the end of this chapter. (Use the form contained in Appendix B, Figure B.3). A sample nutrient analysis printout is given at the end of this chapter in Figures 6.9 and 6.10.

Some of the most revealing information to be learned in a nutrient analysis is the source of fat intake in the diet. The average fat consumption in the American diet is between 40 and 50 percent of the total caloric intake; less than 30 percent is recommended. Each gram of carbohydrates and protein supplies the body with four calories, whereas fat provides nine calories per gram consumed. In this regard, just looking at the total amount of grams consumed for each type of food can be very misleading. For example, a person who consumes 160 grams of carbohydrates, 100 grams of fat, and 70 grams of protein has a total intake of 330 grams of food. This indicates that 33 percent of the total grams of food is in the form of fat (100 grams of fat ÷ 330 grams of total food × 100). In reality, the diet consists of almost 50 percent fat calories.

In this sample diet, 640 calories are derived from carbohydrates (160 grams × 4 calories/gram), 280 calories from protein (70 grams × 4 calories/gram), and 900 calories from fat (100 grams × 9 calories/gram), for a total of 1,820 calories. If 900 calories are derived from fat, you can easily observe that almost half of the total caloric intake is in the form of fat (900 ÷ 1,820 × 100 = 49.5 percent).

Realizing that each gram of fat yields nine calories is useful when attempting to determine the fat content of individual foods. All you have to do is multiply the grams of fat by nine and divide by the total calories in that particular food. The percentage is obtained by multiplying the latter figure by 100. For example, if a food label lists a total of 100 calories and 7 grams of fat, the fat content would be 63 percent of total calories. This simple guideline can help you decrease fat intake in your diet. The fat content of selected foods, expressed in grams and as a percent of total calories, is given in Table 6.2.

Table 6.2.
Fat Content of Selected Foods (expressed in grams and as a Percent of Total Calories)

Food	Serving Size	Calories	Fat (g)	Percent of Calories
Avocado	.5 medium	185	19	92
Bacon	2 slc.	86	8	84
Beef, ground (lean)	3 oz.	186	10	48
Beef, round steak	3 oz.	222	13	53
Beef, sirloin	3 oz.	329	27	74
Butter	1 tsp.	36	4	100
Cheese, American	1 oz.	100	8	72
Cheese, cheddar	1 oz.	114	9	71
Cheese, cottage (1% fat)	.5 cup	82	1	11
Cheese, cottage (4% fat)	.5 cup	112	5	40
Cheese, cream	1 oz.	99	8	73
Cheese, muenster	2 oz.	208	17	74
Cheese, parmesan	2 oz.	261	17	61
Cheese, swiss	2 oz.	214	16	67
Chicken, light meat, no skin	3 oz.	141	3	17
Chicken, dark meat, no skin	3 oz.	149	5	30
Egg (hard-cooked)	1	72	5	63
Frankfurter	1	176	16	82
Halibut	3 oz.	144	6	38
Ice Cream (vanilla)	.5 cup	135	7	47
Ice Milk (vanilla)	.5 cup	100	3	27
Lamb leg, roast, trimmed	3 oz.	237	16	61
Margarine	1 tsp.	34	4	100
Mayonnaise	1 tsp.	36	4	100
Milk, skim	1 cup	88	0	—
Milk, low fat (2%)	1 cup	145	5	31
Milk, whole	1 cup	159	9	51
Nuts (brazil)	1 oz.	186	19	92
Salmon, broiled with butter	3 oz.	156	6	35
Sherbet	.5 cup	135	2	12
Shrimp, boiled	3 oz.	99	1	1
Tuna (canned, oil, drained)	3 oz.	167	7	38
Tuna (canned, water, drained)	3 oz.	126	1	1
Turkey, light and dark	3 oz.	162	5	28

Achieving a Balanced Diet

An individual who has completed a nutrient analysis and has given careful consideration to Figures 6.4 and 6.5 (vitamins and minerals) would probably realize that to have a well-balanced diet, a variety of foods must be consumed, accompanied by a decreased daily intake in fats and sweets. Although achieving a balanced diet may seem very complex, the basic guidelines to achieve an optimal diet are given in Figure 6.6. If two simple rules are followed, the diet will most likely have all of the required nutrients for proper

body functions. The rules of this "New American Eating Guide" are:

1. Eat the minimum number of servings required for each one of the four basic food groups:

   (a) four or more servings per day of beans, grains, and nuts;

   (b) four or more servings per day of fruits and vegetables, including one good source of vitamin A (milk and milk products, apricots, cantaloupe, broccoli, carrots, pumpkin, and dark leafy vegetables),

Figure 6.6. *The New American Eating Guide*

NEW AMERICAN EATING GUIDE

Center for Science in the Public Interest

The Center for Science in the Public Interest seeks to improve the public's health by offering reliable information and working for better food and health policies. CSPI is a nonprofit group. Send for a free list of publications and membership information.

What You Can Do

If you would like the government to promote better nutrition, write to your elected officials and to the Commissioner of FDA (Rockville, Md. 20857) and the Secretary of Agriculture (Washington, D.C. 20250).

Introduction

Eating can be a real joy, especially when you know that your diet is keeping you healthy.

Eat foods from each of the four food groups every day. Each food group contains different nutrients that your body needs. But each group has some foods that are better than others. This poster will help you pick the foods that best contribute to good health.

A good diet consists of vegetables, fruits, whole wheat bread and grains, potatoes, beans, lean meat, fish, poultry, and low-fat dairy products. This diet is high in nutrients and low in fat, sugar, salt, and cholesterol.

Pick plenty of ANYTIME foods—they should be the backbone of your diet. They are low in fat (less than 30% of a food's calories) and low in sugar and salt. Grain foods are mostly unrefined, whole grains, and therefore high in fiber and trace minerals.

Next best are the IN MODERATION foods. They contain moderate amounts of either saturated fats* or unsaturated fats*. Some items contain large amounts of fat, but mostly mono-unsaturated or polyunsaturated*. (The small numbers listed after items in the chart denote a food's drawbacks.)

Eat small portions of NOW & THEN foods and eat them less often than the other foods. They are usually high in fat, with large amounts of saturated fats*, or they are very high in added sugar*, salt*, or cholesterol*. Foods that are sometimes high in salt, depending on the manufacturer or recipe, are designated* Try to eat only two NOW & THEN foods a day. Foods that contain low to moderate amounts of fat but are high in sugar, salt, cholesterol, or refined grains*, are usually moved one or sometimes two categories to the right.

You can make a game out of rating your diet by keeping track of the foods you eat for one or several days. ANYTIME foods get one point; IN MODERATION foods do not get any points; and NOW & THEN foods lose one point. If you have a "+" score, congratulations! If you get a "—" score, shape up! BON APPETIT!

1—moderate fat, saturated   2—moderate fat, unsaturated   3—high fat, unsaturated   4—high fat, saturated   5—high in added sugar   6—high in salt or sodium   (6)—may be high in salt or sodium   7—high in cholesterol   8—refined grains

group 1 — Beans, Grains & Nuts (FOUR OR MORE SERVINGS/DAY)

Anytime	In Moderation	Now & Then
bread & rolls (whole grain)	cornbread²	croissant⁴˒⁸
bulghur	flour tortilla⁸	doughnut (yeast-leavened)³˒⁵˒⁸
dried beans & peas (legumes)	granola cereals¹˒²	presweetened breakfast cereals⁵˒⁸
lentils	hominy grits⁸	sticky buns¹˒⁵˒⁸
oatmeal	macaroni and cheese¹˒⁶˒⁸	stuffing (made with butter)⁴˒⁸
pasta, whole wheat	matzoh⁸	
rice, brown	nuts³	
rye bread	pasta, except whole wheat⁸	
sprouts	peanut butter³	
whole grain hot & cold cereals	pizza⁶˒⁸	
whole wheat matzoh	refried beans, commercial¹ or homemade in oil²	
	seeds³	
	soybeans²	
	tofu²	
	waffles or pancakes with syrup⁵˒⁶˒⁸	
	white bread and rolls⁸	
	white rice⁸	

group 2 — Fruits & Vegetables

Anytime	In Moderation	Now & Then
all fruits and vegetables except those listed at right	avocado³	coconut⁴
applesauce (unsweetened)	cole slaw²	pickles⁶
unsweetened fruit juices	cranberry sauce (canned)⁵	
unsalted vegetable juices	dried fruit	
potatoes, white or sweet	french fries, homemade in vegetable oil³ commercial³	
	fried eggplant (vegetable oil)³	
	fruits canned in syrup⁵	
	gazpacho²⁽⁶⁾	
	glazed carrots¹⁽⁶⁾	
	guacamole²	
	potatoes au gratin¹⁽⁶⁾	

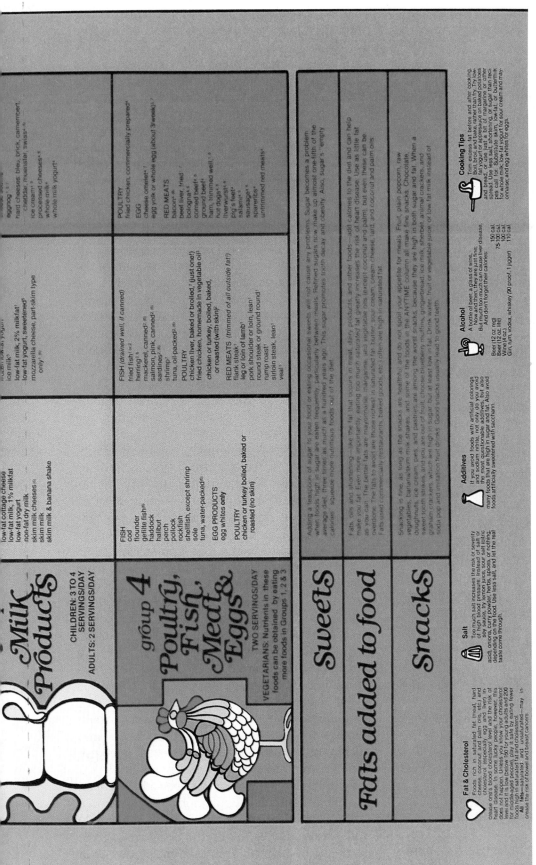

Reprinted from New American Eating Guide poster, available from the Center for Science in the Public Interest, 1501-16th St., N.W., Washington, D.C., for $3.95, copyright 1982.

One serving equals: Group 1 = 1 slice of bread, 1 cup ready-to-eat cereal, ½ cup cooked cereal/pasta/grits, or equivalent; Group 2 = ½ cup cooked or juice, 1 cup raw, or 1 medium-size fruit; Group 3 = 1 cup milk/yogurt, 1½ oz. cheese, 1 cup pudding/ice cream, 2 cups cottage cheese, or equivalent; Group 4 = 2 oz. cooked lean meat/fish/poultry, 2 eggs, or equivalent.

and one good source of vitamin C (cantaloupe, citrus fruit, kiwi fruit, strawberries, broccoli, cabbage, cauliflower, and green pepper);

(c) two or more servings per day of milk products;

(d) two or more servings per day of poultry, fish, meat, and eggs.

2. Obtain a final positive (+) score at the end of each day:

(a) "anytime" foods get one positive point;

(b) "in moderation" foods do not get any points;

(c) "now and then" foods lose one point.

To aid you in balancing your diet, use the log given in Figure 6.7 to record your daily food intake. This record sheet is much easier to keep than the complete dietary analysis. But first, make a copy of Figure 6.6 (or obtain the poster from the Center for Science in the Public Interest — see footnote at the bottom of the figure); post it somewhere visible in the kitchen or keep it accessible at all times.

Figure 6.7 then can be used. Whenever you have something to eat, record the code for the food from the list at the end of this chapter and the +, NP (no points), or − characters in the corresponding spaces provided for each day. If you are on a weight reduction program, also record the caloric content of each food. This information can be obtained from the list of foods contained in Appendix B, the food container itself, or some of the references given at the end of the list of foods. Record the information immediately after each meal so it will be easier to keep track of foods and the amount eaten. If you eat twice the amount of a particular serving, double the calories and record two +, −, or NP characters also.

At the end of the day, evaluate the diet by checking whether you consumed the minimum required servings for each food group, and by adding up the + and − points accumulated. If you met the required servings and ended up with a positive score, you achieved a well-balanced diet for that day.

Vitamin and Mineral Supplementation

Another point of significant interest in nutrition is the unnecessary and sometimes unsafe use of vitamin and mineral supplementation. Even though experts agree that supplements are not necessary, people consume them at a greater rate than ever before. Sales of vitamin and mineral supplements have more than doubled in the last ten years, and are predicted to increase from about $2.6 billion in 1987 to almost $10 billion by 1990. The Food and Drug Administration has indicated that in the United States four of every ten adults take daily supplements, and one in every seven has a nutrient intake of almost eight times the Recommended Dietary Allowances. Research has clearly demonstrated that even when a person consumes as few as 1,200 calories per day, no additional supplementation is needed as long as the diet contains the recommended servings from the four basic food groups.

Although water-soluble vitamins cannot be stored as long as fat-soluble vitamins, they are easily retained for weeks or months in various organs and tissues of the body. Excessive intakes are readily excreted from the body. Fat-soluble vitamins are stored in fatty tissue. Therefore, daily intake of these vitamins is not as crucial. Furthermore, excessive amounts of vitamins A and D can be detrimental to your health. Mineral requirements are provided in sufficient quantities in a normal balanced diet.

For most people, vitamin and mineral supplementation is unnecessary. Iron deficiency (determined through blood testing) is the only exception for women who suffer from heavy menstrual flow. Pregnant and lactating women also may require supplements. In all instances, supplements should be taken under a physician's supervision. Other people who may benefit from supplementation are alcoholics who are not consuming a balanced diet, strict vegetarians, individuals on extremely low-calorie diets, elderly people who don't regularly receive balanced meals, and newborn infants (usually given a single dose of vitamin K to prevent abnormal bleeding).

For healthy people with a balanced diet, supplementation provides no additional health benefits. It will not help a person run faster, jump higher, relieve stress, improve sexual prowess, cure a common cold, or boost energy levels!

Research has shown that not even athletes need vitamin and mineral supplementation or, for that matter, any other special type of diet. The simple truth is that, unless the diet is deficient in basic nutrients, no special, secret, or magic diets will help a person perform better or develop faster as a result of what he/she is eating. As long as the

Figure 6.7. *Daily diet record form*

Name: _____　　Course: _____　　Section: _____　　Date: _____

Code[a]	Food	Amount	Score +, −, or NP[b]	Calories[c]	Number of Servings						
					Beans, Grains, & Nuts	Fruits & Vegetables			Milk Products	Poultry, Meat, Fish, & Eggs
						Vit. A	Vit. C	Other		

Totals

	+ Score			Number of Servings						
Recommended Standard				[d]	4	1	1	2	2	2

Deficiencies

[a,c]See list of nutritive value of selected foods in Appendix B.　　[b]See Figure 6.6: New American Eating Guide.　　[d]Use value obtained from Figure 6.8.

Figure 6.7. *Daily diet record form*

Name: _____ Course: _____ Section: _____ Date: _____

Code[a]	Food	Amount	Score +, −, or NP[b]	Calories[c]	Beans, Grains, & Nuts	Fruits & Vegetables			Milk Products	Poultry, Meat, Fish, & Eggs
						Vit. A	Vit. C	Other		
Totals			+ Score							
Recommended Standard				d	4	1	1	2	2	2
Deficiencies										

Number of Servings

[a,c] See list of nutritive value of selected foods in Appendix B.   [b] See Figure 6.6: New American Eating Guide.   [d] Use value obtained from Figure 6.8.

diet is balanced (meets the daily servings from each of the four food groups), athletes do not need any additional supplements. Even in strength training and body building no additional protein in excess of 20 percent of total daily caloric intake is needed.

The only difference between a sedentary person and a highly trained one is in the total number of calories required on a daily basis. The trained person may consume more calories because of the increased energy expenditure as a result of intense physical training.

The only time that a normal diet should be modified is when an individual is going to participate in long-distance events lasting in excess of one hour (e.g., marathon, triathlon, and road cycling). Athletic performance is increased for these types of events by consuming a regular balanced diet (or a diet low in carbohydrates) along with exhaustive physical training on the fifth and fourth days prior to the event, followed by a diet high in carbohydrates (about 70 percent) and a progressive decrease in training intensity during the last three days before the event.

Another fallacy regarding nutrition is that many people who regularly eat fast foods or sweets think that vitamin and mineral supplementation is needed to balance their diet. The problem in these cases is not that the diet lacks vitamins and minerals but, rather, that the diet is too high in calories, fat, and sodium. Supplementation will not offset such poor eating habits.

If you think that your diet is not balanced, you first have to determine which nutrients are missing from your own nutrient analysis. Then use the "New American Eating Guide" (Figure 6.6) and the vitamin and mineral charts (Figures 6.4 and 6.5), and increase the intake of those foods high in nutrients that are deficient in your diet.

PRINCIPLES OF WEIGHT CONTROL

Achieving and maintaining ideal body weight is a major objective of a good physical fitness and wellness program (the assessment of ideal body weight is explained in Chapter 5). Next to poor cardiovascular fitness, obesity is the most common problem encountered in fitness and wellness assessments. Estimates indicate that only 5 to 10 percent of all people who ever initiate a traditional weight loss program are able to lose the

desired weight, and worse yet, only one in 100 is able to keep the weight off for a significant period of time.

You may ask why the traditional diets have failed. The answer is simply because very few diets teach the importance of lifetime changes in food selection and the role of exercise as the keys to successful weight loss. The diet industry is a multimillion-dollar industry that tries to capitalize on the idea that weight can be lost quickly without taking into consideration the long-term consequences of fast weight loss.

Fad Dieting

There are several reasons why fad diets continue to deceive people and can claim that weight will indeed be lost if all instructions are followed. Most diets are very low in calories or deprive the body of certain nutrients (or both), creating a metabolic imbalance that can even cause death. Under such conditions, a lot of the weight loss is in the form of water and protein and not fat. On a crash diet, nearly 50 percent of the weight loss is in lean (protein) tissue. When the body uses protein instead of a combination of fats and carbohydrates as a source of energy, weight is lost as much as ten times faster. A gram of protein yields half the amount of energy that fat does. In the case of muscle protein, one-fifth of protein is mixed with four-fifths water. In other words, each pound of muscle yields only one-tenth the amount of energy of a pound of fat. As a result, most of the weight loss is in the form of water, which on the scale, of course, looks good. Nevertheless, when regular eating habits are resumed, most of the lost weight comes right back.

Some diets allow the consumption of only certain foods. If people would just realize that there are no "magic" foods that will provide all of the necessary nutrients, and that a person has to eat a variety of foods to be well-nourished, the diet industry would not be as successful. The unfortunate thing about most of these diets is that they create a nutritional deficiency, which at times can be fatal. The reason why some of these diets succeed is because in due time people get tired of eating the same thing day in and day out and eventually start eating less. If they happen to achieve the lower weight, they quickly regain the weight once they go back to old eating habits and do not implement permanent dietary changes.

A few diets recommend exercise along with caloric restrictions, which, of course, is the best method for weight reduction. A lot of the weight lost is due to exercise; hence, the diet has achieved its purpose. Unfortunately, if no permanent changes in food selection and activity level take place, once dieting and exercise are discontinued, the weight is quickly gained back.

Eating Disorders

Anorexia nervosa and bulimia have been classified as physical and emotional problems usually developed as a result of individual, family, or social pressures to achieve thinness. These medical disorders are steadily increasing in most industrialized nations, where low-calorie diets and model-like thinness are encouraged by society. Individuals who suffer from eating disorders have an intense fear of becoming obese, which does not disappear even as they lose extreme amounts of weight.

Anorexia nervosa is a condition of self-imposed starvation to lose and then maintain very low body weight. Approximately nineteen of every twenty anorexics are young women. An estimated one percent of the female population in the United States suffers from this disease. The anorexic seems to fear weight gain more than death from starvation. Furthermore, these individuals have a distorted image of their body and perceive themselves as being fat even when they are critically emaciated.

Although a genetic predisposition may exist, the anorexic patient often comes from a mother-dominated home, with other possible drug addictions in the family. The syndrome may start following a stressful life event and the uncertainty of the ability to cope efficiently. Because the female role in society is changing more rapidly, women seem to be especially susceptible. Life events such as weight gain, start of menstrual periods, beginning of college, loss of a boyfriend, poor self-esteem, social rejection, start of a professional career, or becoming a wife or mother may trigger the syndrome.

The person, who is not always overweight, usually begins a diet and may initially feel in control and happy about the weight loss. To speed up the weight loss process, severe dieting is frequently combined with exhaustive exercise and overuse of laxatives or diuretics, or both. The individual commonly develops obsessive and compulsive behaviors and emphatically denies the condition. There also appears to be a constant preoccupation with food, meal planning, grocery shopping, and unusual eating habits. As weight is lost and health begins to deteriorate, the anorexic feels weak and tired and may realize that there is a problem but will not discontinue starvation and refuses to accept the behavior as abnormal.

Once significant weight loss and malnutrition begin, typical physical changes become more visible. Some of the more common changes exhibited by anorexics are amenorrhea (cessation of menstruation), digestive difficulties, extreme sensitivity to cold, hair and skin problems, fluid and electrolyte abnormalities (which may lead to an irregular heart beat and sudden stopping of the heart), injuries to nerves and tendons, abnormalities of immune function, anemia, growth of fine body hair, mental confusion, inability to concentrate, lethargy, depression, skin dryness, and decreased skin and body temperature.

Many of the changes of anorexia nervosa are by no means irreversible. Treatment almost always requires professional help, and the sooner it is started, the higher are the chances for reversibility and cure. A combination of medical and psychological techniques are used in therapy to restore proper nutrition, prevent medical complications, and modify the environment or events that triggered the syndrome. Seldom are anorexics able to overcome the problem by themselves.

Unfortunately, anorexics exhibit strong denial, and they are able to hide their condition and deceive friends and relatives quite effectively. Based on their behavior, many individuals meet all of the characteristics of anorexia nervosa, but the condition goes undetected because both thinness and dieting are socially acceptable behaviors. Only a well-trained clinician is able to make a positive diagnosis.

Bulimia, a pattern of binge eating and purging, is more prevalent than anorexia nervosa. For many years it was thought to be a variant of anorexia nervosa, but it is now identified as a separate disease. It afflicts primarily young people. Estimates indicate that as many as one in every five women on college campuses is affected by it. Bulimia is also more frequent than anorexia nervosa in males.

Bulimics are usually healthy-looking people, well-educated, near ideal body weight, who enjoy food and often socialize around it. But they are emotionally insecure, rely on others, and lack self-confidence and esteem. Food and maintenance of ideal weight are both important to them.

As a result of stressful life events or simple compulsion to eat, they periodically engage in binge eating that may last an hour or longer, during which they may consume several thousand calories. A feeling of deep guilt and shame follows, along with intense fear of gaining weight. Purging seems to be an easy answer to the problem, and the binging cycle continues without the fear of gaining weight. The most common form of purging is self-induced vomiting, although strong laxatives and emetics are frequently used. Overuse of the latter caused the death of Karen Carpenter in 1983. Near-fasting diets and strenuous bouts of physical activity are also commonly seen in bulimics.

Medical problems associated with bulimia include cardiac arrhythmias, amenorrhea, kidney and bladder damage, ulcers, colitis, and tearing of the esophagus or stomach. Teeth erosion, gum damage, and general muscular weakness also may result.

Unlike anorexics, bulimics realize that their behavior is abnormal and feel great shame for their actions. Fearing social rejection, the binge-purge cycle is carried out primarily in secrecy and during unusual hours of the day. Nevertheless, bulimia can be treated successfully when the person realizes that such destructive behavior is not the solution to life's problems. Hopefully, the change in attitude will grasp the individual before permanent or fatal damage is done.

PHYSIOLOGY OF WEIGHT LOSS

Only a few years ago the principles that govern a weight loss and maintenance program seemed to be pretty clear, but we now know that the final answers are not yet in. The traditional concepts related to weight control have centered on three assumptions: (1) that balancing food intake against output allows a person to achieve ideal weight, (2) that fat people just eat too much, and (3) that it really does not matter to the human body how much (or little) fat is stored. Although there may be some truth to these statements, they are still open to much debate and research.

The Energy-Balancing Equation

The energy-balancing equation basically states that as long as caloric input equals caloric output, the person will not gain or lose weight. If caloric intake exceeds the output, the individual will gain weight. When output exceeds input, weight is lost. This principle is simple, and if daily energy requirements could be accurately determined, it seems reasonable that the conscious mind could be used to balance caloric intake versus output.

Unfortunately, this is not always the case because large individual differences, genetic and lifestyle-related, determine the number of calories required to maintain or lose body weight. Some general guidelines for estimating daily caloric intake according to lifestyle patterns are given in Table 6.3. These are only estimated figures and, as discussed later in this chapter, serves only as a starting point from whence individual adjustments will have to be made.

Perhaps some examples may help explain this. It is well known that one pound of fat equals 3,500 calories. Assuming that the basic daily caloric expenditure for a given person is 2,500 calories, if this person were to decrease the daily intake by 500 calories per day, one pound of fat should be lost in seven days (500 × 7 = 3,500). Research has shown, however (and many dieters have probably experienced), that even when caloric input is carefully balanced against caloric output, weight loss does not always come as predicted. Furthermore, two people with similar measured caloric intake and output will not necessarily lose weight at the same rate.

The most common explanation given by many in the past regarding individual differences in weight loss or weight gain was the variation in human metabolism from one person to the other. We have all seen people who can eat "all day long" and yet not gain an ounce of weight, while others cannot even "dream about food" without gaining weight. Because many experts did not believe that such extreme differences could be attributed to human metabolism alone, several theories have been developed that may better explain these individual variations.

Setpoint Theory

Scientific research has indicated that a weight-regulating mechanism (WRM) located in the hypothalamus of the brain regulates how much the body should weigh. This mechanism has a setpoint that controls both appetite and the amount of fat stored. It is hypothesized that the setpoint works like a thermostat for body fat, maintaining body weight fairly constant because it knows at all times the exact amount of adipose tissue stored in the fat cells. Some people have high settings, and others have low settings.

If body weight decreases (as in dieting), the setpoint senses this change, and, in turn, triggers the WRM to increase the person's appetite or make the body conserve energy to maintain the "set" weight. The opposite may also be true. Some people who consciously try to gain weight have an extremely difficult time in doing so. In this case, the WRM decreases appetite or causes the body to waste energy to maintain the lower weight.

Dieting Can Make You Fat!

Every person has his/her own certain body fat percentage (as established by the setpoint) that the body attempts to maintain. The genetic instinct to survive tells the body that fat storage is vital, and therefore it sets an inherently acceptable fat level. This level remains fairly constant or may gradually climb because of poor lifestyle habits.

For instance, under strict caloric reductions, the body may make extreme metabolic adjustments in an effort to maintain its setpoint for fat. The basal metabolic rate may drop dramatically against a consistent negative caloric balance, and a person may be on a plateau for days or even weeks without losing much weight.

Dietary restriction alone will not lower the setpoint even though weight and fat may be lost. When the dieter goes back to the normal or even below normal caloric intake, at which the weight may have been stable for a long time, the fat loss is quickly regained as the body strives to regain a comfortable fat store.

Let's use a practical illustration. A person would like to lose some body fat and assumes that a stable body weight has been reached at an average daily caloric intake of 1,800 calories (no weight gain or loss occurs at this daily intake). This person now starts a strict low-calorie diet or, even worse, a near-fasting diet in an attempt to achieve rapid weight loss. Immediately the body

activates its survival mechanism and readjusts its metabolism to a lower caloric balance.

After a few weeks of dieting at less than 400 to 600 calories per day, the body can now maintain its normal functions at 1,000 calories per day. Having lost the desired weight, the person terminates the diet but realizes that the original caloric intake of 1,800 calories per day will have to be decreased to maintain the new lower weight.

Therefore, to adjust to the new lower body weight, the intake is restricted to about 1,500 calories per day, but the individual is surprised to find that, even at this lower daily intake (300 fewer calories), weight is gained back at a rate of one pound every one to two weeks. This new lowered metabolic rate, as pointed out in a Swedish study, may take a year or more after terminating the diet to kick back up to its normal level.

From this explanation, it is clear that individuals should never go on very low-calorie diets. Not only will this practice decrease resting metabolic rate, but it will also deprive the body of the basic daily nutrients required for normal physiological functions. Under no circumstances should a person ever engage in diets below 1,200 and 1,500 calories for women and men, respectively.

Remember that weight (fat) is gained over a period of months and years and not overnight. Likewise, weight loss should be accomplished gradually and not abruptly. Daily caloric intakes of 1,200 to 1,500 calories, if properly distributed over the four basic food groups (meeting the daily required servings from each group), will still provide the necessary nutrients. Of course, the individual will have to learn which foods meet the requirements and yet are low in fat, sugar, and calories. This can be learned after a few days of following the "New American Eating Guide" (Figure 6.6) and by looking up, in the Nutritive Value of Selected Foods list contained in Appendix B, the various foods eaten.

Setpoint and Nutrition

Other researchers believe that a second way in which the setpoint may work is by keeping track of the nutrients and calories that are consumed on a daily basis. The body, like a cash register, records the daily food intake, and the brain will not feel satisfied until the calories and nutrients have been "registered."

For some people this setpoint for calories and nutrients seems to work regardless of the amount of physical activity, as long as it is not too exhausting. Numerous studies have shown that hunger does not increase with moderate physical activity. In such cases, people can choose to lose weight by either going hungry or by increasing daily physical (aerobic) activity. The increased number of calories burned through exercise will help decrease body fat.

The most common question that individuals seem to have regarding the setpoint is how it can be lowered so that the body will feel comfortable at a lower fat percentage. Factors that seem to have a direct effect on the setpoint include: (a) aerobic exercise, (b) a diet high in complex carbohydrates, (c) nicotine, and (d) amphetamines. All of these have been shown to decrease the fat thermostat. The last two, however, are more destructive than being overweight, thereby eliminating themselves as reasonable alternatives. (It has been said that as far as the extra strain on the heart is concerned, smoking one pack of cigarettes per day is the equivalent of carrying fifty to seventy-five pounds of excess body fat.) On the other hand, a diet high in fats and refined carbohydrates, near-fasting diets, and perhaps even artificial sweeteners seem to increase the setpoint. Therefore, it looks as though the only practical and effective way to lower the setpoint and lose fat weight is through a combination of aerobic exercise and a diet high in complex carbohydrates and low in fat and sugar.

Because of the effects of proper food management on the body's setpoint, many nutritionists now believe that the total number of calories should not be a concern in a weight control program; rather, the source of those calories should receive attention. In this regard, most of the effort is spent in retraining eating habits, increasing the intake of complex carbohydrates and high-fiber foods, and decreasing the use of refined carbohydrates (sugars) and fats. In addition, a diet is no longer viewed as a temporary tool to aid in weight loss but, rather, as a permanent change in eating behaviors to ensure adequate weight management and health enhancement. The role of increased physical activity must also be considered, because successful weight loss, maintenance, and ideal body composition are seldom achieved without a regular exercise program.

Yellow Fat Versus Brown Fat

For years it has been known that there are two different types of fat — yellow and brown. The proportion of yellow to brown fat could be another factor that influences weight regulation. The average ratio is about 99 percent yellow fat to 1 percent brown fat. The difference between the two is that yellow fat simply stores energy in the form of fat, while brown fat has a high amount of the iron-containing hemoglobin pigment found in red blood cells. The brown cells do not store fat but, rather, have the capacity to produce body heat by burning the fat. Under resting conditions, brown fat produces an estimated 25 percent of the total body heat. According to Dr. George A. Bray of the Los Angeles Medical Center at Harbour University of California, the brown fat can actually produce as much heat as the entire rest of the body.

The fact that brown fat converts food energy to heat may also explain why some individuals simply do not gain weight. Even though the amount of brown fat is genetically determined and cannot be changed throughout life, people with only slightly higher levels may have an advantage when it comes to weight control. It is also possible that some individuals may have more active brown cells that generate more heat. Perhaps you have come across thin people who are warm even when everyone else seems comfortable. In contrast (because one of the basic functions of fat is body heat preservation), obese people who are successful in losing weight but have a lower proportion or less active brown fat may feel cold when it is actually pleasantly warm.

Diet and Metabolism

Fat can be lost by making proper food selection, participating in aerobic exercise and/or restricting calories. When weight loss is pursued by means of dietary restrictions alone, however, there will always be a decrease in lean body mass (muscle protein, along with vital organ protein). The amount of lean body mass lost depends exclusively on the caloric restriction of your diet. In near-fasting diets, up to 50 percent of the weight loss can be lean body mass, and the other 50 percent will be actual fat loss. When diet is combined with exercise, 98 percent of the weight loss will be in the form of fat, and there may actually be an increase in lean tissue. Lean body mass loss is never desirable because it weakens the organs and muscles and slows down the metabolism.

Contrary to some beliefs, metabolism does not decrease with age. It has been shown that basal metabolism is directly related to lean body weight. The greater the lean tissue, the higher the metabolic rate. What happens is that as a result of sedentary living and less physical activity, the lean component decreases and fat tissue increases. The organism, though, continues to use the same amount of oxygen per pound of lean body mass. Because fat is considered metabolically inert from the point of view of caloric use, even at rest the lean tissue uses most of the oxygen. Consequently, as muscle and organ mass decreases, the energy requirements at rest also decrease.

Decreases in lean body mass are commonly seen with aging (because of physical inactivity) and severely restricted diets. The loss of lean body mass may also account for the lower metabolic rate described under the discussion "Dieting Can Make You Fat" and the lengthy period of time that it takes to kick back up. No diets with caloric intakes below 1,200 to 1,500 calories can ensure no loss of lean body mass. Even at this intake, there is some loss unless the diet is combined with exercise. Many formulators of diets have claimed that the lean component is unaltered with their particular diet, but the simple truth is that, regardless of what nutrients may be added to the diet, if caloric restrictions are too severe, there will always be a loss of lean tissue.

Unfortunately, too many people use low-calorie diets, and every time they do so, the metabolic rate keeps slowing down as more lean tissue is lost. It is not uncommon to find individuals in their forties or older who weigh the same as they did when they were twenty and think that they are at ideal body weight. Nevertheless, during this span of twenty years or more, they have "dieted" all too many times without engaging in physical activity. The weight is regained shortly after terminating each diet, but most of that gain is in fat. Perhaps at age twenty they weighed 150 pounds and were only 15 to 16 percent fat. Now at age forty, even though they still weigh 150 pounds, they may be 30 to 40 percent fat. They may believe that they are at ideal body weight and wonder why they are eating very little and still have a difficult time maintaining that weight.

EXERCISE: THE KEY TO SUCCESSFUL WEIGHT LOSS AND MAINTENANCE

Based on the preceding discussion on weight control, it can be easily concluded that exercise is the key to weight loss. Not only will exercise maintain lean tissue, but advocates of the setpoint theory also indicate that exercise resets the fat thermostat to a new lower level. For a lot of people, this change occurs rapidly, but in some instances it may take time. There are overweight individuals who have faithfully exercised on an almost daily basis, sixty minutes at a time, for a whole year before significant weight changes started to occur. Individuals who have a very "sticky" setpoint will have to be patient and persistent.

For individuals who are trying to lose weight, a combination of aerobic and strength-training exercises works best. Aerobic exercise is the key to offset the setpoint, and because of the continuity and duration of these types of activities, many calories are burned in the process. On the other hand, strength-training exercises have the greatest impact in increasing lean body mass. Each additional pound of muscle tissue can raise the basal metabolic rate between 50 and 100 calories per day. Using the conservative estimate of 50 calories per day, an individual who adds five pounds of muscle tissue as a result of strength training would increase the basal metabolic rate by 250 calories per day, or the equivalent of 91,250 calories per year.

Strength training is especially recommended for people who think that they are at optimal body weight, yet the body fat percentage is higher than ideal. Nevertheless, the number of calories burned during an average hour of strength training is significantly less than during an hour of aerobic exercise. Because of the high intensity of weight training, frequent rest intervals are required to recover from each set of exercise. The typical individual engages in actual lifting a total of only ten to twelve minutes of every hour of exercise. Weight loss can occur with a regular weight-training program, but at a much slower rate. However, the benefits of gains in lean tissue are enjoyed in the long run. Guidelines for developing aerobic and strength-training programs are given in Chapters 2 and 3.

Because exercise leads to an increase in lean body mass, it is not uncommon for body weight to remain the same or increase when you initiate an exercise program, while inches and percent body fat decrease. The increase in lean tissue results in an increased functional capacity of the human body. With exercise, most of the weight loss is seen after a few weeks of training, when the lean component has stabilized.

"Skinny" people should also realize that the only healthy manner to increase body weight is through exercise, primarily strength-training exercises. Attempting to gain weight by just overeating will increase the fat component and not the lean component — which is not conducive to better health. Consequently, exercise is the best solution to weight (fat) reduction as well as weight (lean) gain.

Research also has shown that there is no such thing as spot reducing or losing "cellulite" from certain body parts. Cellulite is nothing but plain fat storage. Just doing several sets of daily sit-ups will not help to get rid of fat in the midsection of the body. When fat comes off, it does so from throughout the entire body, not just the exercised area. The greatest proportion of fat may come off the largest fat deposits, but the caloric output of a few sets of sit-ups is practically nil to have a real effect on total body fat reduction. The amount of exercise has to be much longer to have a real impact on weight reduction.

Other common fallacies regarding quick weight loss relate to the use of rubberized sweatsuits, steam baths, and mechanical vibrators. When an individual wears a sweatsuit or steps into a sauna, there is a significant amount of water (and not fat) loss. Sure, it looks nice immediately afterward when you step on the scale, but it is a false loss of weight. As soon as you replace body fluids, the weight comes back quickly.

Wearing rubberized sweatsuits not only increases the rate of body fluid loss, which is vital during prolonged exercise, but it also increases core temperature. Dehydration as a result of these methods leads to impaired cellular function and in extreme cases even death. Similarly, mechanical vibrators are worthless in a weight control program. Vibrating belts and turning rollers may feel good, but they require no effort whatsoever on the part of the muscles. Fat can not be "shaken off"; it has to be burned off in muscle tissue.

Although we now know that a negative caloric balance of 3,500 calories will not always result in an exact loss of one pound of fat, the role of exercise in achieving a negative balance by burning additional calories is significant in weight reduction and maintenance programs. Sadly, some individuals claim that the amount of calories burned during exercise is hardly worth the effort. These individuals believe that it is easier to cut the daily intake by some 200 calories than to participate in some sort of physical activity that would burn the equivalent amount of calories. The only problem is that the willpower to cut those 200 calories lasts only a few weeks, and then the old eating patterns resume. In comparison, if a person gets into the habit of exercising regularly, say three times per week, running three miles per exercise session (about 300 calories burned), this would represent 900 calories in one week, 3,600 in one month, or 43,200 calories per year. This apparently insignificant amount of exercise could mean as many as twelve extra pounds of fat in one year, twenty-four in two, and so on. We tend to forget that our weight creeps up gradually over the years, not just overnight.

Hardly worth the effort? And we have not even taken into consideration the increase in lean tissue, possible resetting of the setpoint, benefits to the cardiovascular system, and, most important, the improved quality of life! There is very little argument that the fundamental reasons for overfatness and obesity are lack of exercise and sedentary living.

LOSING WEIGHT THE SOUND AND SENSIBLE WAY

Dieting has never been fun and never will be. Individuals who have a weight problem and are serious about losing weight will have to make exercise a regular part of their daily life, along with proper food management, and perhaps even sensible adjustments in caloric intake. Some precautions are necessary, because excessive body fat is a risk factor for cardiovascular disease. Depending on the extent of the weight problem, a stress ECG may be required prior to initiating the exercise program. A physician should be consulted in this regard.

Significantly overweight individuals may also have to choose activities in which they will not have to support their own body weight but that will still be effective in burning calories. Joint and muscle injuries are very common among over-weight individuals who participate in weight-bearing exercises such as walking, jogging, and aerobic dancing. Swimming may not be a good exercise either. The increased body fat makes the person more buoyant, and most people do not have the skill level to swim fast enough to get an optimal training effect. The tendency is to just "float" along, limiting the amount of calories burned as well as the benefits to the cardiovascular system.

Some better alternatives are riding a bicycle (either road or stationary), walking in a shallow pool, or running in place in deep water (treading water). The last exercise, quickly gaining in popularity, has proven to be effective in achieving weight reduction without the "pain" and fear of injuries.

How long should each exercise session last? To develop and maintain cardiovascular fitness, twenty to thirty minutes of exercise at the ideal target rate, three to five times per week, is sufficient (see Chapter 2). For weight loss purposes, many experts recommend exercising for an hour at a time, five to six times per week. But a person should not try to increase the duration and frequency of exercise too fast. It is recommended that unconditioned beginners start with about fifteen minutes three times per week, and then gradually increase the duration by approximately five minutes each week and the frequency by one day per week during the next three to four weeks.

Exercising for sixty minutes an average of five to six times per week will not only ensure a high caloric output but, because of the prolonged duration of exercise, will also keep the metabolic rate at a higher level long after the individual has finished the exercise session. Extra calories are still being burned even though the person is done exercising. The longer the duration of exercise in the appropriate cardiovascular target zone, the longer the body will take to return to the basal rate.

One final benefit of exercise as related to weight control is that fat can be burned more efficiently. Because both carbohydrates and fats are sources of energy, when the glucose levels begin to decrease during prolonged exercise, more fat is used as energy substrate. Equally important is the fact that fat-burning enzymes increase with aerobic training. The role of these enzymes is significant, because fat can be lost only by burning it in muscle. As the concentration of the enzymes increases, so does the ability to burn fat.

In addition to exercise and adequate food management, many experts still recommend that individuals take a look at their daily caloric intake and compare it against the estimated daily requirement. Your current daily caloric intake is determined through the nutritional analysis. Although this intake may not be as crucial if proper food management and exercise are incorporated into your daily lifestyle, it is still beneficial in certain circumstances. All too often the nutritional analysis reveals that faithful dieters are not consuming enough calories and actually need to increase the daily caloric intake (combined with an exercise program) to get the metabolism to kick back up to a normal level.

In other cases, knowledge of the daily caloric requirement is needed for successful weight control. The reasons for prescribing a certain caloric figure to either maintain or lose weight are:

1. It takes time to develop new behaviors and some individuals have difficulty changing and adjusting to the new eating habits.

2. Many individuals are in such poor physical condition that it takes them a long time to increase their activity level so as to have a significant impact in offsetting the setpoint and in burning enough calories to aid in body fat loss.

3. Some dieters find it difficult to succeed unless they can count calories.

4. Some individuals will simply not alter their food selection.

All of these people can benefit from a caloric intake guideline, and in many instances a sensible caloric decrease is helpful in the early stages of the weight reduction program. For the latter group, those who will not alter their food selection, a significant increase in physical activity, a negative caloric balance, or a combination of both are the only solutions for successful weight loss.

How to Set Up Your Own Weight Control Program

To write your own weight control program, you will have to determine your typical daily caloric intake, including exercise, required to maintain your current weight. This estimated daily caloric requirement can be determined by using Figure 6.8 and Tables 6.3 and 6.4. Keep in mind that this is only an estimated value, and individual adjustments related to many of the factors discussed in this chapter may be required to establish a more precise value. Nevertheless, the estimated value will provide an initial guideline for weight control or reduction.

The average daily caloric requirement without exercise is based on typical lifestyle patterns, total body weight, and gender. Individuals who hold jobs that require heavy manual labor burn more calories during the day than those who hold sedentary jobs such as working behind a desk. To determine the activity level, refer to Table 6.3 and rate yourself accordingly. Because the number given in this table is per pound of body weight, you will have to multiply your current weight by that number (use the form provided in Figure 6.8). For example, the typical caloric requirement to maintain body weight for a moderately active male who weighs 160 pounds would be 2,400 calories (160 lbs $\times$ 15 cal/lb).

The second step is to determine the average number of calories that are burned on a daily basis as a result of exercise. To obtain this number, you will need to figure out the total number of minutes in which you engage in

Figure 6.8. *Computation form for daily caloric requirement*

A. Current body weight _____

B. Caloric requirement per pound of body weight (use Table 6.3). _____

C. Typical daily caloric requirement without exercise to maintain body weight (A $\times$ B) _____

D. Selected physical activity (e.g., jogging)* _____

E. Number of exercise sessions per week _____

F. Duration of exercise session (in minutes) _____

G. Total weekly exercise time in minutes (E $\times$ F) _____

H. Average daily exercise time in minutes (G $\div$ 7) _____

I. Caloric expenditure per pound per minute (cal/lb/min) of physical activity (use Table 6.4) _____

J. Total calories burned per minute of physical activity (A $\times$ I) _____

K. Average daily calories burned as a result of the exercise program (H $\times$ J) _____

L. Total daily caloric requirement with exercise to maintain body weight (C + K) _____

M. Number of calories to subtract from daily requirement to achieve a negative caloric balance** _____

N. Target caloric intake to lose weight (L − M) _____

* If more than one physical activity is selected, you will need to estimate the average daily calories burned as a result of each additional activity (steps D through K) and add all of these figures to L above.

** Subtract 500 calories if the total daily requirement with exercise (L) is below 3,000 calories. As many as 1,000 calories may be subtracted for daily requirements above 3,000 calories.

Table 6.3.
Average Caloric Requirement Per Pound of Body Weight Based on Lifestyle Patterns and Gender

	Calories per pound	
Activity Rating	Men	Women*
Sedentary — Limited physical activity	13.0	12.0
Moderate physical activity	15.0	13.5
Hard Labor — Strenuous physical effort	17.0	15.0

* Pregnant or lactating women: Add three calories to these values.

Table 6.4.
Caloric Expenditure of Selected Physical Activities
(calories per pound of body weight per minute of activity)

Activity*	Cal/lb/min	Activity	Cal/lb/min
Archery	0.030	Rowing (vigorous)	0.090
Badminton		Running	
Recreation	0.038	11.0 min/mile	0.070
Competition	0.065	8.5 min/mile	0.090
Baseball	0.031	7.0 min/mile	0.102
Basketball		6.0 min/mile	0.114
Moderate	0.046	Deep water[a]	0.100
Competition	0.063	Skating (moderate)	0.038
Cycling (level)		Skiing	
5.5 mph	0.033	Downhill	0.060
10.0 mph	0.050	Level (5 mph)	0.078
13.0 mph	0.071	Soccer	0.059
Bowling	0.030	Strength Training	0.050
Calisthenics	0.033	Swimming (crawl)	
Dance		20 yds/min	0.031
Moderate	0.030	25 yds/min	0.040
Vigorous	0.055	45 yds/min	0.057
Golf	0.030	50 yds/min	0.070
Gymnastics		Table Tennis	0.030
Light	0.030	Tennis	
Heavy	0.056	Moderate	0.045
Handball	0.064	Competition	0.064
Hiking	0.040	Volleyball	0.030
Judo/Karate	0.086	Walking	
Racquetball	0.065	4.5 mph	0.045
Rope Jumping	0.060	Shallow pool	0.090
		Wrestling	0.085

* Values are only for actual time engaged in the activity.
[a] Treading water (estimated value)
Adapted from:

    Allsen, P. E., J. M. Harrison, and B. Vance. *Fitness for Life: An Individualized Approach.* Dubuque, IA: Wm. C. Brown, 1984.
    Bucher, C. A., and W. E. Prentice. *Fitness for College and Life.* St. Louis: Times Mirror/Mosby College Publishing, 1985.
    Consolazio, C. F., R. E. Johnson, and L. J. Pecora. *Physiological measurements of Metabolic Functions in Man.* New York: McGraw-Hill, 1963.
    Hockey, R. V. *Physical Fitness: The Pathway to Healthful Living.* St. Louis: Times Mirror/Mosby College Publishing, 1985.

physical activity on a weekly basis and then determine the daily average exercise time. For instance, a person cycling at thirteen miles per hour, five times per week, for thirty minutes each time, exercises a total 150 minutes per week (5 × 30). The average daily exercise time would be twenty-one minutes (150 ÷ 7, rounded off to the lowest unit).

Next, using Table 6.4, determine the energy requirement for the activity (or activities) chosen for the exercise program. In the case of cycling (thirteen miles per hour), the requirement is .071 calories per pound of body weight per minute of activity (cal/lb/min). A man with a body weight of 160 pounds, would burn 11.4 calories each minute (body weight × .071 or 160 × .071). In twenty-one minutes, he would burn approximately 240 calories (21 × 11.4).

The third step is to determine the estimated total caloric requirement, with exercise, needed to maintain body weight. This value is obtained by adding the typical daily requirement (without exercise) and the average calories burned through exercise. In our example, it would be 2,640 calories (2,400 + 240).

If a negative caloric balance is recommended to lose weight, this person would have to consume less than 2,640 daily calories to achieve the objective. Because of the many different factors that play a role in weight control, the previous value is only an estimated daily requirement. Furthermore, to lose weight, it would be difficult to say that exactly one pound of fat would be lost in one week if daily intake were reduced by 500 calories (500 × 7 = 3,500 calories, or the equivalent of one pound of fat). Nevertheless, the estimated daily caloric figure provides a target guideline for weight control. Periodic readjustments are necessary because there can be significant differences among individuals, and the estimated daily requirement will change as you lose weight and modify your exercise habits.

The recommended number of calories to be subtracted from the daily intake to obtain a negative caloric balance depends on the typical daily requirement. At this point, the best recommendation is to moderately decrease the daily intake, never below 1,200 calories for women and 1,500 for men. A good rule to follow is to restrict the intake by no more than 500 calories if the daily requirement is below 3,000 calories. For caloric requirements in excess of 3,000, as many as 1,000 calories per day may be subtracted from the total intake. Remember also that the daily distribution should be approximately 60 percent carbohydrates (mostly complex carbohydrates), less than 30 percent fat, and about 15 percent protein.

The time of day when food is consumed may also play a role in weight reduction. A study conducted at the Aerobics Research Center in Dallas, Texas, indicated that when on a diet, weight is lost most effectively if the majority of the calories is consumed before 1:00 p.m. and not during the evening meal. This center recommends that when a person is attempting to lose weight, a minimum of 25 percent of the total daily calories should be consumed for breakfast, 50 percent for lunch, and 25 percent or less at dinner.

Other experts have indicated that if most of your daily calories are consumed during one meal, the body may perceive that something is wrong and will slow down your metabolism so that it can store a greater amount of calories in the form of fat. Also, eating most of the calories in one meal causes you to go hungry the rest of the day, making it more difficult to adhere to the diet.

The principle of consuming most of the calories earlier in the day seems to be helpful not only in losing weight but also in the management of atherosclerosis. According to research, the time of the day when most of the fats and cholesterol are consumed can have an impact on blood lipids and coronary heart disease. Peak digestion time following a heavy meal takes place about seven hours after that meal. If most lipids are consumed during the evening meal, digestion peaks while the person is sound asleep, at a time when the metabolism is at its lowest rate. Consequently, the body may not be able to metabolize fats and cholesterol as effectively, leading to higher blood lipids and increasing the risk for atherosclerosis and coronary heart disease.

To monitor daily progress, you may use a form similar to Figure 6.7. Meeting the basic requirements from each food group should be given top priority. The caloric content for each food is found in the Nutritive Value of Selected Foods list in Appendix B. The information should be recorded immediately after each meal to obtain the most precise record. According to the person's progress, adjustments can be made in the typical daily requirement or the exercise program, or both.

TIPS TO HELP CHANGE BEHAVIOR AND ADHERE TO A LIFETIME WEIGHT MANAGEMENT PROGRAM

Achieving and maintaining ideal body composition is by no means an impossible task, but it does require desire and commitment. If adequate weight management is to become a priority in life, people must realize that some retraining of behavior is crucial for success. Modifying old habits and developing new positive behaviors take time. The following list of management techniques has been successfully used by individuals to change detrimental behavior and adhere to a positive lifetime weight control program. People are not expected to use all of these strategies, but they should note those that apply and that will help them in developing a retraining program.

1. *Make a commitment to change.* The first ingredient to modify behavior is the desire to do so. The reasons for change must be more important than those for carrying on with present lifestyle patterns. People must accept the fact that there is a problem and decide by themselves whether they really want to change. If a sincere commitment is there, the chances for success are already enhanced.

2. *Set realistic goals.* Most people with a weight problem would like to lose weight in a relatively short time, but they fail to take into consideration the reality that the weight problem developed over a span of several years. A sound weight reduction and maintenance program can be accomplished only by establishing new lifetime eating and exercise habits, both of which take time to develop.

   In setting a realistic long-term goal, short-term objectives should also be planned. The long-term goal may be a decrease in body fat to 20 percent of total body weight. The short-term objective may be a one percent decrease in body fat each month. Such objectives allow for regular evaluation and help maintain motivation and renewed commitment to achieve the long-term goal.

3. *Incorporate exercise into the program.* Selecting enjoyable activities, places, times, equipment, and people to work with enhances adherence to exercise. Details on developing a complete exercise program are found in Chapters 2 (cardiovascular), 3 (strength), and 4 (flexibility).

4. *Develop healthy eating patterns.* Eating three regular meals per day consistent with the body's nutritional requirements is best. People should also learn to differentiate between hunger and appetite. Hunger is the actual physical need for food. Appetite is a desire for food, usually triggered by factors such as stress, habit, boredom, depression, food availability, or just the thought of food itself. Eating only when there is a physical need is wise weight management. In this regard, developing and sticking to a regular meal pattern helps control hunger.

5. *Avoid automatic eating.* Many people associate certain daily activities with eating. For example, people eat while cooking, watching television, reading, talking on the telephone, or visiting with neighbors. Most of the time, the foods consumed in such situations lack nutritional value or are high in sugar and fat.

6. *Stay busy.* People tend to eat more when they sit around and do nothing. Keeping the mind and body occupied with activities not associated with eating helps decrease the desire to eat. Some suggestions are walking, cycling, playing sports, gardening, sewing, or visiting a library, a museum, or a park. People should develop other skills and interests or try something new and exciting to break the routine of life.

7. *Plan your meals ahead of time.* Wise shopping is required to accomplish this objective (by the way, shopping should be done on a full stomach, because this will decrease impulsive buying of unhealthy foods — and then snacking on the way home). Whole-grain breads and cereals, fruits and vegetables, low-fat milk and dairy products, lean meats, fish, and poultry should be included.

8. *Cook wisely.* The use of fat and refined foods should be decreased in food preparation.
   a. Trim all visible fat off meats, remove skin off poultry prior to cooking.
   b. Skim the fat off gravies and soups.
   c. Bake, broil, and boil instead of frying.
   d. Use butter, cream, mayonnaise, and salad dressings sparingly.

e. Avoid shellfish, coconut oil, palm oil, and cocoa butter.

f. Prepare plenty of bulky foods.

g. Add whole-grain breads and cereals, vegetables, and legumes to most meals.

h. Try fruits for dessert.

i. Beware of soda pop, fruit juices, and fruit-flavored drinks.

j. Drink plenty of water — at least six glasses a day.

9. *Do not serve more food than can or should be eaten.* If the food portions are measured and serving dishes are kept away from the table, less food is consumed, seconds are more difficult to obtain, and appetite is decreased because food is not visible. People (including children) should not be forced to eat when they are satisfied and have had a healthy, nutritious serving.

10. *Learn to eat slowly and at the table only.* Eating is one of the pleasures of life, and we should take time to enjoy it. Eating on the run is detrimental because the body is not given sufficient time to "register" nutritive and caloric consumption, and overeating usually occurs before the fullness signal is perceived. Always eating at the table also forces people to take time out to eat and decreases snacking between meals, primarily because of the extra time and effort required to sit down and eat. When done eating, people should not sit around the table but, rather, clean up and put the food away to avoid unnecessary snacking.

11. *Avoid social binges.* Social gatherings are a common environment for self-defeating behavior. People should not feel pressured to eat or drink — or rationalize — in these situations; instead, low-calorie foods should be chosen, and people should entertain themselves with other activities such as dancing and talking.

12. *Beware of raids on the refrigerator and the cookie jar.* When these "raids" occur, the person should attempt to take control of the situation, stop and think about what is taking place. For those who have difficulty in avoiding such raids, environmental management is recommended. High-calorie, high-sugar, and high-fat foods should not be brought into the house. If they are, they ought to be stored in places where they are difficult to get to or are less visible. If they are unseen or not readily available, there will be less temptation. Keeping them in places such as the garage and basement may be sufficient to discourage many people from taking the time and effort to get them. By no means should treats be completely eliminated, but all things should be done in moderation.

13. *Practice adequate stress management techniques.* Many people snack and increase food consumption when confronted with stressful situations. Eating is not a stress-releasing activity and can in reality aggravate the problem if weight control is an issue. Several stress management techniques are discussed in Chapter 9.

14. *Monitor changes and reward accomplishments.* Feedback on fat loss, lean tissue gain, and weight loss is a reward in itself. Awareness of changes in body composition also helps reinforce new behaviors. Furthermore, being able to exercise uninterruptedly for fifteen, twenty, thirty, sixty minutes, or swimming a certain distance or running a mile is an accomplishment that deserves recognition. When certain objectives are met, rewards that are not related to eating are encouraged. Buying new clothing, a tennis racquet, a bicycle, exercise shoes, or something else that is special and would have not been acquired otherwise, is encouraged.

15. *Think positive.* Negative thoughts about how difficult it might be to change past behaviors should be avoided, replaced by thoughts of the benefits that will be reaped, such as feeling, looking, and functioning better, plus enjoying better health and improving the quality of life. Negative environments and people who will not be supportive likewise should be avoided. Those who do not have the same desires or encourage self-defeating behaviors should be avoided.

CONCLUSION

There is no simple and quick way to take off excessive body fat and keep it off for good. Weight management is accomplished through a lifetime commitment to physical activity and adequate food selection. When engaged in a weight (fat) reduction program, people may also have to moderately decrease caloric intake and implement appropriate strategies to modify unhealthy eating behaviors.

During the process of behavior modification, it is almost inevitable to relapse and engage in past negative behaviors. Making mistakes is human and does not necessarily mean failure. Failure comes to those who give up and do not use previous experiences to build upon and, in turn, develop appropriate skills that will prevent self-defeating behaviors in the future. "If there is a will, there is a way," and those who persist will reap the rewards.

Bibliography

Adams, T. D., et al. *Fitness for Life*. Salt Lake City: Intermountain Health Care, 1983.

Bennett, W., and J. Gurin. "Do Diets Really Work?" *Science* 42-50, March 1982.

"Brown Fat is Good Fat." *Health Letter*. December 11, 1981.

"Brown Fat/White Fat." *Aviation Medical Bulletin*. June 1981.

Christian, J. L., and J. L. Greger. *Nutrition for Living*. Menlo Park, CA: Benjamin/Cummings Publishing, 1988.

Cumming, C., and V. Newman. *Eater's Guide: Nutrition Basis for Busy People*. Englewood Cliffs, NJ: Prentice-Hall, 1981.

"Dangerous Dieting." *Health Letter*. July 25, 1980.

Fitness Monitoring Preventive Medicine Clinic. *Interpreting Your Nutritional Analysis*. Lake Geneva, WI: Clinic. 1984.

Girdano, D. A., D. Dusek, and G. S. Everly. *Experiencing Health*. Englewood Cliffs, NJ: Prentice-Hall, 1985.

Hafen, B. Q., A. L. Thygerson, and K. J. Frandsen. *Behavioral Guidelines for Health & Wellness*. Englewood, CO: Morton Publishing, 1988.

Hoeger, W. W. K. *The Complete Guide for the Development & Implementation of Health Promotion Programs*. Englewood, CO: Morton Publishing, 1987.

"How to Balance Your Diet." *Fit* 46-47, April 1983.

Kirschmann, J. D. *Nutrition Almanac*. New York: McGraw-Hill, 1984.

McArdle, W. D., F. I. Katch, and V. L. Katch. *Exercise Physiology: Energy, Nutrition and Human Performance*. Philadelphia: Lea & Febiger, 1986.

Morgan, B. L. G. *The Lifelong Nutrition Guide*. Englewood Cliffs, NJ: Prentice-Hall, 1983.

Remington, D., A. G. Fisher, and E. A. Parent. *How to Lower Your Fat Thermostat*. Provo, UT: Vitality House International, 1983.

"The Fallacies of Taking Supplementation." *Tufts University Diet & Nutrition Letter*. July 1987.

"Use a Variety of Fibers." *Health Letter*. March 1982.

"Vitamin Information for Patients." *Medical Times* 35, November 1982.

Whitney, E. N., and E. V. N. Hamilton. *Understanding Nutrition*. St. Paul: West Publishing, 1987.

Wolf, M. D. "The Battle Against Body Fat." *Fitness Management* 3(3):48-49, 1987.

Figure 6.9. *Computerized nutritional analysis. Sample food list* *

NUTRITIONAL ANALYSIS
based on Appendix B of the textbook
LIFETIME PHYSICAL FITNESS & WELLNESS: A PERSONALIZED PROGRAM
by Werner W. K. Hoeger
Morton Publishing Company, 1989

John Doe   Date: 02-15-1989
Age: 18
Body Weight: 184 lbs (83.5 kg)
Activity Rating: Sedentary

Food Intake Day One

Food	Amount	Calo-ries	Pro-tein gm	Fat gm	Sat Fat gm	Cho-les-terol mg	Car-bohy-drate gm	Cal-cium mg	Iron mg	Sodium mg	Vit A I.U.	Thi-amin mg	Ribo-fla-vin mg	Nia-cin mg	Vit C mg
Pancakes	2 (6 in. diam.)	338	10.4	10	2.0	72	50	148	1.8	620	180	0.24	0.32	1.8	0
Butter	1 tsp	36	0.0	4	0.4	12	0	1	0.0	46	160	0.00	0.00	0.0	0
Syrup(maple)	2 tbsp.	100	0.0	0	0.0	0	26	66	0.4	6	0	0.00	0.00	0.0	0
Milk whole	1 c	159	9.0	9	5.1	34	12	288	0.1	120	350	0.07	0.40	0.2	2
Bacon/cooked	2 slices	86	3.8	8	2.7	30	1	2	0.5	153	0	0.08	0.05	0.8	0
Bacon/lettuce/tomato sand.	1 sandwich	327	11.6	19	4.7	21	31	84	2.5	661	426	0.42	0.28	4.1	12
Cola	12 oz.	144	0.0	0	0.0	0	37	27	0.0	30	0	0.00	0.00	0.0	0
Pickles/dill	1 large	15	0.9	0	0.0	0	3	35	1.4	1,928	140	0.00	0.03	0.0	8
Potato/french fried	10 strips	214	3.4	10	1.7	0	28	12	1.0	5	0	0.10	0.06	2.4	16
Chocolate/M&M's plain	1.7 oz.	238	3.2	10	5.6	0	32	80	0.9	41	51	0.02	0.12	0.3	0
Lettuce/head	1 c sm. chunks	10	0.7	0	0.0	0	2	15	0.4	7	250	0.05	0.05	0.2	5
Tomatoes/raw	.5 med	10	0.5	0	0.0	0	2	6	0.3	2	410	0.03	0.02	0.3	11
Dressing/blue cheese	2 tbsp.	154	1.4	16	3.8	8	2	24	0.0	16	64	0.00	0.04	0.0	0
Spaghetti/sauce/cheese	2 c	520	17.6	18	4.0	20	74	160	4.6	1,910	2,160	0.50	0.36	4.6	26
Milk skim	1 c	88	9.0	0	0.3	5	12	296	0.1	126	10	0.09	0.44	0.2	2
Apple pie	1 pc. (3.5 in.)	302	2.6	13	3.5	120	45	9	0.4	355	40	0.02	0.02	0.5	1
Ice Cream/vanilla	.5 c	135	3.0	7	4.4	27	14	97	0.1	42	295	0.03	0.14	0.1	1
Totals Day One		2,876	77.1	124	38.2	349	371	1,350	14.4	6,067	4,536	1.6	2.3	15.5	84

*Software available through Morton Publishing Company.

Figure 6.10. *Computerized nutritional analysis. Sample daily analysis, average, and recommended dietary allowance comparison* *

NUTRITIONAL ANALYSIS: DAILY ANALYSIS, AVERAGE, AND
RECOMMENDED DIETARY ALLOWANCE (RDA) COMPARISON

	Calo- ries	Pro- tein gm	Fat %	Sat Fat %	Cho- les- terol mg	Car- bohy- drate %	Cal- cium mg	Iron mg	Sodium mg	Vit A I.U.	Thi- amin mg	Ribo- fla- vin mg	Nia- cin mg	Vit C mg
Day One	2,876	77.1	38	12	349	51	1,350	14.4	6,067	4,536	1.6	2.3	15.5	84
Day Two	2,480	60.6	30	12	480	60	1,076	10.1	2,747	5,938	1.0	1.8	15.3	42
Day Three	3,432	91.1	39	14	499	51	1,533	16.6	4,619	1,843	1.4	1.9	17.5	22
Three Day Average	2,929	76.3	36	13	443	53	1,320	13.7	4,477	4,106	1.4	2.0	16.1	49
RDA	2,392*	66.8	<30	<10	<300	50>	1,200	18.0	2,392	5,000	1.4	1.7	18.0	60

*Estimated caloric value based on gender, current body weight, and activity rating (does not include additional calories burned through a physical exercise program).

OBSERVATIONS

Daily caloric intake should be distributed in such a way that 50 to 60 percent of the total calories come from carbohydrates and less than 30 percent of the total calories from fat. Protein intake should be about .8 to 1.5 grams per kilogram of body weight or about 15 to 20 percent of the total calories. Pregnant women need to consume an additional 30 grams of daily protein, while lactating women should have an extra 20 grams of daily protein, or about 25 and 22 percent of total calories, respectively (these additional grams of protein are already included in the RDA values for pregnant and lactating women). Saturated fats should constitute less than 10 percent of the total daily caloric intake.

Please note that the daily listings of food intake express the amount of carbohydrates, fat, saturated fat, and protein in grams. However, on the daily analysis and the RDA, only the amount of protein is given in grams. The amount of carbohydrates, fat, and saturated fat are expressed in percent of total calories. The final percentages are based on the total grams and total calories for all days analyzed, not from the average of the daily percentages.

If your average intake for protein, fat, saturated fat, cholesterol, or sodium is high, refer to the daily listings and decrease the intake of foods that are high in those nutrients. If your diet is deficient in carbohydrates, calcium, iron, vitamin A, thiamin, riboflavin, niacin, or vitamin C, refer to the statements below and increase your intake of the indicated foods, or consult Appendix B in the textbook Lifetime Physical Fitness & Wellness: A Personalized Program.

Caloric intake may be too high.

Total fat intake is too high.

Saturated fat intake is too high, which increases your risk for coronary heart disease.

Dietary cholesterol intake is too high. An average consumption of dietary cholesterol above 300 mg/day increases the risk for coronary heart disease. Do you know your blood cholesterol level?

Iron intake is low. Iron containing foods include organ meats such as liver, lean meats, poultry, eggs, seafood, dried peas/beans, nuts, whole and enriched grains, and green leafy vegetables.

Sodium intake is high.

Vitamin A intake is low. Foods high in vitamin A include skim milk fortified with vit. A, cheese, butter, fortified margarine, eggs (yolk), liver, and dark green/yellow fruits and vegetables.

Niacin intake is low. Good sources of niacin include liver and organ meats, meats, fish, poultry, whole grains, enriched breads, dried beans and peas, nuts, and green leafy vegetables.

Vitamin C (ascorbic acid) intake is low. Fruits and vegetables in general (such as citrus fruits, tomatoes, cabbage, broccoli) are high in vitamin C.

*Software available through Morton Publishing Company.

Cardiovascular Disease Risk Reduction

Cardiovascular disease is the leading cause of death in the United States, accounting for nearly one-half of the total mortality rate in 1988. The disease refers to any pathological condition that affects the heart and the circulatory system (blood vessels). Some examples of cardiovascular diseases are coronary heart disease, peripheral vascular disease, congenital heart disease, rheumatic heart disease, atherosclerosis, strokes, high blood pressure, and congestive heart failure.

Although heart and blood vessel disease is still the number one health problem in the country, the incidence has declined by 36 percent in the last twenty years. The primary cause for this dramatic decrease has been health education. More people are now aware of the risk factors for cardiovascular disease and are making significant changes in their lifestyles to lower their own potential risk of suffering from this disease.

The major form of cardiovascular disease is coronary heart disease (CHD), a condition in which the arteries that supply the heart muscle with oxygen and nutrients are narrowed by fatty deposits such as cholesterol and triglycerides. The heart and its coronary vessels are depicted in Figure 7.1. Narrowing of the coronary arteries diminishes the blood supply to the heart muscle, which eventually can lead to a heart attack. CHD is the single leading cause of death in the United States, accounting for approximately one-third of all deaths, and more than half of all cardiovascular deaths. Oddly enough, almost all of the risk factors for CHD are preventable and reversible, and risk reduction can be accomplished by the individual.

CORONARY HEART DISEASE RISK PROFILE

Although genetic inheritance plays a role in the development of CHD, the most important determinant in whether an individual will suffer from this disease is the person's own personal lifestyle. In this regard, CHD risk factor analyses are administered to evaluate the impact of an individual's lifestyle and the genetic endowment as potential factors contributing to the development of coronary disease. The specific objectives of a CHD risk factor analysis are: (a) to screen individuals who may be at high risk for the disease, (b) to educate regarding the leading risk factors that lead to its development, (c) to implement programs aimed at risk reduction, and (d) to use the analysis as a starting point to ascertain changes induced by the intervention program.

The leading risk factors that contribute to the development of CHD have been identified. They are listed in Table 7.1. A self-assessment CHD risk factor analysis is given in Figure 7.2. This CHD risk factor analysis was constructed in such a way that it can be used by someone who has limited or no medical information concerning his/her state of cardiovascular health, as well as by a person who has had a thorough medical examination. Because the guidelines for zero risk are outlined for each factor, this self-assessment risk factor analysis can be used as a valuable tool in CHD risk factor management.

For example, a person who fills out the form would know that ideal blood pressure is around 120/80 or lower; that risk is reduced by smoking less or quitting altogether; and that total cholesterol/HDL-cholesterol ratio for men should be 4.5

Figure 7.1. *The heart and its coronary arteries.*

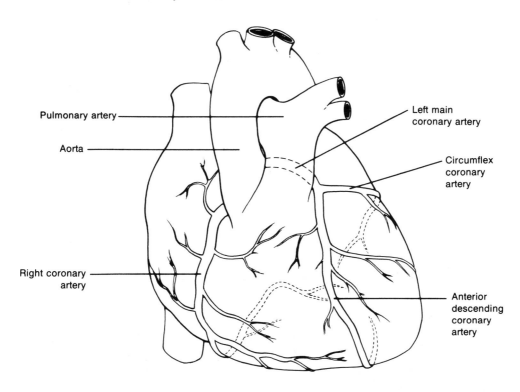

Table 7.1.
Maximal Number of Risk Points Assigned to the Various Coronary Heart Disease Risk Factors

Risk Factors	Maximal Risk Points
Total cholesterol/HDL-cholesterol ratio	10
Stress electrocardiogram	8
Smoking	8
Personal history of heart disease	8
Blood pressure	8
Cardiovascular endurance	6
Diabetes	6
Body composition (percent fat)	4
Family history of heart disease	4
Tension and stress	4
Age	4
Resting electrocardiogram	3
Triglycerides	2
Estrogen use	2

or lower (4.0 or lower for women), if unknown, basic nutritional guidelines are given; and so on (the role of HDL-cholesterol in heart disease protection is discussed later in this chapter).

To provide a meaningful CHD risk score, a weighing system was developed according to the impact that each risk factor has on the development of the disease.* This weighing system was developed based on current research available in this area, and according to the work done at leading preventive medicine facilities in the United States. The most significant risk factors are given the heaviest numeric weight.

For example, the total cholesterol/HDL-cholesterol ratio seems to be the best predictor for CHD development. Consequently, up to ten risk points are assigned to a "very high risk" ratio. On the other hand, the least heavily weighted risk factors are estrogen use and triglycerides; a

* The weighing system for the coronary heart disease risk factor analysis has been adapted with permission from: Hoeger, W. W. K. *The Complete Guide for the Development of Health Promotion Programs.* Englewood, CO: Morton Publishing, 1987.

Figure 7.2 *Self-assessment coronary heart disease risk factor analysis*

					Score
1. Cardiovascular Endurance (Max. VO_2 expressed in ml/kg/min)	**Men** 55+ 50-54 45-49 40-44 <39	**Women** 46+ 41-45 36-40 31-35 <30	. . . .	0 1.5 3 4.5 6	☐

2. Resting and Stress Electrocardiograms (ECG)	Add scores for both ECGs **ECG** Normal Equivocal Abnormal	**Resting** (0) (1) (3)	**Stress** (0) (4) (8)	0 1-5 3-11	☐

3. Total Cholesterol/HDL-Cholesterol Ratio (If unknown, answer question 5)	**Men** <4.5 4.6-5.5 5.6-6.5 6.6-7.7 7.8>	**Women** <4.0 4.1-5.0 51.-6.0 6.1-7.2 7.3>	. . . .	0 3 5 7 10	☐

4. Triglycerides (If unknown, answer question 5)	<100 101-145 146-190 191-235 236>	. . . .	0 0.5 1 1.5 2	☐

5. Diet (Do not answer if questions 3 and 4 have been answered)	Does your regular diet include (high score if all apply): One or more daily servings of red meat; 7 or more eggs/week; daily butter, cheese, whole milk, sweets, and alcohol	8-12	
	Four to six servings of red meat/week, 4-6 eggs per week, margarine, 1 or 2% milk, some cheese, sweets, and alcohol	3-7	
	Fish (no hard shell), poultry, red meat less than three times/week, less than 3 eggs/week, skim milk and skim milk products, moderate sweets and alcohol	0	☐

6. Diabetes/Glucose	<120 121-128 129-136 137-144 145-149 150> Diabetics add another 3 points	. . . .	0 1 1.5 2 2.5 3 3	☐

7. Blood Pressure	Score applies to each reading (e.g. 144/88 score = 4) **Systolic** <120 (0) 121-130 (1) 131-140 (2) 141-150 (3) 151> (4)	**Diastolic** <80 (0) 81- 90 (1) 91- 98 (2) 99-106 (3) 107> (3)	. . . .	0 1-2 2-4 3-6 4-8	☐

8. Body Composition (Percent Fat)	**Men** <12% 12-17% 18-22% 23-27% 28%>	**Women** <17% 18-22% 23-27% 28-32% 33%>	. . . .	0 1 2 3 4	☐

Subtotal Risk Score: ☐

Figure 7.2 *Self-assessment coronary heart disease risk factor analysis (continued)*

Subtotal Risk Score (from previous page): ☐

9. Smoking	Lifetime nonsmoker	0
	Ex-smoker over one year	0
	Ex-smoker less than one year	1
	Smoke less than 1 cigarette/day	1
	Nonsmoker, but live or work in smoking environment	2
	Pipe, cigar smoker, or chew tobacco	2
	Smoke 1-9 cigarettes/day	3
	Smoke 10-19 cigarettes/day	4
	Smoke 20-29 cigarettes/day	5
	Smoke 30-39 cigarettes/day	6
	Smoke 40 or more cigarettes/day	8 ☐

10. Tension and Stress	Are you:	
	Hardly ever tense	0
	Sometimes tense	1
	Often tense	2
	Nearly always tense	3
	Always tense	4 ☐

11. Personal History	Have you ever had a heart attack, stroke, coronary disease, or any known heart problem:	
	During the last year	8
	1-2 years ago	5
	2-5 years ago	3
	More than 5 years ago	2
	Never suffered from heart disease	0 ☐

12. Family History	Have any of your blood relatives (parents, uncles, brothers, sisters, grandparents) suffered from cardiovascular disease (heart attack, strokes, bypass surgery):	
	One or more before age 50	4
	One or more between 51 and 60	2
	One or more after age 60	1
	None have suffered from cardiovascular disease	0 ☐

13. Age	29 or younger	1
	30-39	1
	40-49	2
	50-59	3
	60>	4 ☐

14. Estrogen Use (Birth control pills and certain hormone drugs)	Are you:	
	35 or older and using estrogen	2
	Any age and used estrogen for over 5 years	2
	35 and younger and used estrogen for less than 5 years	1
	Do not use estrogen	0 ☐

Total Risk Score: ☐

Risk Categories

Very low	5 or less points
Low	Between 6 and 15 points
Moderate	Between 16 and 25 points
High	Between 26 and 35 points
Very High	36 or more points

maximum of two risk points is assigned to these two factors.

Each risk factor also is given a zero risk level, or the level at which a particular factor does not increase the risk for disease. Based on the actual test results, a person receives a score anywhere from zero to the maximum number of points for each factor. When the risk points obtained from all of the risk factors are totaled, the final number is used to rate an individual in one of five overall risk categories for potential development of coronary heart disease.

A "very low" CHD risk category is used to indicate the lowest risk group for developing heart disease based on age and gender. The "low" CHD risk category indicates that a person is taking good care of his/her cardiovascular health but that small improvements can be made (unless all of the risk points come from age and family history). "Moderate" CHD risk calls for definite improvements in lifestyle to decrease the risk for disease, and possible medical treatment. A final score in the "high" or "very high" CHD risk category indicates a very strong probability of developing heart disease within the next three to five years. It requires immediate implementation of a personal risk reduction program, including medical, nutritional, and exercise intervention prescribed by professional staff.

An important concept in CHD risk management is that, with the exception of age, family history of heart disease, and certain ECG abnormalities, all of the other risk factors are preventable and reversible. To aid in the implementation of a lifetime risk reduction program, the leading risk factors for coronary heart disease will now be discussed, along with the general recommendations for risk reduction.

CARDIOVASCULAR ENDURANCE

Cardiovascular endurance has been defined as the ability of the heart, lungs, and blood vessels to deliver adequate amounts of oxygen to the cells to meet the demands of prolonged physical activity. The level of cardiovascular endurance (or fitness) is most commonly given by the maximal amount of oxygen (in milliliters) that every kilogram (2.2 pounds) of body weight is able to

utilize per minute of physical activity (ml/kg/ min). As maximal oxygen uptake increases, so does the efficiency of the cardiovascular system.

Even though cardiovascular endurance is not the most significant factor in terms of the maximal number of risk points assigned (6 points for a poor level of fitness, as compared to 10 for a very high total cholesterol/HDL-cholesterol ratio; see Table 7.1), improving cardiovascular endurance through aerobic exercise has perhaps the greatest impact in overall heart disease risk reduction.

Although specific recommendations can be followed to improve each individual risk factor, engaging in a regular aerobic exercise program has shown to control most of the major risk factors that lead to heart disease. Aerobic exercise will help: (a) increase cardiovascular endurance, (b) decrease and control blood pressure, (c) decrease body fat, (d) decrease blood lipids (cholesterol and triglycerides), (e) improve HDL-cholesterol, (f) help control diabetes, (g) increase and maintain good heart function and improve in many cases certain ECG abnormalities, (h) motivate toward smoking cessation, (i) decrease tension and stress, and (j) prevent a personal history of heart disease. In the words of Dr. Kenneth H. Cooper, pioneer of the aerobic movement in the United States, the evidence of the benefits of aerobic exercise in the reduction of heart disease is "far too impressive to be ignored."

Caution should be taken, however, not to ignore the other risk factors. Although aerobically fit individuals have a lower incidence of cardiovascular disease, a regular aerobic exercise program by itself is not an absolute guarantee for a lifetime free of cardiovascular problems. Poor lifestyle habits such as smoking, eating excessive fatty/salty/sweet foods, excess body fat, and high levels of stress increase cardiovascular risk and will not always be completely eliminated through aerobic exercise. Overall risk factor management is the best guideline to minimize the risk for cardiovascular disease. Yet, aerobic exercise, if carried out properly, is one of the most important aspects in the prevention and reduction of cardiovascular problems. The basic principles for cardiovascular exercise prescription were given in Chapter 2.

BLOOD PRESSURE (HYPERTENSION)

There are some 60,000 miles of blood vessels running through the human body. As the heart forces the blood through these vessels, the fluid is under pressure. Hence, blood pressure is but a measure of the force exerted against the walls of the vessels by the blood flowing through them. Blood pressure is measured in milliliters of mercury and is usually expressed in two numbers. Ideal blood pressure should be 120/80 or below. The higher number reflects the pressure exerted during the forceful contraction of the heart or systole (therefore, the name "systolic" pressure), and the lower pressure is taken during the heart's relaxation, or diastolic phase, when no blood is being ejected. Figure 7.3 illustrates blood pressure assessment using a mercury gravity manometer.

The procedures for blood pressure assessment are outlined in Appendix D. If blood pressure equipment is available, you should take the opportunity to assess your blood pressure in the near future.

When Is Blood Pressure Considered Too High?

A few years ago, a systolic pressure of 100 plus your age was the acceptable standard. This is no longer the case. Hypertension has been viewed as the point at which the pressure doubles the mortality risk. This pressure has been determined to be about 160/96. Traditionally, the upper limits of normal were established at 140/90, a reading that by today's standards is considered by many as borderline hypertension. Readings between 140/90 and 160/96 (either number being in that range) were classified as mild hypertension. Statistical evidence, however, clearly indicates that blood pressure readings above 140/90 increase the risk of disease and premature death. Consequently, in 1986 the American Heart Association revised its standards and now considers all blood pressures over 140/90 as hypertension.

Although the threshold for hypertension has been set at 140/90, many experts believe that the lower the blood pressure, the better. Even if the pressure is around 90/50, as long as that person does not have any symptoms of low blood

pressure or hypotension, he/she does not need to be concerned. Typical hypotension symptoms are dizziness, lightheadedness, and fainting.

Blood pressure may also fluctuate during a regular day. Many factors affect blood pressure, and one single reading may not be a true indicator of your real pressure. For example, physical activity and stress increase blood pressure, while rest and relaxation decrease it. Consequently, several measurements should be made before a diagnosis of elevated pressure is suggested.

Based on 1988 estimates by the American Heart Association, almost 60 million adults in the United States are hypertensive. As a disease, hypertension has been referred to as the silent killer. It does not hurt; it does not make you feel sick; and unless you check it, years may go by before you even realize that you have a problem. Elevated blood pressure is a risk factor not only for coronary heart disease but also for congestive heart failure, strokes, and kidney failure.

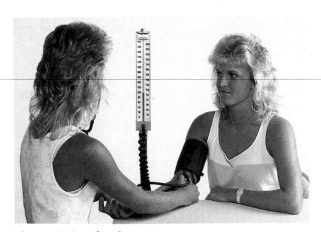

Figure 7.3. *Blood pressure assessment*

What Makes Hypertension A Killer?

All inner walls of arteries are lined by a layer of smooth endothelial cells. The nature of this lining is such that blood lipids cannot penetrate it and build up unless the cells are damaged. High blood pressure is thought to be a leading factor contributing to destruction of this lining. As blood pressure rises, so does the risk for atherosclerosis or the development of fatty-cholesterol deposits in the walls of the arteries. The higher the pressure, the greater is the damage to the arterial wall, allowing faster occlusion of the vessels, especially if serum cholesterol is also elevated. Occlusion of the coronary vessels decreases the blood supply to the heart muscle and can lead to heart attacks. When brain arteries are involved, strokes may follow.

A clear example of the role of elevated pressure in the development of atherosclerosis can be seen by comparing blood vessels in the human body. Even when significant atherosclerosis is present throughout major arteries in the body, fatty plaques are rarely seen in the pulmonary artery, which goes from the right heart to the lungs. The pressure in this artery is normally below 40 mmHg, and at such low pressure significant deposits do not occur. This is one of the reasons why people with low blood pressure have a lower incidence of cardiovascular disease.

Constantly elevated blood pressure also causes the heart to work much harder. Initially the heart does well, but in time this constant strain results in a pathologically enlarged heart and subsequent congestive heart failure. Furthermore, high blood pressure damages blood vessels to the kidneys and eyes, leading to eventual kidney failure and loss of vision.

How Can Hypertension Be Controlled?

Ninety percent of all hypertension has no definite cause. This type of hypertension, referred to as *essential hypertension,* is treatable. Aerobic exercise, weight reduction, a low-sodium/high-potassium diet, stress reduction, smoking cessation, a decrease in blood lipids, a lower caffeine and alcohol intake, and antihypertensive medication have all been used effectively in treating essential hypertension. The other 10 percent is caused by pathological conditions such as narrowing of the kidney arteries, glomerulonephritis (a kidney disease), tumors of the adrenal glands, and narrowing of the aortic artery. With this type of hypertension, the pathological cause has to be treated first in order to correct the blood pressure problem.

Antihypertensive medications are often the first choice of treatment modality, but they also produce multiple side effects, such as lethargy, somnolence, sexual difficulties, increased blood cholesterol and glucose levels, lower potassium levels, and elevated uric acid levels. Often, a physician may end up treating these side effects as much as the hypertension problem itself. Because of the multiple side effects, approximately 50 percent of the patients will stop taking the medication within the first year of treatment.

Perhaps one of the most significant factors contributing to elevated blood pressure is excessive sodium in the diet (salt is sodium chloride and contains approximately 40 percent sodium). Water retention increases with high sodium intake. As water retention increases, so does the blood volume, which, in turn, drives the pressure up. On the other hand, high intake of potassium seems to regulate water retention and therefore appears to lower the pressure slightly.

Although sodium is essential for normal physiological functions, only 200 mg, or one-tenth of a teaspoon of salt, is required on a daily basis. Even under the most strenuous conditions, such as jobs and sports participation where heavy sweating is involved, the greatest amount of sodium required by the organism seldom exceeds 3,000 mg per day. Yet, in the typical American diet, sodium intake ranges between 6,000 and 20,000 mg per day! No wonder hypertension is so prevalent today.

In underdeveloped countries and Indian tribes where no salt is used in cooking or added later, and the only sodium consumed comes from food in its natural form, daily intake seldom exceeds 2,000 mg. Blood pressure among these people does not increase with age, and hypertension is practically unknown. These findings seem to indicate that the human body may be able to handle 2,000 mg per day, but higher intakes than that on a regular basis may cause a gradual rise in blood pressure over the years.

Many people ask themselves: Where does all the sodium come from? The answer is found in Table 7.2. Most individuals do not realize the amount of sodium contained in various foods, and the list in Table 7.2 does not even include the salt added at the table. Although you may not have a blood pressure problem now, you need to be concerned about sodium intake. Otherwise blood pressure may sneak up on you.

New research studies have also indicated that there may be a link between hypertension and calcium and magnesium deficiencies. The connection between calcium and hypertension isn't quite clear, but national dietary surveys have

Table 7.2.
Sodium, Potassium, Calcium, and Magnesium Levels of Selected Foods

Food	Serving Size	Sodium (mg)	Potassium (mg)	Calcium (mg)	Magnesium (mg)
Apple	1 med.	1	182	10	6
Asparagus	1 cup	2	330	26	24
Avocado	1/2	4	680	11	39
Banana	1 med.	1	440	8	33
Bologna	3 oz.	1,107	133	6	12
Bouillon Cube	1	960	4	0	0
Cantaloupe	1/4	17	341	20	22
Carrot (raw)	1	34	225	27	12
Cheese					
American	2 oz.	614	93	376	16
Cheddar	2 oz.	342	56	408	16
Muenster	2 oz.	356	77	406	16
Parmesan	2 oz.	1,056	53	672	24
Swiss	2 oz.	148	64	410	16
Chicken (light meat)	6 oz.	108	700	20	20
Corn (canned)	1/2 cup	195	80	4	15
Corn (natural)	1/2 cup	3	136	2	29
Frankfurter	1	627	136	4	5
Haddock	6 oz.	300	594	66	41
Hamburger (reg)	1	500	321	63	25
Lamb (leg)	6 oz.	108	700	18	22
Milk (whole)	1 cup	120	351	288	33
Milk (skim)	1 cup	126	406	296	28
Orange	1 med.	1	263	54	13
Orange Juice	1 cup	1	200	26	27
Peach	1 med.	2	308	14	9
Pear	1 med.	2	130	13	9
Peas (canned)	1/2 cup	200	82	22	20
Peas (boiled-natural)	1/2 cup	2	178	18	24
Pizza (cheese - 14" diam.)	1/8	456	85	110	25
Potato	1 med.	6	763	14	75
Potato Chips	10	150	226	8	25
Potato (french fries)	10	5	427	12	40
Pork	6 oz.	96	438	17	25
Roast Beef	6 oz.	98	448	15	27
Salami	3 oz.	1,047	170	12	5
Salmon (canned)	6 oz.	198	756	262	50
Salt	1 tsp.	2,132	0	14	7
Soups					
Chicken Noodle	1 cup	979	55	17	5
Clam Chowder					
(New England)	1 cup	914	146	43	7
Cream of Mushroom	1 cup	955	98	191	5
Vegetable Beef	1 cup	1,046	162	12	6
Soy Sauce	1 tsp.	1,123	22	13	2
Spaghetti (tomato sauce and cheese)	6 oz.	648	276	54	20
Strawberries	1 cup	1	244	31	16
Tomato (raw)	1 med.	3	444	12	11
Tuna (drained)	3 oz.	38	255	7	0

linked calcium deficiency to high blood pressure. Magnesium supplementation has been used effectively to lower blood pressure in patients suffering from hypertensive encephalopathy and in patients affected by diuretic-induced low magnesium levels. But no evidence at this point shows a decrease in blood pressure in patients with normal magnesium levels.

When treating high blood pressure, prior to using medication (unless elevation is extremely high), many sports medicine physicians prefer a combination of aerobic exercise, weight loss, and sodium reduction. In most instances this treatment modality will bring blood pressure under control.

The link between hypertension and obesity has been well-established. Not only does blood volume increase with excess body fat, but every additional pound of fat requires an estimated extra mile of blood vessels to feed this tissue. Furthermore, blood capillaries are constricted by the adipose tissue as these vessels run through them. As a result, the heart muscle must work harder to pump the blood through a longer, constricted network of blood vessels.

The role of aerobic exercise in the treatment of hypertensive patients is becoming more important each day. On the average, cardiovascularly fit individuals have lower blood pressures than unfit people. Several well-documented studies have shown that nearly 90 percent of hypertensive patients who initiate an aerobic exercise program can expect a significant decrease in blood pressure after only a few months of training. These changes, however, are not maintained if aerobic exercise is discontinued.

The best tip, though, is to use a preventive approach. It is a lot easier to keep blood pressure under control than try to bring it down once it is elevated. Blood pressure should be checked regularly, regardless of whether elevation is present. Regular physical exercise, weight control, a low-salt diet, smoking cessation, and stress management are the basic guidelines for blood pressure control. Those who suffer from hypertension should not stop using the medication unless their personal physician so indicates. Remember — high blood pressure kills people if not treated properly. Combining the medication with the other treatment modalities may eventually lead to a reduction or complete elimination of the drug therapy.

BODY COMPOSITION

As discussed in Chapter 5, body composition refers to the ratio of lean body weight to fat weight. If too much fat is accumulated, the person is considered to be obese. Obesity has been long recognized as a primary risk factor for coronary heart disease. Until a few years ago, experts believed that the disease was actually brought on by some of the other risk factors that usually deteriorate with increased body fat such as higher cholesterol and triglycerides, hypertension, diabetes, lower level of cardiovascular fitness). Recent evidence, however, suggests that excess body fat, in and of itself, is a serious coronary risk factor. Even when all of the other risk factors are in good range, individuals with body fat percentages higher than the "ideal" standard have a higher incidence of coronary disease.

Attaining ideal body composition is important not only in decreasing cardiovascular risk but also in achieving a better state of health and wellness. The only positive thing that can be said about excess body fat accumulation is that it can be lost through a combination of adequate nutrition and exercise. Dieting by itself very seldom works. If you have a weight problem and you desire to achieve ideal weight, three things must take place: (a) an increase in the level of physical activity; (b) a diet low in fat, alcohol, and sweets, and high in complex carbohydrates and fiber; and (c) a moderate reduction in total caloric intake that will still provide all of the necessary nutrients to sustain normal physiological body functions. Additional recommendations for weight reduction and weight control were discussed in Chapter 6.

TOTAL CHOLESTEROL/HDL-CHOLESTEROL RATIO

The term *blood lipids* (fats) is used mainly in reference to cholesterol and triglycerides. These lipids are carried in the bloodstream by molecules of protein known as high-density lipoproteins, low-density lipoproteins, very low-density lipoproteins, and chylomicrons. A significant elevation in blood lipids has long been associated with heart and blood vessel disease.

Cholesterol has received considerable attention in the last few years. This fatty or lipid substance is essential for certain metabolic functions in the body. But high levels of blood cholesterol contribute to the formation of the atherosclerotic plaque, or the buildup of fatty tissue in the walls of the arteries. In the case of the heart, as the plaque builds up, it obstructs the coronary vessels. Because these arteries supply the heart muscle (myocardium) with oxygen and nutrients, a myocardial infarction or heart attack will follow when obstruction occurs. Unfortunately, the heart disguises its problems quite effectively, and typical symptoms of heart disease, such as angina pectoris or chest pain, do not start until the arteries are about 75 percent occluded; in many cases, the first symptom is sudden death. Figure 7.4 illustrates the condition of the heart in a heart attack.

Only a few years ago the general recommendation was to keep total blood cholesterol levels below 200 mg/dl (milligrams per deciliter). For individuals age thirty and younger it is now recommended that the total cholesterol count should not exceed 180 mg/dl. Even though these guidelines should be followed, the crucial factor seems to be the way in which cholesterol is "packaged" or carried in the bloodstream rather than the total amount present.

Cholesterol is primarily transported in the form of high-density lipoprotein cholesterol (HDL-cholesterol) and low-density lipoprotein cholesterol (LDL-cholesterol). The high-density molecules have a high affinity for cholesterol and tend to attract cholesterol, which is then carried to the liver to be metabolized and excreted. They act as "scavengers," removing cholesterol from the body, and thus preventing plaque formation in the arteries. LDL-cholesterol, on the other hand, tends to release cholesterol, which may then penetrate the lining of the arteries, enhancing the process of atherosclerosis. Figures 7.5 and 7.6 depict the atherosclerotic process.

From the previous discussion, it can easily be seen that the more HDL-cholesterol present, the better. HDL-cholesterol, the so called "good cholesterol," offers a certain degree of protection against heart disease. Many authorities now believe that the ratio of total cholesterol to HDL-cholesterol is a better indicator of potential risk

Figure 7.4. *Heart attack (myocardial infarction): A result of acute reduction in the blood flow through a coronary vessel*

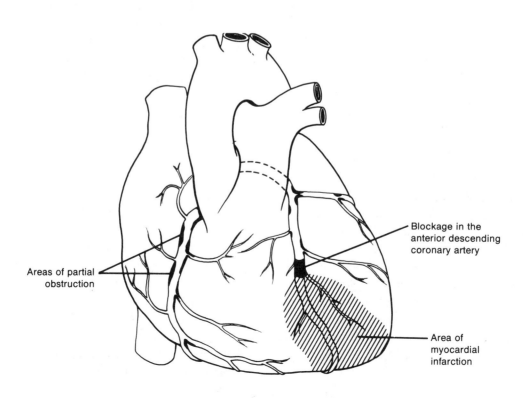

Areas of partial obstruction

Blockage in the anterior descending coronary artery

Area of myocardial infarction

for cardiovascular disease than is the total value by itself. It is generally accepted that a 4.5 or lower ratio (total cholesterol/HDL-cholesterol) is excellent for men, and 4.0 or lower is best for women.

For instance, 50 mg/dl of HDL-cholesterol as compared to 200 mg/dl of total cholesterol yields a ratio of 4.0 (200/50 = 4.0). The lower the ratio, the greater is the protection. In another instance, a person's total cholesterol could also be 200 mg/dl, but if the HDL-cholesterol is only 20 mg/dl, the ratio would be 10.0. Such a ratio is extremely dangerous and very conducive to atherosclerosis and coronary disease.

New evidence also indicates that low levels of HDL-cholesterol could be the best predictor of coronary heart disease, and seems to be more significant than the total value itself. Researchers at the 1988 annual American Heart Association meeting indicated that people with low total cholesterol (less than 200 mg/dl) and also low HDL-cholesterol (under 35 to 40 mg/dl) may have three times the heart disease risk of those with high cholesterol but with good HDL-cholesterol levels. Another researcher presented data on 797 patients whose total cholesterol was less than 200 mg/dl. Their work showed that 60 percent of the patients had heart disease, and almost 75 percent of this group had HDL-cholesterol levels below 40 mg/dl.

Although on the average a person absorbs about 225 mg of cholesterol daily, the body actually manufactures more cholesterol than is consumed in the diet. Approximately 700 mg of cholesterol per day are produced from saturated fats. These fats are found primarily in meats and dairy products but are seldom found in foods of plant origin. Poultry and fish also contain less saturated fat than beef. Unsaturated fats are mainly of plant origin and cannot be converted to cholesterol. There are individual differences as to how much cholesterol can be manufactured by the body. Some people can have higher-than-normal intakes of saturated fats and still maintain normal blood levels, while others with a lower intake can have abnormally high levels.

If the total cholesterol/HDL-cholesterol ratio is higher than ideal, certain guidelines should be followed to lower the ratio. Initially, total cholesterol levels should be lowered. This can be accomplished by lowering the LDL-cholesterol component. This type of cholesterol increases proportionally with the amount of saturated fat and cholesterol intake in the regular diet. Table 7.3 gives the cholesterol and saturated fat content of selected foods.

Total fat consumption on a daily basis should not exceed 30 percent of the total caloric intake, and less than half of the fat consumed should be in the form of saturated fat (about 10 percent of the total caloric intake). The average intake of cholesterol also should be limited to less than 300 mg per day. LDL-cholesterol can be further lowered by losing excess body fat and using medication.

As a general rule of thumb, the following dietary guidelines are recommended to lower LDL-cholesterol levels:

1. Limit egg consumption to less than three eggs per week.

2. Eat red meats fewer than three times per week, and avoid organ meats (e.g., liver and kidneys), sausage, bacon, hot dogs, and canned meats.

3. Consume low-fat milk (1 percent or less, preferably) and low-fat dairy products.

4. Avoid shellfish, coconut oil, palm oil, and cocoa butter.

5. Achieve ideal body weight.

The second factor involved in improving the ratio is to increase the HDL-cholesterol component. HDL-cholesterol is genetically determined, and women have higher values than men. This is probably one of the reasons why heart disease is less common among women. Research has indicated that increases in HDL-cholesterol values are almost completely dependent upon a regular aerobic exercise program. There is a clear relationship between HDL-cholesterol and aerobic exercise. The greater the amount of exercise, the higher the HDL-cholesterol. A cardiovascular exercise program, if properly prescribed, should yield positive results. A combination of adequate nutrition and aerobic exercise is the best prescription for achieving a "zero risk" ratio.

Several additional factors can lower the HDL-cholesterol levels. Beta-blocker type medications (used in treating heart disease and hypertension), tobacco usage, and birth control pills all have a negative effect on HDL-cholesterol levels. A combination of two or three of these is even worse.

Table 7.3.
Cholesterol and Saturated Fat Content of Selected Foods

Food	Serving Size	Cholesterol (mg)	Saturated Fat (gr)
Avocado	1/8 med.	—	3.2
Bacon	2 slc.	30	2.7
Beans (all types)	any	—	—
Beef — Lean, fat trimmed off	3 oz.	75	6.0
Beef — Heart (cooked)	3 oz.	150	1.6
Beef — Liver (cooked)	3 oz.	255	1.3
Butter	1 tsp.	12	0.4
Caviar	1 oz.	85	—
Cheese — American	2 oz.	54	11.2
Cheese — Cheddar	2 oz.	60	12.0
Cheese — Cottage (1% fat)	1 cup	10	0.4
Cheese — Cottage (4% fat)	1 cup	31	6.0
Cheese — Cream	2 oz.	62	6.0
Cheese — Muenster	2 oz.	54	10.8
Cheese — Parmesan	2 oz.	38	9.3
Cheese — Swiss	2 oz.	52	10.0
Chicken (no skin)	3 oz.	45	0.4
Chicken — Liver	3 oz.	472	1.1
Chicken — Thigh, Wing	3 oz.	69	3.3
Egg (yolk)	1	250	1.8
Frankfurter	2	90	11.2
Fruits	any	—	—
Grains (all types)	any	—	—
Halibut, Flounder	3 oz.	43	0.7
Ice Cream	1/2 cup	27	4.4
Lamb	3 oz.	60	7.2
Lard	1 tsp.	5	1.9
Lobster	3 oz.	170	0.5
Margarine (all vegetable)	1 tsp.	—	0.7
Mayonnaise	1 tbsp.	10	2.1
Milk — Skim	1 cup	5	0.3
Milk — Low Fat (2%)	1 cup	18	2.9
Milk — Whole	1 cup	34	5.1
Nuts	1 oz.	—	1.0
Oysters	3 oz.	42	—
Salmon	3 oz.	30	0.8
Scallops	3 oz.	29	—
Sherbet	1/2 cup	7	1.2
Shrimp	3 oz.	128	0.1
Trout	3 oz.	45	2.1
Tuna (canned — drained)	3 oz.	55	—
Turkey — Dark Meat	3 oz.	60	0.6
Turkey — Light Meat	3 oz.	50	0.4
Vegetables (except avocado)	any	—	—

Figure 7.5. *The atherosclerotic process*

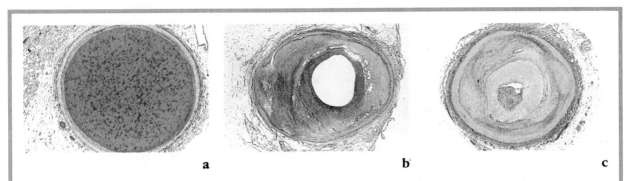

a   b   c

Cross-section of normal artery (a); lumen significantly narrowed by fibrous lesion (b); progression of lesion shown in (b), with almost complete obstruction of the artery (c).

From *The Atherosclerotic Process.* The American Heart Association. Reproduced by permission.

Figure 7.6. *Comparison of a normal healthy artery (a) and diseased arteries (b and c)*

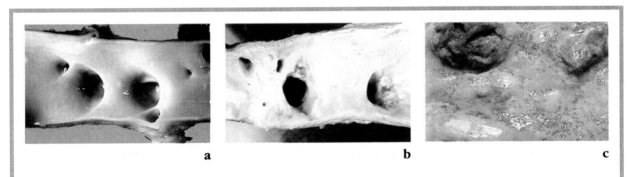

a   b   c

Illustrations a and b are reproduced by permission, *The Atherosclerotic Process,* American Heart Association. Illustration c reproduced by permission from "If You Smoke" slide show by Gordon Hewlett.

TRIGLYCERIDES

Triglycerides are also known as free fatty acids. In combination with cholesterol, they accelerate the formation of plaque. Triglycerides are carried in the bloodstream primarily by very low-density lipoproteins (VLDL) and chylomicrons. These fatty acids are found in poultry skin, lunch meats, and shellfish, but they are manufactured mainly in the liver from refined sugars, starches, and alcohol. High intake of alcohol and sugars (honey included) will significantly increase triglyceride levels. Thus, they can be lowered by decreasing the consumption of the above-mentioned foods, along with weight reduction (if overweight) and

aerobic exercise. An optimal blood triglyceride level is lower than 100 mg/dl.

Individuals who have never had a blood chemistry test should probably have one done in the near future. An initial test is always useful to establish a baseline for future reference. Make sure that the blood test does include the HDL-cholesterol component, because some clinics and hospitals still do not include this factor in their regular analyses. Although no definite guidelines have yet been given, as long as a person follows an initial normal baseline test and adheres to the recommended dietary and exercise guidelines, a blood analysis every three to five years prior to age thirty-five should suffice. After age thirty-five, a blood lipid test should be conducted every year in conjunction with a regular preventive medicine physical examination.

DIABETES

Diabetes is a condition in which the blood glucose is unable to enter the cells because of insufficient insulin production by the pancreas. Several studies have shown that the incidence of cardiovascular disease among diabetic patients is quite high. Cardiovascular disease is also the leading cause of death among these patients.

Individuals with chronically elevated blood glucose levels may also have problems in metabolizing fats. This, in turn, can increase susceptibility to atherosclerosis, increasing the risk for coronary disease and other conditions such as vision loss and kidney damage. Fasting blood glucose levels over 120 mg/dl may be an early sign of diabetes and should be brought to the attention of a physician. Many health care practitioners consider blood glucose levels around 150 to 160 mg/dl as borderline diabetes.

Although there is a genetic predisposition to diabetes, adult-onset diabetes is closely related to obesity. In most cases, this condition can be corrected by following a special diet, a weight loss program, and exercise. If you have elevated blood glucose levels, you should consult your physician and let him/her decide on the best approach to treat this condition.

RESTING AND STRESS ELECTROCARDIOGRAMS

The electrocardiogram, or ECG, can provide a valuable indication of the heart's function. It is a record of the electrical impulses that stimulate the heart to contract. In the actual reading of an ECG, five general areas are interpreted: heart rate, the heart's rhythm, the heart's axis, enlargement or hypertrophy of the heart, and myocardial infarction or heart attack.

On a standard twelve-lead ECG, ten electrodes are placed on the person's chest. From these ten electrodes, twelve "pictures" or leads of the electrical impulses are studied as they travel through the heart muscle (myocardium) from twelve different positions. By looking at the tracings of an ECG, abnormalities in the functioning of the heart can be identified. Based on the findings, the ECG may be interpreted as normal, equivocal, or abnormal. Because not all problems will be identified by an ECG, a normal tracing is not an absolute problem-free guarantee, nor does an abnormal tracing necessarily mean the presence of a serious condition.

ECGs are taken at rest, during stress of exercise, and during recovery. A stress ECG is also known as a *maximal exercise tolerance test* (see Figure 7.7). Similar to a high-speed road test on a car, a stress ECG reveals the heart's tolerance to high-intensity exercise. It is a much better test than a resting ECG to discover coronary heart disease. It is also used to determine cardiovascular fitness levels, to screen persons for preventive and cardiac rehabilitation programs, to detect abnormal blood pressure response during exercise, and to establish actual or functional maximal heart rate for exercise prescription purposes. The recovery ECG also becomes an important diagnostic tool in monitoring the return of the heart's activity to normal conditions. Figures 7.7 and 7.8 show normal and abnormal ECGs, respectively.

Although not every adult who wishes to start an exercise program needs a stress ECG, the following criteria can be used to determine when this type of test should be administered:

1. Adults forty-five years or older.
2. Individuals with a total cholesterol level above 200 mg/dl, or a total cholesterol/HDL-cholesterol ratio above 4.0 for women and 4.5 for men.
3. Individuals with a HDL-cholesterol level below 35 mg/dl.
4. Hypertensive and diabetic patients.
5. Cigarette smokers.
6. Individuals with a family history of coronary heart disease, syncope, or sudden death before age sixty.
7. All individuals with symptoms of chest discomfort, dysrhythmias, syncope, or chronotropic incompetence (a heart rate that increases slowly during exercise and never reaches maximum).

The predictive value of a stress ECG has been questioned at times, but at present it is the most practical, inexpensive, noninvasive procedure available in diagnosing latent coronary heart disease. The sensitivity of the test is increased as the

Figure 7.7. *Normal electrocardiogram. (P wave = atrial depolarization, QRS complex = ventricular depolarization, T wave = ventricular repolarization)*

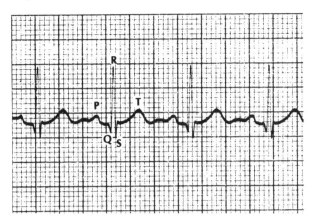

Figure 7.8. *Abnormal electrocardiogram showing a depressed S-T segment (commonly seen during exercise in patients with coronary disease)*

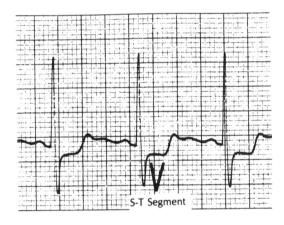

severity of the disease increases. Test protocols, number of leads, electrocardiographic criteria, and the competence of the technicians administering the test further increase its sensitivity. Therefore, it remains a highly useful tool in identifying those who are at high risk for exercise-related sudden death.

SMOKING

Cigarette smoking is the single largest preventable cause of illness and premature death in the United States. Smoking has been linked to cardiovascular (see Figure 7.9) disease, cancer, bronchitis, emphysema, and peptic ulcers. In relation to coronary disease, it speeds up the process of atherosclerosis and the risk of sudden death following a myocardial infarction increases threefold.

Smoking causes the release of nicotine and some 1,200 other toxic compounds into the bloodstream. Similar to hypertension, many of these substances are destructive to the inner membrane that protects the walls of the arteries. As mentioned before, once the lining is damaged, cholesterol and triglycerides can be readily deposited in the arterial wall. As the plaque builds up, blood flow significantly decreases as obstruction of the arteries occurs.

Furthermore, smoking enhances the formation of blood clots, which can completely obstruct an artery that already has been narrowed as a result of atherosclerosis. In addition, carbon monoxide, a byproduct of cigarette smoke, significantly decreases the oxygen-carrying capacity of the blood. A combination of obstructed arteries, decreased oxygen, and the presence of nicotine in the heart muscle greatly increases the risk for a serious heart problem.

Figure 7.9. *Comparison of normal and atherosclerotic arteries at the base of the brain*

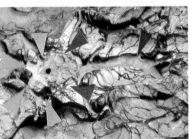
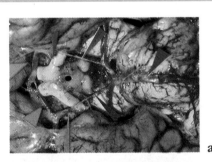

(a) A healthy artery. (b) Obstruction of the same artery by fatty substances in a chronic smoker.

Smoking also increases heart rate, blood pressure, and the irritability of the heart, which can trigger fatal cardiac arrhythmias. Another harmful effect is a decrease in HDL-cholesterol (the "good type" that helps control blood lipids). Without question, smoking actually causes a much greater risk of death from heart disease than from lung disease.

Pipe and cigar smoking and chewing tobacco also increase the risk for heart disease. Even if no smoke is inhaled, certain amounts of toxic substances can be absorbed through the mouth membranes and end up in the bloodstream. Individuals who use tobacco in any of these three forms also have a much greater risk for cancer of the oral cavity.

Cigarette smoking, a poor total cholesterol/HDL-cholesterol ratio, and high blood pressure are the three most significant risk factors for coronary disease. Nevertheless, the risk for both cardiovascular disease and cancer starts to decrease the moment you quit. The risk approaches that of a lifetime nonsmoker in ten and fifteen years, respectively, following cessation. A more thorough discussion of the harmful effects of cigarette smoking, the benefits of quitting, and a complete program for smoking cessation are outlined in Chapter 10.

TENSION AND STRESS

Tension and stress have become a normal part of every person's life. Everyone has to deal with goals, deadlines, responsibilities, and pressures in daily living. Almost everything in life (whether positive or negative) is a source of stress. It is not the stressor itself, however, that creates the health hazard; rather, it is the individual's response to it that may pose a health problem.

There are basically two types of behavior. *Type A behavior,* on the one hand, is typical of a person who is hard-driving, high-strung, overly competitive, and easily irritated. *Type B behavior,* on the other hand, is characteristic of a relaxed, easygoing, casual person who sometimes even appears apathetic toward life. A person exhibiting Type A behavior (high stress) is at higher risk for coronary disease than a Type B person. These individuals actually become ill because of their inability to deal with increasing amounts of stress.

The way in which the human body responds to stress is by increasing the amount of catecholamines (hormones) to prepare the body for the "fight or flight" mechanism. These hormones increase heart rate, blood pressure, and blood glucose levels, preparing the individual to take action. If the person "fights or flees," the increased levels of catecholamines are metabolized and the body is able to return to a "normal" state. But if a person is under constant stress and unable to take action (such as in the death of a close relative or friend, loss of a job, trouble at work, financial insecurity) the catecholamines will remain elevated in the bloodstream. The person cannot relax and will experience a constant low-level strain on the cardiovascular system that could manifest itself in the form of heart disease.

Additionally, when a person is in a stressful situation, the coronary arteries that feed the heart muscle constrict (clamp down), reducing the oxygen supply to the heart. If significant arterial occlusion attributable to atherosclerosis is present, abnormal rhythms of the heart or even a heart attack may follow.

Individuals who could be classified as Type A and feel that they are under a lot of stress and do not cope well with it, need to begin to take appropriate measures to reduce the effects of stress in their lives. Type A behavior is mostly a learned behavior. One of the best recommendations to overcome stress is to identify the sources of stress and learn how to cope with those events. Even slight changes in behavioral responses can slide individuals along the continuum so that they become more Type B and less Type A. These people need to take control of themselves and examine and act upon the things of greatest importance in their lives. Less significant or meaningless details should be ignored.

Physical exercise has been found to be one of the best ways to relieve stress. When a person engages in physical activity, excess catecholamines are metabolized, and the body is able to return to a normal state. Exercise also increases muscular activity, which causes muscular relaxation upon completion of physical activity. Many executives in large cities are choosing the evening hours for their physical activity programs, stopping after work at the health or fitness club. In this way they are able to "burn up" the excess tension accumulated during the day and better enjoy the evening hours. This has proven to be one of the best stress management techniques. Additional information on stress management techniques is presented in Chapter 9.

PERSONAL AND FAMILY HISTORY

Individuals who have suffered from cardiovascular problems are at higher risk than those who have never had a problem. People with such a history should be strongly encouraged to maintain the other risk factors at as low a level as possible. Because most risk factors are reversible, this practice significantly decreases the risk for future problems. The longer it has been since the incidence of the cardiovascular problem, the lower the risk for recurrence.

The genetic predisposition toward heart disease has been clearly demonstrated and seems to be gaining in importance each day. All other factors being equal, a person who has had blood relatives who suffered from heart disease prior to age sixty runs a greater risk than someone who has no such history. The younger the age at which the incident happened to the relative, the greater is the risk for the disease.

In many cases there is no way of knowing whether a true genetic predisposition or simply poor lifestyle habits led to a particular problem. Quite possibly, a person may have been physically inactive, been overweight, smoked, and had bad dietary habits, leading to a heart attack, and therefore all blood relatives would fall in the same family history category. Because there is no definite way of telling them apart, a person with a family history of heart problems should keep a close watch on all other factors and maintain them at as low a risk level as possible. In addition, an annual blood chemistry analysis is strongly recommended to make sure that the body is handling blood lipids properly.

AGE

Age is a risk factor because of the greater incidence of heart disease among older people. This tendency may be induced partly by an increased risk from the other factors resulting from changes in lifestyle as we get older (e.g., less physical activity, poor nutrition, obesity).

Young people, however, should not think that heart disease will not affect them. The disease process begins early in life. This was clearly shown among American soldiers who died during the Korean and Vietnam conflicts. Autopsies conducted on soldiers killed at twenty-two years of age and younger revealed that approximately 70 percent showed early stages of atherosclerosis. Other studies have found elevated blood cholesterol levels in children as young as ten years old.

Although the aging process cannot be stopped, it can certainly be slowed down. It often has been said that certain individuals in their sixties or older possess the bodies of twenty-year-olds. The opposite also holds true: Twenty-year-olds are sometimes in such poor condition and health that they almost seem to have the bodies of sixty-year-olds. Adequate risk factor management and positive lifestyle habits are the best ways to slow down the natural aging process.

ESTROGEN USE

Only recently were estrogens (found in oral contraceptives and certain other drugs) added to the list of risk factors for coronary disease. Estrogens cause an increase in blood pressure, enhance the clotting mechanism of the blood, and also decrease HDL-cholesterol (the "good guys"). High blood pressure by itself will increase the susceptibility to atherosclerosis. If in addition to that, HDL-cholesterol is reduced, a greater amount of fats can be deposited in the arteries (even worse among women smokers, as smoking also decreases HDL-cholesterol). As plaque builds up, complete obstruction may occur from a blood clot enhanced by the use of estrogen. It is therefore recommended that women at moderate, high, or very high risk for heart disease consult their physician in this regard.

A FINAL WORD ON CORONARY RISK REDUCTION

As was mentioned at the beginning of this chapter, most of the risk factors for coronary heart disease are reversible and preventable. The fact that a person has a family history of heart disease and possibly some of the other risk factors because of neglectful lifestyle does not signify by any means that this person is doomed. The objective of this chapter was to provide guidelines and recommendations to decrease the risk of suffering from cardiovascular disease (particularly coronary heart disease).

A healthier lifestyle — free of cardiovascular problems — is something that you can pretty much control by yourself. You are encouraged to be persistent. Willpower and commitment are necessary to develop positive patterns that will eventually turn into healthy habits conducive to total well-being. Only you can act by taking control of your lifestyle and thereby reaping the benefits of wellness.

Bibliography

American Heart Association. *Coronary Risk Handbook:* Estimating Risk of Coronary Heart Disease in Daily Practice. Dallas: AHA, 1973.

American Heart Association. *Heart Facts.* Dallas: AHA, 1988.

Blair, S. N., N. N. Goodyear, L. W. Gibbons, and K. H. Cooper. "Physical Fitness and Incidence of Hypertension in Healthy Normotensive Men and Women." *JAMA* 252:487-490, 1984.

Blair, S. N., K. H. Cooper, L. W. Gibbons, L. R. Gettman, S. Lewis, and N. N. Goodyear. "Changes in Coronary Heart Disease Risk Factors Associated with Increased Treadmill Time in 753 Men." *American Journal of Epidemiology* 3:352-359, 1983.

Cooper, K. H. *The Aerobics Way.* New York: Mount Evans and Co., 1977.

Cooper, K. H. *The Aerobics Program for Total Well-Being.* New York: Mount Evans and Co., 1982.

Cooper, K. H. *Running Without Fear.* New York: Mount Evans and Co., 1985.

Diethrich, E. B. *The Arizona Heart Institute's Heart Test.* New York: International Heart Foundation, 1981.

Gibbons, L. W., S. Blair, K. H. Cooper, and M. Smith. "Association Between Coronary Heart Disease Risk Factors and Physical Fitness in Healthy Adult Women." *Circulation* 5:977-983, 1983.

Guss, S. B. *Heart Attack Risk Score.* Cardiac Alert, 1983.

Hoeger, W. W. K. *Ejercicio, Salud y Vida [Exercise, Health and Life].* Caracas, Venezuela: Editorial Arte, 1980.

Hoeger, W. W. K. "Self-Assessment of Cardiovascular Risk." *Corporate Fitness & Recreation* 5(6):13-16, 1986.

Hoeger, W. W. K. *The Complete Guide for the Development & Implementation of Health Promotion Programs.* Englewood, CO: Morton Publishing, 1987.

How Good is "Good" Cholesterol? *Health Letter.* April 9, 1982.

Hubert, H. B., M. Feinleib, P. M. MacNamara, and W. P. Castelli. "Obesity as an Independent Risk Factor for Cardiovascular Disease: A 26-year Follow-up of Participants in the Framingham Heart Study." *Circulation* 5:968-977, 1983.

Johnson, L. C. *Interpreting Your Test Results.* Lake Geneva, WI: Fitness Monitoring Preventive Medicine Clinic, 1981.

Kannel, W. B., D. McGee, and T. Gordon. "A General Cardiovascular Risk Profile: The Framingham Study." *American Journal of Cardiology* 7:46-51, 1976.

Kostas, G. "Three Nutrients May Help Control Blood Pressure." *Aerobics News* 1(7):6, 1986.

Multiple Risk Factor Intervention Trial Research Group. "Risk Factor Changes and Mortality Results." *JAMA* 248:1465-1477, 1982.

Neufeld, H. N., and U. Gouldbourt. "Coronary Heart Disease: Genetic Aspects." *Circulation.* 5:943-954, 1983.

Page, L. B. "On Making Sense of Salt and Your Blood Pressure." *Executive Health.* August 1982.

Van Camp, S. P. "The Fixx Tragedy: A Cardiologist's Perspective." *Physician & Sportsmedicine* 12:153-155, 1984.

Wiley, J. A., and T. C. Camacho. "Lifestyle and Future Health: Evidence from the Alameda County Study." *Preventive Medicine* 9:1-21, 1980.

Cancer Prevention

The human body has approximately 100 trillion cells, and under normal conditions these cells reproduce themselves in an orderly manner. The growth of cells occurs so that old, worn-out tissue can be replaced and injuries can be repaired. In some instances, however, certain cells grow in an uncontrolled and abnormal manner. Some cells will grow into a mass of tissue called a tumor, which can be either *benign or malignant;* a malignant tumor is considered to be a cancer. Cancer cells grow for no reason and multiply uncontrollably, destroying normal tissue. The rate at which cancer cells grow varies from one type to another. Certain types grow fast, while others may take much longer.

More than 100 types of cancer can develop in any tissue or organ of the body. Cancer probably starts with the abnormal growth of one cell, which can then multiply into billions of cancerous cells. It takes approximately one billion cells, or the equivalent of a one-centimeter tumor, before cancer can be detected. Through *metastasis* (the movement of bacteria or body cells from one part of the body to another), cells break away from a malignant tumor and migrate to other parts of the body, where they can cause new cancer. Although most cancer cells are destroyed by the immune system, it only takes one abnormal cell to lodge elsewhere and start a new cancer. In contrast, benign tumors do not invade other tissue. They can interfere with normal bodily functions, but, they rarely cause death. Figure 8.1 depicts the growth of cancer cells.

Figure 8.1. *Cancer cells dividing erratically and crowding out normal cells.*

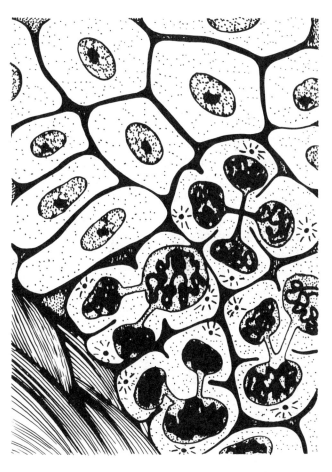

Illustration courtesy of American Cancer Society (contained in *Youth Looks at Cancer.* New York: American Cancer Society, p. 4, 1982).

CANCER RISK

The 1987 report by the National Center for Health Statistics indicated that 22.4 percent of all deaths in the United States was caused by cancer. It is the second leading cause of death in the country and the leading cause among children between the ages of three and fourteen. About 494,000 people died from the disease in 1988, and approximately 985,000 new cases were expected the same year. The 1988 statistical estimates of cancer incidence and deaths by sex and site are given in Figure 8.2 (these estimates exclude nonmelanoma skin cancer and carcinoma in situ). Estimates also indicated that 75 million Americans, based on the total 1988 population, would suffer from cancer in their lifetime. This translates to approximately three of every four families.

As with coronary heart disease, cancer is largely a preventable disease. As much as 80 percent of all human cancers are related to lifestyle or environmental factors including diet, tobacco use, excessive use of alcohol, overexposure to sunlight, and exposure to occupational hazards. Most of these cancers could be prevented through positive lifestyle habits. The proportion of cancers related to environmental factors was carefully studied in the Birmingham and West Midland region of England. The report indicated that only six percent of cancers in men and two percent in women originated in the workplace. Approximately 85 to 90 percent were lifestyle-related (see Table 8.1).

Equally important is the fact that cancer is now viewed as the most curable of all chronic diseases. Over half of all cancers are curable. More than five million Americans who had a history of cancer were alive in 1988. Close to three million of them were considered cured. The biggest factor in fighting cancer today is health education. People need to be informed regarding the risk factors for cancer and the guidelines for early detection.

Figure 8.2. *Cancer incidence and deaths by site and gender: 1988 estimates*

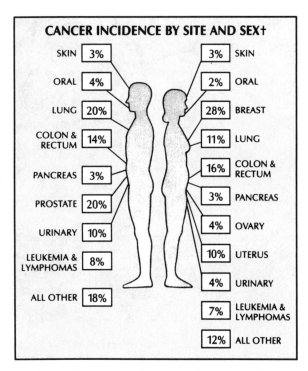

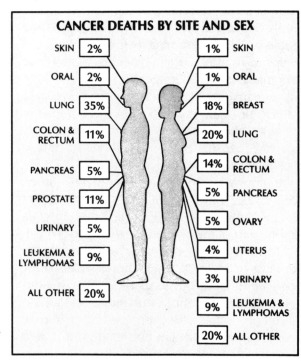

†Excluding non-melanoma skin cancer and carcinoma in situ.

From *Cancer Facts & Figures.* New York: American Cancer Society, 1988.

Table 8.1.
Cancer Deaths from Presumed and Environmental Factors in the Birmingham and West Midland Region of England, 1968-1972

	Percentages of Cancer	
Factor	Males	Females
Tobacco*	30	7
Tobacco/alcohol*	5	3
Sunlight*	10	10
Occupation*	6	2
Radiation*	1	1
Iatrogenic*	1	1
Other "Lifestyle" Factors**	30	63
Congenital**	2	2
Unknown	15	11

* Defined environmental factors.
** Presumed environmental factors.
Adapted from Higginson, J., and C. S. Muir. "Environmental Carcinogenesis: Misconceptions and Limitations to Cancer Control" *JNCL* 63(6):1291-1297, 1979.

GUIDELINES FOR CANCER PREVENTION

The most effective way to protect against cancer is by changing negative lifestyle habits and behaviors that have been practiced for years. The American Cancer Society has issued the following recommendations in regard to cancer prevention:

1. *Dietary changes.* The diet should be low in fat and high in fiber, with ample amounts of vitamins A and C from natural sources. Cruciferous vegetables are encouraged in the diet; alcohol should be used in moderation; and obesity should be avoided.

   High fat intake has been linked primarily to breast, colon, and prostate cancers. Low fiber intake seems to increase the risk of colon cancer. Foods high in vitamins A and C may help decrease the incidence of larynx, esophagus, and lung cancers. Conversely, salt-cured, smoked, and nitrite-cured foods should be avoided; these foods have been linked to cancer of the esophagus and stomach. Vitamin C seems to help decrease the formation of nitrosamines (cancer-causing substances that are formed when cured meats are eaten). Cruciferous vegetables (cauliflower, broccoli, Brussels sprouts, and kohlrabi) should be included in the diet, because

they seem to decrease the risk for developing certain cancers.

Alcohol should be used in moderation. Alcoholism increases the risk of certain cancers, especially when combined with tobacco smoking or smokeless tobacco. In combination, they significantly increase the risk of mouth, larynx, throat, esophagus, and liver cancers. According to some research, the synergistic action of heavy use of alcohol and tobacco yields a fifteen-fold increase in cancer of the oral cavity.

Maintenance of ideal body weight is also recommended. Obesity has been associated with colon, rectum, breast, prostate, gallbladder, ovary, and uterine cancers.

2. *Abstinence from cigarette smoking.* It has been reported that 83 percent of all lung cancer and 30 percent of all cancers are attributed to smoking. Smokeless tobacco also increases the risk of mouth, larynx, throat, and esophagus cancers. About 148,000 annual cancer deaths are attributed to the use of tobacco. Cigarette smoking by itself is a major health hazard. When considering all related deaths, cigarette smoking is responsible for 300,000 unnecessary deaths per year. The average life expectancy for a chronic smoker is seven years less than for a nonsmoker.

3. *Avoid sun exposure.* Sunlight exposure is a major factor in the development of skin cancer. Almost 100 percent of the 500,000 nonmelanoma skin cancer cases reported annually in the United States are related to sun exposure. Sun screen lotion should be used at all times when the skin is going to be exposed to sun light for extended periods of time. Tanning of the skin is the body's natural reaction to cell damage taking place as a result of excessive sun exposure.

4. *Avoid estrogen use, radiation exposure, and occupational hazard exposure.* Estrogen use has been linked to endometrial cancer, but it can be taken safely under careful medical supervision. Radiation exposure also increases cancer risk. Many times, however, the benefits of X-ray use outweigh the risk involved, and most medical facilities use the lowest dose possible to decrease the risk to a minimum. Occupational hazards, such as asbestos fibers, nickel and uranium dusts, chromium compounds, vinyl chloride, and

bischlormethyl ether, increase cancer risk. The risk of occupational hazards is significantly magnified by the use of cigarette smoking.

The contribution of many of the other much publicized factors is not as significant as the above factors. Intentional food additives, saccharin, processing agents, pesticides, and packaging materials in current use in the United States and other developed countries appear to have a minimal impact on the incidence of cancer.

Genetics plays a role in susceptibility in only two percent of all cancers. Most of it is seen in the early childhood years. Some cancer can be viewed as a combination of genetic and environmental liability. Genetics may act to enhance environmental risks for certain types of cancers. The biggest carcinogenic exposure in the workplace is cigarette smoke. But environment means more than pollution and smoke. It includes diet, lifestyle-related events, viruses, and physical agents such as X-rays and sun exposure.

Equally important is the fact that through early detection, many cancers can be controlled or cured. The real problem is the spreading of cancerous cells. Once spreading occurs, it becomes very difficult to wipe out the cancer. It is therefore crucial to practice effective prevention or at least to catch cancer when the possibility of cure is greatest. Herein lies the importance of proper periodic screening for prevention and for early detection.

The following are the seven notable warning signals for cancer. Every individual should become familiar with these warning signals and bring them to the attention of a physician if any of them are present:

1. Change in bowel or bladder habits.
2. A sore that does not heal.
3. Unusual bleeding or discharge.
4. Thickening or lump in breast or elsewhere.
5. Indigestion or difficulty in swallowing.
6. Obvious change in wart or mole.
7. Nagging cough or hoarseness.

In addition to the seven warning signals, The American Medical Association has developed a questionnaire to help alert people to symptoms that may indicate a serious health problem. This questionnaire is given at the end of this chapter,

in Figure 8.4. Although in most cases nothing is seriously wrong, if any of the described symptoms arise, a physician should be consulted as soon as possible. Furthermore, the Guidelines for Screening Recommendations by the American Cancer Society, outlined in Table 8.2, should be included in regular physical examinations as a part of a cancer prevention program.

There is also growing evidence that the body's auto-immune system may play a role in preventing cancer. Studies have indicated that exercise improves the auto-immune system. In contrast, high levels of tension and stress and poor coping skills may have a negative impact on this system and consequently reduce the body's effectiveness in dealing with the various cancers. Other recent research has indicated that moderately intense, long-term athletic participation lowers the risk for breast and reproductive system cancers. The possible link may be related to the finding that highly trained athletes possesses lower estrogen levels.

Scientific evidence and testing procedures for prevention and early detection of cancer do change. Results of new clinical and epidemiologic studies constantly provide new information about cancer prevention and detection. The purpose of cancer prevention programs is to educate and guide individuals toward a lifestyle that will aid them in the prevention or early detection of malignancy. Treatment of cancer should always be left to specialized physicians and cancer clinics.

CANCER QUESTIONNAIRE: ASSESSING YOUR RISKS*

This simple self-testing questionnaire was designed by the Texas Division of the American Cancer Society to help people assess their risk for cancer. Some people may have more than the average risk of developing certain cancers. These people will be identified by risk factors for certain common types of cancer. They are the major risk factors and by no means represent the only ones that might be involved. The following are

---

* Cancer Questionnaire: Assessing Your Risks obtained from the Texas Division of the American Cancer Society and reproduced with permission. (NOTE: This questionnaire is not available nation wide; distribution is limited to Texas residents only).

Table 8.2.
Guidelines for Cancer Screening

Test	Patient age	Frequency
Breast physical examination	20-40 Over 40	Every 3 yrs Annually
Breast self-examination	Over 20	Monthly
Chest X-ray	No specific recommendation	No specific recommendation
Digital rectal examination	Over 40	Annually
Endometrial tissue examination	At menopause[a]	At menopause
Mammography	35-40 40-49 Over 50	One baseline Every 1-2 yrs Annually
Pap smear	20-65 and sexually active teenagers	2 consecutive yrs, then every 3 yrs
Pelvic examination	20-40 Over 40 At menopause	Every 3 yrs Annually
Sigmoidoscopy	Over 50	2 consecutive yrs, then every 3-5 yrs
Sputum cytology	No specific recommendation	No specific recommendation
Stool guaiac	Over 50	Annually
Health counseling and cancer check-up[b]	Over 20 Over 40	Every 3 yrs Every yr

[a] Recommended for obese women with a history of involuntary infertility, failure of ovulation, abnormal uterine bleeding, or estrogen therapy.
[b] To include examinations for cancers of the thyroid, testicles, prostate, ovaries, lymph nodes, oral region, and skin.
From *Guidelines for the Cancer-Related Checkup: Recommendations and Rationale*. New York: American Cancer Society, July/August 1980. Reproduced by permission.

the instructions given to people who take this questionnaire:

Read each question concerning each site and its specific risk factors. Be honest in your responses. Place the number in parenthesis (risk points) in the correct space provided to the left of each question. For example, Question #2 on lung cancer: if you are fifty-three years old (age fifty to fifty-nine), enter 5 (risk points) as your score on the left. At the end of each site, total your number of points for that particular site. [The final number of points should also be recorded in Figure 8.3 and in Appendix A, Figure A.1.]

Men should complete the questions for lung, colon-rectum, and skin cancer. For women, three additional major cancer sites for women are included, with space to enter the score totals.

Check your own risks against the answers contained on this questionnaire. Individual numbers

for specific questions are not to be interpreted as a precise measure of relative risk, but the totals for a given site should give you a general indication of your risk. An explanation of the risk factors for each type of cancer follows the questionnaire. You are advised to discuss the results with your physician if you are at higher risk.

Lung Cancer

_____ 1. Sex

    a. Male (2)
    b. Female (1)

_____ 2. Age

    a. 39 or younger (1)
    b. 40–49 (2)
    c. 50–59 (5)
    d. 60+ (7)

_____ 3. Smoking status

    a. Smoker (8)

    b. Nonsmoker (1)

_____ 4. Type of smoking

    a. Current cigarettes or little cigars (10)

    b. Pipe and/or cigar, but not cigarettes (3)

    c. Ex-cigarette smoker (2)

_____ 5. Amount of cigarettes smoked per day

    a. 0 (1)

    b. Less than ½ pack per day (5)

    c. ½–1 pack (9)

    d. 1–2 packs (15)

    e. 2+ packs (20)

_____ 6. Type of cigarette*

    a. High tar/nicotine (10)

    b. Medium T/N (9)

    c. Low T/N (7)

    d. Nonsmoker (1)

_____ 7. Duration of smoking

    a. Never smoked (1)

    b. Ex-smoker (3)

    c. Up to 15 years (5)

    d. 15–25 years (10)

    e. 25+ years (20)

_____ 8. Type of industrial work

    a. Mining (3)

    b. Asbestos (7)

    c. Uranium and radioactive products (5)

_____ Total

Colon-Rectum Cancer

_____ 1. Age

    a. 39 or younger (10)

    b. 40–59 (20)

    c. 60+ (50)

_____ 2. Has anyone in your immediate family ever had:

    a. Colon cancer (20)

    b. One or more polyps of the colon (10)

    c. Neither (1)

_____ 3. Have you ever had:

    a. Colon cancer (100)

    b. One or more polyps of the colon (40)

    c. Ulcerative colitis (20)

    d. Cancer of the breast or uterus (10)

    e. None (1)

_____ 4. Bleeding from the rectum (other than obvious hemorrhoids or piles)

    a. Yes (75)

    b. No (1)

_____ Total

Skin Cancer

_____ 1. Frequent work or play in the sun:

    a. Yes (10)

    b. No (1)

_____ 2. Work in mines, around coal tars, or around radioactivity:

    a. Yes (10)

    b. No (1)

_____ 3. Complexion — fair and/or light skin:

    a. Yes (10)

    b. No (1)

_____ Total

Breast Cancer

_____ 1. Age

    a. 20–34 (10)

    b. 35–49 (40)

    c. 50+ (90)

---

* High T/N: 20 mg + Tar/1.3 + mg. nicotine.
  Medium T/N: 16-19 mg. Tar/1.1-1.2 nicotine
  Low T/N: 15 mg. or less Tar/1.0 mg. or less nicotine.

_____ 2. Race group

    a. Oriental (5)
    b. Black (20)
    c. White (25)
    d. Mexican American (10)

_____ 3. Family history

    a. Mother, sister, aunt, or grand-mother with breast cancer (30)
    b. None (10)

_____ 4. Your history

    a. Previous lumps or cysts (25)
    b. No breast disease (10)
    c. Previous breast cancer (100)

_____ 5. Maternity

    a. 1st pregnancy before 25 (10)
    b. 1st pregnancy after 25 (15)
    c. No pregnancies (20)

_____ Total

Cervical Cancer

(Lower portion of uterus. These questions do not apply to a woman who has had a total hysterectomy.)

_____ 1. Age group

    a. Younger than 25 (10)
    b. 25–39 (20)
    c. 40–54 (30)
    d. 55+ (30)

_____ 2. Race

    a. Oriental (10)
    b. Puerto Rican (20)
    c. Black (20)
    d. White (10)
    e. Mexican American (20)

_____ 3. Number of pregnancies

    a. 0 (10)
    b. 1 to 3 (20)
    c. 4 and over (30)

_____ 4. Viral infections

    a. Herpes and other viral infections or ulcer formations on the vagina (10)
    b. Never (1)

_____ 5. Age at first intercourse

    a. Before 15 (40)
    b. 15–19 (30)
    c. 20–24 (20)
    d. 25 and over (10)
    e. Never (5)

_____ 6. Bleeding between periods or after intercourse

    a. Yes (40)
    b. No (1)

_____ Total

Endometrial Cancer

(Body of uterus. These questions do not apply to a woman who has had a total hysterectomy.)

_____ 1. Age group

    a. 39 or younger (5)
    b. 40–49 (20)
    c. 50+ (60)

_____ 2. Race

    a. Oriental (10)
    b. Black (10)
    c. White (20)
    d. Mexican American (10)

_____ 3. Births

    a. None (15)
    b. 1 to 4 (7)
    c. 5 or more (5)

_____ 4. Weight

    a. 50 or more pounds overweight (50)
    b. 20–49 pounds overweight (15)
    c. Underweight for height (10)
    d. Normal (10)

_____ 5. Diabetes (elevated blood sugar)

    a. Yes (3)
    b. No (1)

_____ 6. Estrogen hormone intake

    a. Yes, regularly (15)
    b. Yes, occasionally (12)
    c. None (10)

7. Abnormal uterine bleeding
   a. Yes (40)
   b. No (1)

8. Hypertension (high blood pressure)
   a. Yes (3)
   b. No (1)

_____ Total

CANCER QUESTIONNAIRE INTERPRETATION

The following interpretation of the cancer questionnaire is to summarize, explain new evidence, and provide valuable information on the individual risk that a person may have for each type of cancer. Potential cancer risk is based on individual lifestyle and medical history.

Lung Cancer

1. *Sex.* Men have a higher risk of lung cancer than women, equating them for type, amount, and duration of smoking. Because more women are smoking cigarettes for a longer duration than previously, their incidence of lung and upper respiratory tract (mouth, tongue, and larynx) cancer is increasing.

2. *Age.* The occurrence of lung and upper respiratory tract cancer increases with age.

3. *Smoking status.* Cigarette smokers have up to twenty times or even greater risk than nonsmokers. The rates for ex-smokers who have not smoked for ten years approach those of nonsmokers.

4. *Type of smoking.* Pipe and cigar smokers are at a higher risk for lung cancer than nonsmokers. Cigarette smokers are at a much higher risk than nonsmokers or pipe and cigar smokers. All forms of tobacco, including chewing, markedly increase the user's risk of developing cancer of the mouth.

5. *Amount of cigarettes smoked per day.* Males who smoke less than one-half pack per day have five times higher lung cancer rates than nonsmokers. Males who smoke one to two packs per day have fifteen times higher lung cancer rates than nonsmokers. Those who smoke more than two packs per day are twenty times more likely to develop lung cancer than nonsmokers.

6. *Type of cigarette.* Smokers of low-tar/nicotine cigarettes have slightly lower lung cancer rates.

7. *Duration of smoking.* The frequency of lung and upper respiratory tract cancer increases with the duration of smoking.

8. *Type of industrial work.* Exposures to materials used in the industries mentioned in the questionnaire have been demonstrated to be associated with lung cancer. Smokers who work in these industries may have greatly increased risks. Exposure to materials in other industries may also carry a higher risk.

TOTAL RISK:

24 or less . . . . . You have a low risk for lung cancer (low risk category).

25-49 . . . . You may be a light smoker and would have a good chance of kicking the habit (light risk).

50-74 . . . . As a moderate smoker, your risks of lung and upper respiratory tract cancer are increased. If you stop smoking now, these risks will decrease (moderate risk).

75 or over . . . . As a heavy cigarette smoker, your chances of getting lung and upper respiratory tract cancer are greatly increased. Your best bet is to stop smoking now — for the health of it. See your doctor if you have a nagging cough, hoarseness, persistent pain, or a sore in the mouth or throat (high risk).

Colon-Rectum Cancer

1. *Age.* Colon cancer occurs more frequently after age fifty.

2. *Family predisposition.* Colon cancer is more common in families with a previous history of this disease.

3. *Personal history.* Polyps and bowel diseases are associated with colon cancer.

4. *Rectal bleeding.* Rectal bleeding may be a sign of colorectal cancer.

TOTAL RISK:

29 or less . . . . . You are at a low risk for colon-rectum cancer.

30-69 . . . . This is a moderate risk category. Testing by your physician may be indicated.

70 or over . . . . This is a high-risk category. You should see your physician for the following tests: digital rectal exam, guaiac slide test, and proctoscopic exam.

In addition to the risk factors mentioned in the questionnaire, a diet high in fat and low in fiber, as well as a history of breast or endometrial cancer, also increase the risk for colon-rectum cancer.

Skin Cancer

1. *Sun exposure.* Excessive ultraviolet light causes cancer of the skin. Protect yourself with a sun screen medication.

2. *Work environment.* Working in mines, around coal tar, or around radioactive materials can cause cancer of the skin.

3. *Complexion.* Persons with light complexions need more protection than others.

TOTAL RISK:

Numerical risks for skin cancer are difficult to state. For instance, a person with a dark complexion can work longer in the sun and be less likely to develop cancer than a light-complected person. Furthermore, a person wearing a long-sleeved shirt and wide-brimmed hat may work in the sun and be less at risk than a person who wears a bathing suit for only a short period. The risk greatly increases with age.

If you answer yes to any question, you need to protect your skin from the sun or any other toxic material. Changes in moles, warts, or skin sores are very important and should be seen by your doctor.

Breast Cancer

1. *Age.* The risk for breast cancer significantly increases after age fifty.

2. *Race.* Breast cancer occurs more frequently in white women than any other groups.

3. *Family history.* The risk for breast cancer is higher in women with a family history of this type of cancer. The risk is even higher if more than one family member has developed breast cancer, and is also enhanced by the closeness in terms of immediacy (e.g., mother, sister, aunt, or grandmother).

4. *Personal history.* A previous history of breast or ovarian cancer would indicate a greater risk.

5. *Maternity.* The risk is greater in women who have never had children and in women who bear children after age thirty.

TOTAL RISK:

Under 100 . . . . Low-risk women should practice monthly breast self-examination (BSE) and have their breasts examined by a doctor as a part of a cancer-related check-up.

100–199 . . . . . . Moderate-risk women should practice monthly BSE and have their breasts examined by a doctor as part of a cancer-related check-up. Periodic breast X-rays should be included as your doctor may advise.

200 or over . . . High-risk women should practice monthly BSE and have the above examinations more often. (See your doctor for the recommended frequency of breast physical examinations and X-ray examinations related to you.)

Other possible risk factors for breast cancer not listed in the questionnaire are a diet high in fat, onset of menstruation prior to age thirteen, chronic cystic disease, and ionizing radiation.

Cervical Cancer

1. *Age.* The highest occurrence is in the forty and over age group. The numbers represent relative rates of cancer for different age groups. A forty-five-year-old woman has a risk three times higher than a twenty-year-old.

2. *Race.* Puerto Ricans, Blacks, and Mexican Americans have higher rates of cervical cancer.

3. *Number of pregnancies.* Women who have delivered more children have a higher occurrence.

4. *Viral infections.* Viral infections of the cervix and vagina are associated with cervical cancer.

5. *Age at first intercourse.* Women with earlier intercourse and with more sexual partners are at a higher risk.

6. *Bleeding.* Irregular bleeding may be a sign of uterine cancer.

TOTAL RISK:

40–69 . . . . This is a low-risk group. Ask your doctor for a pap test. You will be advised how often you should be tested after your first test.

70–99 . . . . In this moderate-risk group, more frequent pap tests may be required.

100 or over . . . You are in a high-risk group and should have a pap test (and pelvic exam) as advised by your doctor.

Endometrial Cancer

1. *Age.* Endometrial cancer is seen in older age groups. The numbers accompanying the age groups represent relative rates of endometrial cancer at different ages. A fifty-year-old woman has a risk twelve times higher than a thirty-five-year-old woman.

2. *Race.* Caucasians have a higher occurrence.

3. *Births.* The fewer children one has delivered, the greater the risk of endometrial cancer.

4. *Weight.* Women who are overweight are at greater risk.

5. *Diabetes.* Cancer of the endometrium is associated with diabetes.

6. *Estrogen use.* Cancer of the endometrium may be associated with prolonged continuous estrogen hormone intake. This occurs in only a small number of women. You should consult your physician before starting or stopping any estrogen medication.

7. *Abnormal bleeding.* Women who do not have cyclic regular menstrual periods are at greater risk.

8. *Hypertension.* Cancer of the endometrium is associated with high blood pressure.

TOTAL RISK:

45–59 . . . . You are at low risk for developing endometrial cancer.

60–99 . . . . Your risks are slightly higher (moderate risk). Report any abnormal bleeding immediately to your doctor. Tissue sampling at menopause is recommended.

100 or over . . . Your risks are much greater (high risk). See your doctor for tests as appropriate.

Additional risk factors that may be associated with endometrial cancer, not included in the questionnaire, are infertility, a prolonged history of failure to ovulate, and menopause after age fifty-five.

OTHER CANCER SITES

Risk factors and prevention techniques for other types of cancer not contained in the cancer questionnaire have also been outlined in The American Cancer Society *Cancer Book* and in a series of pamphlets on "Facts on Cancer" (one each for selected cancer sites). These types of cancer are listed next, along with the risk factors associated with each type and preventive techniques to help decrease risk. Unlike the previous questionnaire, no numeric weights for the various risk factors have been assigned. As you read the information, however, rate yourself on a scale from 1 to 3 (1 = low risk, 2 = moderate risk, 3 = high risk) for each cancer site, and record your results in Figure 8.3.

Prostate Cancer

The prostate gland is actually a cluster of smaller glands that encircles the top section of the urethra (urinary channel) at the point where it leaves the bladder. The function of the prostate is not quite clear, but the muscles of these small glands help squeeze prostatic secretions into the urethra.

1. The highest incidence of prostate cancer is found in men over age fifty-five. The incidence is also higher among blacks than whites, and more married than single men develop this type of cancer.

2. A history of venereal disease. Herpes Simplex Virus Type 2 and Cytomegalovirus (herpes virus) have been linked to prostate cancer.

3. A history of prostate infections (more than two).

4. A diet high in fat may also increase risk.

PREVENTION AND WARNING SIGNALS

Prostate cancer is difficult to control because the causes are not known. Death rates can be decreased through early detection and awareness of the warning signals. Detection, made by a rectal exam of the gland, should be conducted once a year after the age of forty. Possible warning signals include: difficulties in urination (especially at night), painful urination, blood in the urine, and constant pain in the lower back or hip area.

Testicular Cancer

Testicular cancer accounts for only 1 percent of all male cancers, but it is the most common type of cancer in men between the ages of twenty-five and thirty-five. The incidence is slightly higher in whites than blacks, and it is rarely seen in middle-aged and older men. The malignancy rate of testicular tumors is 96 percent, but this type of cancer is highly curable if it is diagnosed early.

RISK FACTORS

1. An undescended testicle not corrected before age six.

2. Atrophy of the testicle following mumps or virus infection.

3. A family history of testicular cancer.

4. Recurrent injury to the testicle.

5. Abnormalities of the endocrine system (e.g., high hormone levels of pituitary gonadotropin or androgens).

6. Incomplete testicular development.

PREVENTION AND WARNING SIGNALS

The incidence of testicular cancer is quite high in males born with an undescended testicle. Therefore, this condition should be corrected early in life. Parents of infant males should make sure that the child is checked by a physician to ensure that the testes have descended into the scrotum. Testicular self-examination (TSE) once a month following a warm bath or shower (when the scrotal skin is relaxed) is recommended. Each testicle is gently examined by rolling it between the thumb and fingers. The individual should feel for a firm lump about the size of a pea. Although most lumps are noncancerous, if a lump is detected, a physician should be promptly consulted.

Some of the warning signs associated with testicular cancer are: a small lump on the testicle, slight enlargement (usually painless) and change in consistency of the testis, sudden build-up of blood or fluid in the scrotum, groin and lower abdominal pain or discomfort accompanied by a sensation of dragging and heaviness, breast enlargement or tenderness, and enlarged lymph glands.

Early diagnosis of testicular cancer is essential because this type of cancer spreads rapidly to other parts of the body. As no early symptoms or pain are associated with testicular cancer in most cases, individuals do not usually see a physician for months following the discovery of a lump or a slightly enlarged testis. Unfortunately, this delay allows almost 90 percent of testicular cancers to metastasize before a diagnosis is made.

Pancreatic Cancer

The pancreas is a thin gland that lies behind the stomach. This gland releases insulin and pancreatic juice. Insulin regulates blood sugar; pancreatic juice contains enzymes that aid in food digestion.

POSSIBLE RISK FACTORS

1. The incidence increases between the ages of thirty-five and seventy but is significantly higher around the age of fifty-five.

2. Cigarette smoking.

3. High cholesterol diet.

4. Exposure to unspecified environmental agents.

Detection of pancreatic cancer is difficult because (a) no symptoms are evoked in the early disease process, and (b) advanced disease symptoms are similar to those of other diseases. Warning signals that may be related to pancreatic cancer include: pain in the abdomen or lower back, jaundice, loss of weight and appetite, nausea, weakness, agitated depression, loss of energy and feeling weary, dizziness, chills, muscle spasms, double vision, and coma.

Kidney and Bladder Cancer

The kidneys are the organs that filter the urine, and the bladder stores and empties the urine. Most of these two types of cancers are caused by environmental factors. Bladder cancer occurs most frequently between the ages of fifty and seventy. Eighty percent of bladder cancers are seen in men, and the incidence is twice as high in white males as in black males.

RISK FACTORS

1. Congenital abnormalities of either organ (these conditions are detected by a physician).
2. Exposure to certain chemical compounds such as aniline dyes, naphthalenes, or benzidines.
3. Heavy cigarette smoking.
4. A history of schistosomiasis (a parasitic bladder infection).
5. Frequent urinary tract infections, particularly after the age of fifty.

PREVENTION AND WARNING SIGNALS

Avoidance of cigarette smoking and occupational exposure to cancer-causing chemicals is important to decrease risk. Bloody urine, especially repeated occurrences, is always an important warning sign requiring immediate evaluation.

Oral Cancer

Oral cancer includes the mouth, lips, tongue, salivary glands, pharynx, larynx, and floor of the mouth. Most of these cancers seem to be related to cigarette smoking and excessive alcohol consumption.

RISK FACTORS

1. Heavy smoking and/or drinking.
2. Broken or ill-fitting dentures.
3. A broken tooth that irritates the inside of the mouth.
4. Chewing and dipping tobacco.
5. Excessive sun exposure (lip cancer)

PREVENTION AND WARNING SIGNALS

Regular examinations and good dental hygiene help in the prevention and early detection of oral cancer. Warning signals may include the following: a nonhealing sore or white patch in the mouth, the presence of a lump, problems with chewing and swallowing, and constant feeling of having "something" in the throat. A person with any of the previous conditions should be evaluated by a physician or dentist. A tissue biopsy is normally conducted to diagnose the presence of cancer.

Esophageal and Stomach Cancer

The incidence of gastric cancer in the United States has decreased by about 40 percent in the last thirty years. Cancer experts attribute this drastic decrease to changes in dietary habits and increased use of refrigeration. This type of cancer is more common in men, and the incidence is also higher among black males than whites.

RISK FACTORS

1. A diet high in starch and low in fresh fruits and vegetables.
2. Increased consumption of salt-cured, smoked, and nitrate-cured foods.
3. Stomach acid imbalance.
4. A history of pernicious anemia.
5. Chronic gastritis or gastric polyps.
6. A family history of these types of cancer.

PREVENTION AND WARNING SIGNALS

Prevention is accomplished primarily by increasing dietary intake of complex carbohydrates and fiber and decreasing the intake of cured, smoked, and nitrate-cured foods. In addition, regular guiac testing for occult blood (hemoccult test) is recommended. Warning signals for this type of cancer include: indigestion for two weeks or longer, blood in the stools, vomiting, and rapid weight loss.

Ovarian Cancer

The ovaries, part of the female reproductive system, produce and release the egg and the hormone estrogen. Ovarian cancer develops more frequently after menopause, and the highest incidence is seen between the ages of fifty-five and sixty-four.

RISK FACTORS

1. Women over fifty years old are at higher risk.

2. A history of ovarian problems.

3. Extensive history of menstrual irregularities.

4. A family history of ovarian cancer.

5. A personal history of breast, bowel, or endometrial cancer.

6. Nulliparity (not having given birth).

PREVENTION AND WARNING SIGNALS

In most cases, there are no signs or symptoms related to ovarian cancer. Therefore, regular pelvic examinations to detect signs of enlargement or other abnormalities are highly recommended. Some warning signals that may occur with ovarian cancer are: an enlarged abdomen, abnormal vaginal bleeding, unexplained digestive disturbances in women over forty, and normal-sized ovaries (premenopause size) after menopause has occurred.

Thyroid Cancer

The thyroid gland, located in the lower portion of the front of the neck, helps regulate growth and metabolism. Thyroid cancer among women occurs almost twice as often as in men, and the incidence is also higher in whites than blacks.

RISK FACTORS

1. Risk increases with age.

2. Radiation therapy of the head and neck region received in childhood or adolescence.

3. A family history of thyroid cancer.

PREVENTION AND WARNING SIGNALS

Regular inspection for thyroid tumors is done by palpation of the gland and surrounding areas during a physical examination. Thyroid cancer is slow-growing; therefore, this malignancy is highly treatable. Nevertheless, any unusual lumps in front of the neck should be promptly reported to a physician. Although thyroid cancer is quite asymptomatic, warning signals (besides a lump) may include: difficulty in swallowing, choking, labored breathing, and persistent hoarseness.

Liver Cancer

The incidence of liver cancer in the United States is very low. Men are more prone to liver cancer, and the disease is more common after the age of sixty.

RISK FACTORS

1. A history of cirrhosis of the liver.

2. A history of hepatitis B virus.

3. Exposure to vinyl chloride (industrial gas used in manufacturing plastics) and aflatoxin (natural food contaminant).

4. Heavy alcohol consumption.

PREVENTION AND WARNING SIGNALS

Prevention is accomplished primarily by avoiding the risk factors and being aware of warning signals. Possible signs and symptoms are: a lump or pain in the upper right abdomen (which may radiate into the back and the shoulder), fever, nausea, rapidly deteriorating health, jaundice, and liver tenderness.

Leukemia

Leukemia is a type of cancer that interferes with blood-forming tissues (bone marrow, lymph nodes, and spleen), characterized by the production of too many immature white blood cells. Consequently, people afflicted by leukemia cannot fight infection effectively. For the most part, the causes of leukemia are unknown, although suspected risk factors have been identified.

RISK FACTORS

1. Inherited susceptibility, but not directly transmitted from parent to child.

2. An increased incidence among children with Down Syndrome (mongolism) and a few other genetic abnormalities.

3. Excessive exposure to ionizing radiation.

4. Environmental exposure to chemicals such as benzene.

PREVENTION AND WARNING SIGNALS

Detection is not easy because early symptoms may be attributed to less serious ailments. Early warning signals include: fatigue, pallor, weight loss, easy bruising, nose bleeds, paleness, loss of appetite, repeated infections, hemorrhages, night sweats, bone and joint pain, and fever. At a more advanced stage, fatigue increases, hemorrhages become more severe, pain and high fever continue, and swelling of the gums and various skin disorders occur.

Lymphomas

Lymphomas are cancers that afflict the lymphatic system, which consists of lymph nodes throughout the body and a connecting network of vessels that link these nodes. The lymphatic system participates in the body's immune reaction to foreign cells, substances, and infectious agents.

RISK FACTORS

As with leukemia, the causes of lymphomas are unknown at this time. Some researchers suspect that a particular form of herpes virus, referred to as Epstein-Barr virus, is active in the initial stages of lymphosarcomas. Other researchers hypothesize that certain external factors may alter the immune system, making it more susceptible to the development and multiplication of cancer cells.

PREVENTION AND WARNING SIGNALS

Prevention of lymphomas is limited because little is known regarding its causes. Enlargement of a lymph node or cluster of lymph nodes is the initial sign of lymphoma. Other signs and symptoms may be: an enlarged spleen or liver, weakness, fever, back or abdominal pain, nausea and/or vomiting, unexplained weight loss, unexplained itching and sweating, or fever at night that lasts for a prolonged period of time.

WHAT CAN YOU DO?

If you are at high risk for any of the cancer sites, you are advised to discuss any particular problems with your physician. An ounce of prevention is worth a pound of cure! Although cardiovascular disease is the number one killer in the country, cancer is the number one fear. Keep in mind that 60 to 80 percent of all cancer is preventable, and about 50 percent is curable. Because most cancers are lifestyle-related, awareness of the risk factors and implementation of the screening guidelines (Table 8.2), along with the basic recommendations for cancer prevention, will significantly decrease cancer risk. The main purpose of the information provided in this chapter is to educate and help you initiate your own fight against cancer.

Bibliography

American Cancer Society. *Guidelines for the Cancer-Related Checkup: Recommendations and Rationale.* New York: ACS, 1980.

American Cancer Society, Texas Division. *Cancer: Assessing Your Risk.* Dallas: ACS, 1982.

American Cancer Society. *Cancer Book.* New York: ACS, 1986.

American Cancer Society. *1988 Cancer Facts and Figures.* New York: ACS, 1988.

American Cancer Society. [Pamphlets on Facts on "Selected" Cancer Sites.] New York: ACS. (published between 1978 and 1983).

Greenwald, P. "Assessment of Risk Factors for Cancer." *Preventive Medicine* 9:260-263, 1980.

Hammond, E. C., and H. Seidman. "Smoking and Cancer in the United States." *Preventive Medicine* 9:169-173, 1980.

Higginson, J. "Proportion of Cancers Due to Occupation." *Preventive Medicine* 9:180-188, 1980.

Rothman, K. J. "The Proportion of Cancer Attributable to Alcohol Consumption." *Preventive Medicine* 9:174-179, 1980.

Weisburger, J. H., D. M. Hegsted, G. B. Gori, and B. Lewis. "Extending the Prudent Diet to Cancer Prevention." *Preventive Medicine* 9:297-304, 1980.

Williams, C. L. "Primary prevention of cancer beginning in childhood." *Preventive Medicine* 9:275-280, 1980.

Williams, P. A. "A Productive History and Physical Examination in the Prevention and Early Detection of Cancer." *Cancer* 47:1146-1150, 1981.

Figure 8.3. *Cancer profile form*

Name: _____ Date: _____

Cancer Site	Total Points		Risk Category
	Men	Women	
Lung	_____	_____	_____
Colon-Rectum	_____	_____	_____
Skin	_____	_____	_____
Breast		_____	_____
Cervical		_____	_____
Endometrial		_____	_____
Prostate	_____		_____
Testicular	_____		_____
Pancreatic	_____	_____	_____
Kidney and Bladder	_____	_____	_____
Oral	_____	_____	_____
Esophageal and Stomach	_____	_____	_____
Ovarian		_____	_____
Thyroid	_____	_____	_____
Liver	_____	_____	_____
Leukemia	_____	_____	_____
Lymphomas	_____	_____	_____

Figure 8.4. *Early warning signs of possible serious illness**

Many serious illnesses begin with apparently minor or localized symptoms that, if they are recognized early, can alert you to act in time for the disease to be cured or controlled. In most cases, of course, nothing is seriously wrong. **If you experience any of the following symptoms, discuss the problem with your physician without delay.** Check only conditions that apply.

☐ 1. Rapid loss of weight — more than about 4 kg (10 lbs) in ten weeks — without apparent cause.

☐ 2. A sore, scab, or ulcer, either in the mouth or on the body, that fails to heal within a period of about three weeks.

☐ 3. A skin blemish or mole that begins to bleed or itch, or that changes color, size, or shape.

☐ 4. Severe headaches that develop for no obvious reason.

☐ 5. Sudden attacks of vomiting, without preceding nausea.

☐ 6. Fainting spells for no apparent reason.

☐ 7. Visual problems such as seeing "haloes" around lights, or intermittently blurred vision, especially in dim light.

☐ 8. Increasing difficulty with swallowing.

☐ 9. Hoarseness without apparent cause, which lasts for a week or more.

☐ 10. A "smoker's" cough or any other nagging cough that has been getting worse.

☐ 11. Blood in coughed-up phlegm, or sputum.

☐ 12. Constantly swollen ankles.

☐ 13. A bluish tinge to the lips, the insides of the eyelids, or the nailbeds.

☐ 14. Extreme shortness of breath for no apparent reason.

☐ 15. Vomiting of blood or a substance that resembles coffee grounds.

☐ 16. Persistent indigestion or abdominal pain.

☐ 17. A marked change in normal bowel habits, such as alternating attacks of diarrhea and constipation.

☐ 18. Bowel movements that look black and tarry.

☐ 19. Rectal bleeding.

☐ 20. Unusually cloudy, pink, red, or smoky-looking urine.

☐ 21. In men, discomfort or difficulty when urinating.

☐ 22. In men, discharge from the tip of the penis.

☐ 23. In women, a lump or unusual thickening of a breast or any alteration in breast shape such as flattening, bulging, or puckering of skin.

☐ 24. In women, bleeding or unusual discharge from the nipple.

☐ 25. In women, vaginal bleeding or "spotting" that occurs between usual menstrual periods or after menopause.

*Reproduced by permission from *Family Medical Guide* by The American Medical Association. New York: Random House, 1982.

Stress Assessment
And Management Techniques

Learning to live and get ahead today is practically impossible without stress. To work under pressure has become the rule rather than the exception for most people to succeed in an unpredictable world that changes with every new day. As a result, stress has become one of the most common problems that we face. According to 1986 estimates, the annual cost of stress and stress-related diseases in the United States exceeds $100 billion — a direct result of health care costs, lost productivity, and absenteeism.

Although excessive stress is one of the factors related to twentieth-century patterns of life that is detrimental to human health, it is also a factor that can be self-controlled. Most people have accepted stress as a normal part of daily living, and even though everyone has to deal with it, few seem to understand it and know how to cope effectively. Stress should not be completely avoided; a certain amount is necessary for an optimal level of health, performance, and well-being. It is difficult to succeed and have fun in life without "hits, runs, and errors."

Just what is stress? Dr. Hans Selye, one of the foremost authorities on stress, defined stress as the nonspecific response of the human organism to any demand that is placed upon it. The term "nonspecific" indicates that the body will react in a similar fashion regardless of the nature of the event that led to the stress response. In simpler terms, stress is the mental, emotional, and physiological response of the body to any situation that is new, threatening, frightening, or exciting.

The response of the human body to stress has been the same ever since man was first put on the earth. Stress prepares the organism to react to the stress-causing event (also referred to as the stressor). The problem, though, arises from the manner in which we react to stress. Many people thrive under stress, while others under similar circumstances are unable to handle it. The individual's reaction to the particular stress-causing agent determines whether stress is positive or negative.

The way in which we react to stress has been defined by Dr. Selye as either "eustress" or "distress." In both cases, the nonspecific response is almost the same. In the case of eustress, health and performance continue to improve even as stress increases. Distress, in contrast, refers to the unpleasant or harmful stress under which health and performance begin to deteriorate. This relationship between stress and performance is illustrated in Figure 9.1.

Every person does need an optimal level of stress that is most conducive to adequate health and performance. But when stress levels reach the mental, emotional, and physiological limits, stress becomes distress and the person no longer functions effectively. Chronic distress increases the risk for many health disorders, including coronary heart disease, hypertension, eating disorders, ulcers, diabetes, asthma, depression, migraine headaches, sleep disorders, and chronic fatigue. It may even play a role in the development of certain types of cancers. Recognizing this turning point and overcoming the problem quickly and efficiently are crucial to maintain emotional and physiological stability.

Figure 9.1. *Relationship between stress and health and performance*

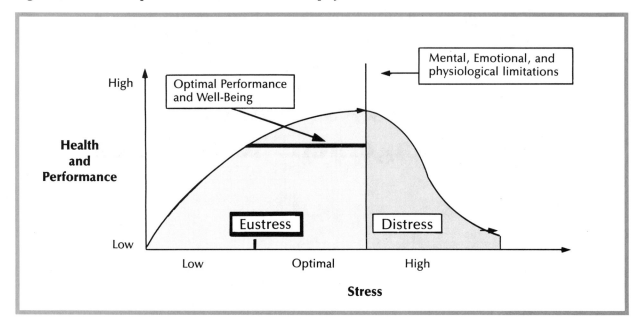

SOURCES OF STRESS

During recent years, several instruments have been developed to assess sources of stress in life. One of the most common instruments used is the Life Experiences Survey (see Figure 9.2). It identifies life changes within the last twelve months that may have an impact on a person's physical and psychological well-being. The survey is divided into two sections. Section 1 is to be completed by all respondents. This section contains a list of forty-seven life events, plus three blank spaces for other events experienced that are not listed in the survey. Section 2 contains an additional ten questions designed for students only (students should fill out both sections).

The format of the survey requires the subjects to rate the extent to which the life events that they experienced had a positive or negative impact on their life at the time they occurred. The ratings are on a seven-point scale. A rating of negative three (−3) indicates an extremely undesirable impact. A rating of zero (0) suggests neither a positive nor a negative impact. A rating of positive three (+3) indicates an extremely desirable impact. After determining the life events that have taken place, the negative and the positive points are added separately. Both scores should be expressed as positive numbers (e.g., positive ratings: 2, 1, 3, 3 = 9 points positive score; negative ratings: −3, −2, −2, −1, −2 = 10 points negative

score). A final "total life change" score can be obtained by adding both the positive score and negative score together as positive numbers (e.g., total life change score: 9 + 10 = 19 points).

Because negative as well as positive changes can produce a nonspecific response, the total life change score gives a good indication of total life stress. Most research in this area, however, indicates that the negative change score is a better predictor for potential physical or psychological illness than the total change score. More research is necessary before the role of total change and the role of the ratio of positive to negative stress can be established. Therefore, only the negative score is used as a part of the stress profile. To obtain a stress rating, refer to Table 9.1, which presents the various stress categories established for college students. Report your total number of negative points and the stress category in Figure 9.5 and in Appendix A.

BEHAVIOR PATTERNS

Common life events are not the only source of stress in life. All too often, stress is brought on by the individual as a result of behavior patterns. Individuals can be categorized as having one of two types of behavior patterns: Type A or Type B. Each type has several characteristics that are used

Figure 9.2. *The Life Experiences Survey*

Section 1		
1. Marriage		−3 −2 −1 0 +1 +2 +3
2. Detention in jail or comparable institution		−3 −2 −1 0 +1 +2 +3
3. Death of spouse		−3 −2 −1 0 +1 +2 +3
4. Major change in sleeping habits (much more or much less sleep)		−3 −2 −1 0 +1 +2 +3
5. Death of close family member:		
a. mother		−3 −2 −1 0 +1 +2 +3
b. father		−3 −2 −1 0 +1 +2 +3
c. brother		−3 −2 −1 0 +1 +2 +3
d. sister		−3 −2 −1 0 +1 +2 +3
e. grandmother		−3 −2 −1 0 +1 +2 +3
f. grandfather		−3 −2 −1 0 +1 +2 +3
g. other (specify)		−3 −2 −1 0 +1 +2 +3
6. Major change in eating habits (much more or much less food intake)		−3 −2 −1 0 +1 +2 +3
7. Foreclosure on mortgage or loan		−3 −2 −1 0 +1 +2 +3
8. Death of close friend		−3 −2 −1 0 +1 +2 +3
9. Outstanding personal achievement		−3 −2 −1 0 +1 +2 +3
10. Minor law violations (traffic tickets, disturbing the peace, etc.)		−3 −2 −1 0 +1 +2 +3
11. Male: Wife's/girlfriend's pregnancy		−3 −2 −1 0 +1 +2 +3
12. Female: Pregnancy		−3 −2 −1 0 +1 +2 +3
13. Changed work situation (different work responsibility, major change in working conditions, working hours, etc.)		−3 −2 −1 0 +1 +2 +3
14. New job		−3 −2 −1 0 +1 +2 +3
15. Serious illness or injury of close family member:		
a. father		−3 −2 −1 0 +1 +2 +3
b. mother		−3 −2 −1 0 +1 +2 +3
c. sister		−3 −2 −1 0 +1 +2 +3
d. brother		−3 −2 −1 0 +1 +2 +3
e. grandfather		−3 −2 −1 0 +1 +2 +3
f. grandmother		−3 −2 −1 0 +1 +2 +3
g. spouse		−3 −2 −1 0 +1 +2 +3
h. other (specify)		−3 −2 −1 0 +1 +2 +3
16. Sexual difficulties		−3 −2 −1 0 +1 +2 +3
17. Trouble with employer (in danger of losing job, being suspended, demoted, etc.)		−3 −2 −1 0 +1 +2 +3
18. Trouble with in-laws		−3 −2 −1 0 +1 +2 +3
19. Major change in financial status (a lot better off or a lot worse off)		−3 −2 −1 0 +1 +2 +3
20. Major change in closeness of family members (increased or decreased closeness)		−3 −2 −1 0 +1 +2 +3
21. Gaining a new family member (through birth, adoption, family member moving in, etc.)		−3 −2 −1 0 +1 +2 +3
22. Change of residence		−3 −2 −1 0 +1 +2 +3
23. Marital separation from mate (due to conflict)		−3 −2 −1 0 +1 +2 +3
24. Major change in church activities (increased or decreased attendance)		−3 −2 −1 0 +1 +2 +3
25. Marital reconciliation with mate		−3 −2 −1 0 +1 +2 +3
26. Major change in number of arguments with spouse (a lot more or a lot less arguments)		−3 −2 −1 0 +1 +2 +3
27. Married Male: Change in wife's work outside the home (beginning work, ceasing work, changing to a new job, etc.)		−3 −2 −1 0 +1 +2 +3

(continued)

From Sarason, I.G., et al. "Assessing the Impact of Life Changes: Development of the Life Experiences Survey." *Journal of Consulting and Clinical Psychology* 46:932-946, 1978. Copyright 1978 by the American Psychological Association. Reprinted by permission of the publisher and the author.

Figure 9.2. *The Life Experiences Survey (continued)*

28. Married Female: Change in husband's work (loss of job, beginning new job, retirement, etc.)	–3 –2 –1 0 +1 +2 +3
29. Major change in usual type and/or amount of recreation	–3 –2 –1 0 +1 +2 +3
30. Borrowing more than $10,000 (buying home, business, etc.)	–3 –2 –1 0 +1 +2 +3
31. Borrowing less than $10,000 (buying car, TV, getting school loan, etc.)	–3 –2 –1 0 +1 +2 +3
32. Being fired from job	–3 –2 –1 0 +1 +2 +3
33. Male: Wife/girlfriend having abortion	–3 –2 –1 0 +1 +2 +3
34. Female: Having abortion	–3 –2 –1 0 +1 +2 +3
35. Major personal illness or injury	–3 –2 –1 0 +1 +2 +3
36. Major change in social activities, e.g., parties, movies, visiting (increased or decreased participation)	–3 –2 –1 0 +1 +2 +3
37. Major change in living conditions of family (building new home, remodeling, deterioration of home, neighborhood, etc.)	–3 –2 –1 0 +1 +2 +3
38. Divorce	–3 –2 –1 0 +1 +2 +3
39. Serious injury or illness of close friend	–3 –2 –1 0 +1 +2 +3
40. Retirement from work	–3 –2 –1 0 +1 +2 +3
41. Son or daughter leaving home (due to marriage, college, etc.)	–3 –2 –1 0 +1 +2 +3
42. Ending of formal schooling	–3 –2 –1 0 +1 +2 +3
43. Separation from spouse (due to work, travel, etc.)	–3 –2 –1 0 +1 +2 +3
44. Engagement	–3 –2 –1 0 +1 +2 +3
45. Breaking up with boyfriend/girlfriend	–3 –2 –1 0 +1 +2 +3
46. Leaving home for the first time	–3 –2 –1 0 +1 +2 +3
47. Reconciliation with boyfriend/girlfriend	–3 –2 –1 0 +1 +2 +3
48. Others _____	–3 –2 –1 0 +1 +2 +3
49. _____	–3 –2 –1 0 +1 +2 +3
50. _____	–3 –2 –1 0 +1 +2 +3

Section 2

51. Beginning a new school experience at a higher academic level (college, graduate school, professional school, etc.)	–3 –2 –1 0 +1 +2 +3
52. Changing to a new school at the same academic level (undergraduate, graduate, etc.)	–3 –2 –1 0 +1 +2 +3
53. Academic probation	–3 –2 –1 0 +1 +2 +3
54. Being dismissed from dormitory or other residence	–3 –2 –1 0 +1 +2 +3
55. Failing an important exam	–3 –2 –1 0 +1 +2 +3
56. Changing a major	–3 –2 –1 0 +1 +2 +3
57. Failing a course	–3 –2 –1 0 +1 +2 +3
58. Dropping a course	–3 –2 –1 0 +1 +2 +3
59. Joining a fraternity/sorority	–3 –2 –1 0 +1 +2 +3
60. Financial problems concerning school (in danger of not having sufficient money to continue)	–3 –2 –1 0 +1 +2 +3

Table 9.1.
Stress Ratings for the Life Experiences Survey*

Category	Negative Score		Total Score	
	Men	**Women**	**Men**	**Women**
Poor	13+	15+	27+	27+
Fair	7-12	8-14	17-26	18-26
Average	6	7	16	17
Good	1-5	1-6	5-15	6-16
Excellent	0	0	1-4	1-5

*Adapted from Sarason, I. G. et al. "Assessing the Impact of Life Changes: Development of the Life Experiences Survey." *Journal of Consulting and Clinical Psychology* 46: 932-946, 1978.

in classifying people into one of these behavioral patterns. Several attempts have been made to develop an objective scale to properly identify the Type A individuals, but these questionnaires are not as valid and reliable as researchers would like them to be. Consequently, the primary assessment tool used to determine behavioral type has been the Structured Interview method.

During the Structured Interview, a person is asked to reply to questions that describe Type A and Type B behavior patterns. The interviewer notes the responses to the questions and also his/her mental, emotional, and physical behaviors while replying to each question.

Based on the answers and the behaviors exhibited, the interviewer rates the person along a continuum, ranging from Type A to Type B. Along this continuum, behavioral patterns are classified into five categories: A-1, A-2, X (a mix of Type A and Type B), B-3, and B-4. The Type A-1 exhibits all of the Type A characteristics, whereas the Type B-4 demonstrates a relative absence of the Type A behaviors. The Type A-2 does not produce a complete Type A pattern, and the Type B-3 exhibits only a few Type A characteristics.

Type A behavior is characteristic primarily of a hard-driving, overambitious, aggressive, at times hostile, and overly competitive person. These individuals often set their own goals, are self-motivated, try to accomplish many tasks at the same time, are excessively achievement-oriented, and have a high degree of time urgency. In contrast, the Type B behavior is characteristic of a calm, casual, relaxed, and easy-going individual. The Type B person takes one thing at a time, does not feel pressured or hurried, and seldom sets his/her own deadlines.

Over the years, research studies have indicated that individuals classified as Type A are under

much more stress and have a significantly higher incidence of coronary heart disease. Based on these findings, Type A individuals have been counseled to decrease their stress level by modifying many of their Type A behaviors.

Most experts agree that Type A behavior is learned. Consequently, if people can learn to identify the sources of stress and make changes in their behavioral responses, they can move down along the continuum and respond more like Type B persons. The debate, however, has centered on which Type A behaviors should be changed, because not all of them are undesirable.

Experts have known that individuals having predominantly Type A behavior are more coronary-prone and that behavioral changes are needed to decrease the risk for disease. But new scientific evidence indicates that not *all* of the typical Type A people are at a higher risk for disease. Type A individuals who commonly exhibit behaviors of anger and hostility seem to be at higher risk for disease. Therefore, many behavioral modification counselors now work primarily on changing the latter behaviors to prevent the incidence of disease.

For years it also has been known that many individuals perform well under pressure. Although they are typically classified as Type A, they do not experience any of the detrimental effects of stress. These people have recently been referred to by Drs. Robert and Marilyn Kriegel as having Type C behavior. Type C individuals are just as highly stressed as Type A but do not seem to be at higher risk for disease than Type B. The keys to successful Type C performance seem to be commitment, confidence, and control. These people are highly committed to what they are doing, have a great deal of confidence in their ability to do their work, and can be in constant control of their actions. In addition, Type C people love and enjoy their work and maintain themselves in top physical condition to be able to meet the mental and physical demands of their work.

STRESS VULNERABILITY

Researchers have now been able to identify a number of factors that can affect the way in which people handle stress. How they deal with these factors can actually increase or decrease their vulnerability to stress. The questionnaire in Figure 9.3 contains a list of these factors. It has been designed to help you determine your vulnerability quotient. The questionnaire will also help you identify particular areas in which improvements can be made to help you cope more efficiently.

As you take this test, you will notice that most of the items describe situations and behaviors that are within your own control. On the test you will rate yourself on a scale from 1 (almost always) to 5 (never), according to how each particular statement applies to you. The final stress vulnerability rating is obtained by totaling the individual ratings and subtracting 20 from the total score. Interpretation of the final score is given at the bottom of Figure 9.3. To make yourself less vulnerable to stress, modify the behaviors on which you gave yourself a rating of 3 or higher. Start by modifying those behaviors that are easiest to change before undertaking some of the most difficult ones. After completing the questionnaire, be sure to record the results on Figure 9.5 and in Appendix A.

STRESS MANAGEMENT TECHNIQUES

It is obvious that the ability to handle stress varies among individuals. If you feel that stress is definitely a problem in your life and that it is interfering with your optimal health and performance, several stress management techniques have been developed to help you cope better.

The initial step, of course, is to recognize that there is a problem. Many people either do not want to accept the fact that they are under too much stress or they fail to recognize some of the

typical symptoms of distress. Noting some of the stress-related symptoms will help you respond more objectively and initiate an adequate coping response. A list of symptoms that people experience when stress becomes distress is given in Figure 9.4. By going through this list, most of us will probably recognize some of our own bodily responses when we are confronted with a stressful event.

When people experience stress-related symptoms, initially they should try to identify and remove the stressor or stress-causing agent. This is not as simple as it may seem, because in some situations elimination of the stressor is impossible, or a person may not even know the exact causing agent. If the cause is unknown, it may be helpful to keep a log of the time and days when the symptoms occur, as well as the events that transpire before and after the onset of symptoms.

For instance, a couple had noted that every afternoon around six o'clock, the wife became very nauseated and experienced a significant amount of abdominal pain. After seeking professional help, the couple was instructed to keep a log of daily events. It soon became clear that the symptoms did not occur on weekends but always started just before the husband came home from work.

Following some personal interviews with the couple, it was determined that the wife felt a lack of attention from her husband and subconsciously responded by becoming ill to the point at which she required personal care and affection from her husband. Once the stressor is identified, appropriate changes in behavior can be initiated to correct the situation.

In many instances, however, the stressor cannot be removed. For example, the death of a close family member, the first year on the job, an intolerable boss, and a change in work responsibility, are all situations in which very little or nothing can be done to eliminate the stress-causing agent. Nevertheless, stress can be managed through the use of adequate relaxation techniques.

The body responds to stress by activating the "fight or flight" mechanism (see Figure 9.6), which prepares a person to take action by stimulating the vital defense systems. This stimulation originates in the hypothalamus and the pituitary gland in the brain. The hypothalamus activates the sympathetic nervous system, and the pituitary activates the release of catecholamines

Figure 9.3. *Stress Vulnerability Scale*

The following scale has been designed to rate your vulnerability to stress. Rate each item from 1 (almost, always) to 5 (never), according to how each particular statement applies to you. Make sure to mark each item. If a particular item doesn't apply to you, circle 1 (for example, if you don't smoke, circle 1).

Item		Score
1.	I eat at least one hot, balanced meal a day.	1 2 3 4 5
2.	I get seven to eight hours of sleep at least four nights a week.	1 2 3 4 5
3.	I give and receive affection regularly.	1 2 3 4 5
4.	I have at least one relative within fifty miles on whom I can rely.	1 2 3 4 5
5.	I exercise to the point of perspiration at least twice a week.	1 2 3 4 5
6.	I limit myself to less than half a pack of cigarettes a day.	1 2 3 4 5
7.	I take fewer than five alcoholic drinks a week.	1 2 3 4 5
8.	I am at the appropriate weight for my height.	1 2 3 4 5
9.	I have an income adequate to meet basic expenses.	1 2 3 4 5
10.	I get strength from my religious beliefs.	1 2 3 4 5
11.	I regularly attend club or social activities.	1 2 3 4 5
12.	I have a network of friends and acquaintances.	1 2 3 4 5
13.	I have one or more friends to confide in about personal matters.	1 2 3 4 5
14.	I am in good health (including eyesight, hearing, teeth).	1 2 3 4 5
15.	I am able to speak openly about my feelings when angry or worried.	1 2 3 4 5
16.	I have regular conversations with the people I live with about domestic problems — for example, chores and money.	1 2 3 4 5
17.	I do something for fun at least once a week.	1 2 3 4 5
18.	I am able to organize my time effectively.	1 2 3 4 5
19.	I drink fewer than three cups of coffee (or other caffeine-rich drinks) a day.	1 2 3 4 5
20.	I take some quiet time for myself during the day.	1 2 3 4 5

To obtain your final score, add up all of the numbers that you circled and subtract 20.

Total Score: _____ – 20 = _____ Points

Stress Vulnerability Rating

0-10 Points ....Excellent. Excellent resistance to stress
11-30 Points ....Good. Very little vulnerability to stress
31-50 Points ....Fair. Some vulnerability to stress
51-80 Points ....Poor. Seriously vulnerable to stress

Figure 9.4. *Common symptoms of stress*

☐ Headaches	☐ Dizziness
☐ Muscular aches (mainly neck, shoulders, and back)	☐ Depression
	☐ Irritation
☐ Grinding teeth	☐ Anger
☐ Nervous tic, finger tapping, toe tapping	☐ Frustration
	☐ Hostility
☐ Increased sweating	☐ Fear, panic, anxiety
☐ Increase or loss of appetite	☐ Stomach pain, flutters
☐ Insomnia	☐ Nausea
☐ Nightmares	☐ Cold, clammy hands
☐ Fatigue	☐ Poor concentration
☐ Dry Mouth	☐ Pacing
☐ Stuttering	☐ Restlessness
☐ High blood pressure	☐ Rapid heart rate
☐ Tightness or pain in the chest	☐ Low-grade infection
☐ Impotence	☐ Loss of sex drive
☐ Hives	☐ Rash or acne

Figure 9.5. *Stress Profile*

Name: _____

Date   _____   _____   _____

Life Experiences Survey

     Score (negative)   _____   _____   _____

     Stress Rating   _____   _____   _____

Stress Vulnerability Scale

     Final Score   _____   _____   _____

     Rating   _____   _____   _____

Stress Management Technique(s)
to be used   _____   _____   _____

(hormones) from the adrenal glands. These changes increase heart rate, blood pressure, blood flow to active muscles and the brain, glucose levels, oxygen consumption, and strength — all necessary for the body to "fight or flee".

For the body to relax, action must take place. If the person "fights or flees," the body relaxes and stress is dissipated, but if he/she is unable to take action, tension and tightening of the muscles increases. As noted earlier, this increased tension and tightening can be effectively dissipated with the aid of coping techniques.

The several relaxation techniques discussed below reap benefits immediately after performing a given technique, although several months of regular practice may be necessary for complete mastery. Keep in mind that relaxation exercises are not a cure-all panacea. If the exercises outlined in this chapter do not prove effective, a more specialized textbook or professional help should be obtained. In some instances the symptoms that a person is experiencing may not be caused by stress but, rather, may be related to a different medical disorder.

Figure 9.6. *Physiological response to stress: Fight or flight mechanism*

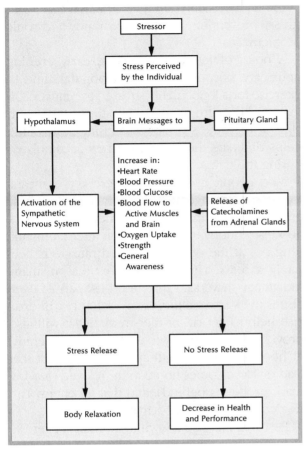

Biofeedback

Clinical application of biofeedback in the treatment of various medical disorders has become popular in the last few years. Besides its successful application in stress management, it is commonly used in the treatment of medical disorders such as essential hypertension, asthma, heart rhythm and rate disturbance, cardiac neurosis, eczematous dermatitis, fecal incontinence, insomnia, and stuttering. Biofeedback as a treatment modality has been defined as follows:[a]

A process in which a person learns to reliably influence physiological responses of two kinds: either responses which are not ordinarily under voluntary control or responses which ordinarily are easily regulated but for which regulation has broken down due to trauma or disease.

In simpler terms, biofeedback is the interaction with the interior self.[b] This interaction allows a person to learn the relationship between the mind and the biological response. The individual can actually "feel" how the thought process influences biological responses (e.g., heart rate, blood pressure, body temperature, muscle tension), and how biological responses also influence the thought process.

An illustration of this process could be the association between a strange noise in the middle of a dark, quiet night and the heart rate response. Initially, the heart rate shoots up because of the stress induced by the unknown noise. The individual may even feel the heart palpitating in the chest. While still uncertain about the noise, the person makes an attempt not to panic in order to prevent a larger increase in heart rate. Upon realizing that all is well, the person can take control and influence the heart rate to come down, or the mind is now able to exert almost complete control over the biological response.

Complex electronic instruments are usually required to conduct biofeedback. The process itself involves a three-stage closed-loop feedback system (see Figure 9.7): (a) a biological response to a stressor is detected and amplified; (b) the response is processed; and (c) the results of the response are immediately fed back to the individual. The person then uses this new input and attempts to voluntarily change the physiological response, which is, in turn, detected, amplified, and processed. The results are then fed back to the subject. The process continues with the intent of teaching the person to reliably influence for the better the physiological response.[c] The most common methods used to measure physiological responses are heart rate, finger temperature, blood pressure equipment, electromyograms, and electroencephalograms.

Although biofeedback has significant applications in the treatment of various medical disorders, including stress, it also requires adequately trained personnel and, in many cases, costly equipment. Therefore, several alternative methods that yield similar results are frequently

[a] Blanchard, E. B., and L. H. Epstein. *A Biofeedback Primer.* Reading, MA: Addison-Wesley, 1978.

[b] Brown, B. *New Mind, New Body.* New York: Harper & Row, 1974.

[c] Andrasik, F., D. Coleman, and L. H. Epstein. "Biofeedback: Clinical and Research Considerations." In *Behavioral Medicine: Assessment and Treatment Strategies.* Edited by D. M. Doleys, R. L. Meredith, and A. R. Ciminero. New York: Plenum Press, 1982.

Figure 9.7. *Biofeedback mechanism*

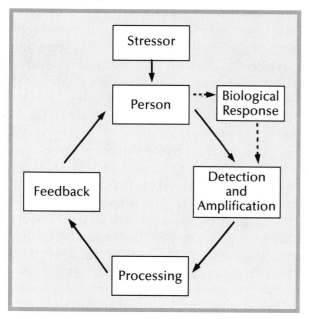

used. For example, research has shown that physical exercise and progressive muscle relaxation, used successfully in stress management, seem to be just as effective as biofeedback in treating essential hypertension.

Exercise as a Means for Stress Reduction

Physical exercise is one of the simplest tools used to control stress. The value of exercise in reducing stress is related to several factors — the principal one being a decrease in muscular tension. For example, a person can be distressed because he/she had a miserable day at work, and the job required eight hours of work in a smoke-filled room with an intolerable boss. To make matters worse, it is late and on the way home the car in front is going much slower than the speed limit. The "fight or flight" mechanism is activated, catecholamines are on the rise, heart rate and blood pressure shoot up, breathing quickens and deepens, muscles tense up, and all systems say "go." But no action can be initiated, nor stress dissipated, because you just cannot hit your boss or the car in front of you.

Instead, a person could surely take action by "hitting" the tennis ball, the weights, the swimming pool, or the jogging trail. By engaging in physical activity, a person is able to reduce the muscular tension and metabolize the increased catecholamines that brought about the physiological changes triggering the "fight or flight"

mechanism. Although exercise will not solve problems at work or take care of slow drivers on the road, it certainly can help a person cope with stress, preventing it from becoming a chronic problem.

A point of interest is that the early evening hours are becoming the most popular time to exercise for a lot of highly stressed executives. On the way home from work, they stop at the health club or the fitness center. Exercising at this time helps dissipate the excessive stress accumulated during the day.

Most people can relate to exercise as a means for stress management by remembering how good they felt the last time they concluded a good, strenuous exercise session after a difficult, long day at the office. A fatigued muscle is definitely a relaxed muscle. For this reason, many individuals have said that "the best part of exercise is the shower afterwards." Not only will exercise help to get rid of the stress, but it will also provide an opportunity to enjoy a better evening. At home, the family will appreciate the fact that Dad or Mom comes home more relaxed (leaving work problems behind), and that all energy can be dedicated to family activities.

Research has also shown that physical exercise requiring continuous and rhythmic muscular activity, such as aerobic exercise, stimulates alpha-wave activity in the brain. These are the same wave patterns commonly seen during periods of meditation and relaxation. Furthermore, during vigorous aerobic exercise lasting thirty minutes or longer, morphine-like substances called endorphins are released from the pituitary gland in the brain. These substances have been known to act not only as painkillers, but they also seem to induce the soothing, calming effect often associated with aerobic exercise.

Another way that exercise helps in reducing stress is by deliberately diverting stress to various body systems. In his book *Stress Without Distress*, Dr. Hans Selye explains that when accomplishing one specific task becomes difficult, a change in activity can be as good or better than rest itself. For example, if a person is having a difficult time with a certain task and does not seem to be getting anywhere, it is better to go jogging or swimming for a while than to sit around and get frustrated. In this manner, the mental strain is diverted to the working muscles, and the one system helps the other to relax.

Another psychologist, Dr. William James, has indicated that when muscular tension is removed from the emotional strain, the emotional strain disappears. In many cases, the change of activity will suddenly clear the mind and help put the pieces together.

Other researchers have found that physical exercise gives people a psychological boost because exercise can (a) reduce feelings of anxiety, depression, frustration, aggression, anger, and hostility; (b) decrease insomnia; (c) provide an opportunity to meet social needs and develop new friendships; (d) allow the person to share common interests and problems; (e) develop discipline; and (f) provide the opportunity to do something enjoyable and constructive that will lead to better health and total well-being.

Beyond the short-term benefits of exercise in reducing stress, another important benefit of a regular aerobic exercise program is the actual strengthening of the cardiovascular system itself. Because the cardiovascular system seems to be most seriously affected by stress, a stronger system should be able to cope more effectively. Good cardiovascular endurance has been shown, for instance, to decrease resting heart rate and blood pressure. Because both heart rate and blood pressure rise in stressful situations, initiating the stress response at a lower baseline will decrease the negative effects of stress. There is little argument that cardiovascularly fit individuals can cope more effectively and are less affected by the stresses of daily living.

Progressive Muscle Relaxation

Progressive muscle relaxation was developed by Dr. Edmund Jacobsen in the 1930s. This technique enables individuals to relearn the sensation of deep relaxation. The technique involves progressive contraction and relaxation of muscle groups throughout the body. Because chronic stress leads to high levels of muscular tension, being closely aware of how it feels to progressively tighten and relax the muscles will release the tension on the muscles and teach the body to relax at will. Being aware of the tension felt during the exercises also helps the person be more alert to signs of distress, because similar feelings are experienced in stressful situations. In everyday life, such feelings can then be used as a cue to implement adequate relaxation exercises.

Relaxation exercises should be conducted in a quiet, warm, well-ventilated room. The recommended exercises and the duration of the routine vary from one author to the next. The important consideration, however, is that the individual pays attention to the sensation felt each time the muscles are tensed and relaxed. The exercises should include all muscle groups of the body. An example of a sequence of progressive muscle relaxation exercises is given below. The instructions for these exercises can be read to the person or memorized or tape-recorded. At least twenty minutes should be set aside to perform the entire sequence. Doing the exercises any faster will defeat their purpose. Ideally, the sequence should be performed twice a day.

The individual performing the exercises must stretch out comfortably on the floor, face up, with a pillow under the knees, and should assume a passive attitude, allowing the body to relax as much as possible. He/she should contract each muscle group in sequence, taking care to avoid any strain. Muscles should be tightened only to about 70 percent of the total possible tension to avoid cramping or some type of injury to the muscle itself. Paying attention to the sensation of tensing up and relaxing is most crucial to produce the relaxation effects. Each contraction is held for about five seconds, and then the muscles are allowed to go totally limp. Sufficient time should be taken to allow for contraction and relaxation before proceeding to the next. The following list of statements given to the participant is an example of a complete progressive muscle relaxation sequence:

1. Point your feet, curling the toes downward, and study the tension in the arches and the top of the feet. Hold this and continue to note the tension, then relax. Repeat a second time.

2. Flex the feet upward toward the face and note the tension in your feet and calves. Hold it . . . and relax. . . . Repeat.

3. Push your heels down against the floor as if burying them in the sand. Hold this and note the tension on the back of the thigh; relax. Repeat one more time.

4. Contract the right thigh by straightening the leg, gently raising the leg off the floor. Hold, and study the tension; relax. . . . Repeat with the left leg; hold and relax. Repeat both legs.

5. Tense the buttocks by raising your hips ever so slightly off the floor. Hold, and note the tension; relax. . . . Repeat.

6. Contract the abdominal muscles. Hold them tight and note the tension; relax. . . . Repeat.

7. Suck in your stomach — try to make it reach your spine. Flatten your lower back to the floor; hold and feel the tension in the stomach and lower back; relax... Repeat.

8. Take a deep breath and hold it . . . then exhale. Repeat. Note your breathing becoming slower and more relaxed.

9. Place your arms on the side of your body and clench both fists. Hold . . . study the tension, and relax. . . . Repeat.

10. Flex the elbow by bringing both hands to the shoulders. Hold this tight and study the tension in the biceps; relax. . . . Repeat.

11. Place your arms flat on the floor, palms up, and push the forearm hard against the floor. Note the tension on the triceps; hold . . . and relax. . . . Repeat the exercise.

12. Shrug your shoulders, raising them as high as possible. Hold and note the tension; relax. . . . Repeat.

13. Gently push your head backward; note the tension in the back of the neck. Hold . . . relax. . . . Repeat.

14. Gently bring the head against the chest, push forward, hold, and note the tension in the neck. Relax. . . . Repeat a second time.

15. Press your tongue toward the roof of your mouth. Hold . . . study the tension; relax. . . Repeat.

16. Press your teeth together. Hold and study the tension; relax. . . . Repeat.

17. Close your eyes tightly. Hold them closed and note the tension. Relax, leaving your eyes closed. Repeat.

18. Wrinkle your forehead. Note the tension; hold . . . and relax. . . . Repeat.

In instances during the daily routine when time is a factor and an individual is not able to go through the entire sequence, only the exercises specific to the area where muscle tension is felt may be performed. Just performing a few exercises is better than none at all. Nevertheless, completing the entire sequence yields the best results.

Breathing Techniques for Relaxation

Breathing exercises can also be used as an antidote to stress. Such exercises have been used for centuries in the Orient and India as a means to develop better mental, physical, and emotional stamina. In breathing exercises, the person concentrates on "breathing away" the tension and inhaling fresh oxygen to the entire body.

Breathing exercises, which can be learned in only a few minutes, require considerably less time than the progressive muscle relaxation exercises. As with any other relaxation technique, a quiet, pleasant, and well-ventilated room should be used to perform the exercise. Three examples of breathing exercises are presented here. Any of these may be performed whenever tension is felt due to stress.

1. *Deep breathing:* Lie with your back flat against the floor; place a pillow under your knees, feet slightly separated, with toes pointing outward (the exercise may also be conducted sitting up in a chair or standing straight up). Place one hand on your abdomen and the other one on your chest. Slowly breathe in and out so that the hand on your abdomen rises when you inhale and falls as you exhale. The hand on the chest should not move much at all. Repeat the exercise about ten times. Next, scan your body for tension, and compare your present tension with that felt at the beginning of the exercise. Repeat the entire process once or twice more.

2. *Sighing:* Using the abdominal breathing technique, breathe in through your nose to a specific count (e.g., 4, 5, 6, etc.). Now exhale through pursed lips to double the intake count (e.g., 8, 10, 12, etc.). Repeat the exercise eight to ten times whenever you feel tense.

3. *Complete natural breathing:* Sit in an upright position or stand straight up. Breathe through your nose and gradually fill your lungs from the bottom up. Hold your breath for several seconds. Now exhale slowly by allowing complete relaxation of the chest and abdomen. Repeat the exercise eight to ten times.

Autogenic Training

Autogenic training is basically a form of self-suggestion, wherein an individual is able to place himself/herself in an autohypnotic state by repeating and concentrating on feelings of heaviness and warmth in the extremities. This technique was developed by Johannes H. Schultz, a German psychiatrist, who noted that hypnotized individuals developed sensations of warmth and heaviness in the limbs and torso. The sensation of warmth is caused by dilation of blood vessels, which increases blood flow to the limbs. The heaviness is felt as a result of muscular relaxation.

When using this technique, the person lies down or sits down in a comfortable position with eyes closed and progressively concentrates on six fundamental stages:

1. **Heaviness**

   My right (left) arm is heavy
   Both arms are heavy
   My right (left) leg is heavy
   Both legs are heavy
   My arms and legs are heavy

2. **Warmth**

   My right (left) arm is warm
   Both arms are warm
   My right (left) leg is warm
   Both legs are warm
   My arms and legs are warm

3. **Heart**

   My heartbeat is calm and regular (repeat four or five times)

4. **Respiration**

   My body breathes itself (repeat four or five times)

5. **Abdomen**

   My abdomen is warm (repeat four or five times)

6. **Forehead**

   My forehead is cool (repeat four or five times)

The autogenic training technique is more difficult to master than any of those previously mentioned. The individual should not move too fast through the entire exercise, because this practice may actually interfere with the learning and relaxation process. Each stage must be mastered before proceeding to the next one.

Meditation

Meditation is a mental exercise that can bring about psychological and physical benefits. The objective of meditation is to gain control over your attention, clearing the mind and blocking out the stressor(s) responsible for the increased tension. This technique, which can also be learned rather quickly, can be used frequently during periods of increased tension and stress.

Initially, the person who is trying to learn to meditate should choose a room that is comfortable, quiet, and free of all disturbances (including telephones). Once the technique is learned, however, the person will be able to meditate just about anywhere. Approximately fifteen minutes, twice a day, are needed to meditate.

1. Sit in a chair in an upright position with the hands resting either in your lap or on the arms of the chair. Close your eyes and focus on your breathing. Allow your body to relax as much as possible. Do not try to consciously relax, because trying means work. Rather, assume a passive attitude and concentrate on your breathing.

2. Allow the body to breathe regularly, at its own rhythm, and repeat in your mind the word "one" every time you inhale and the word "two" every time you exhale. Paying attention to these two words keeps distressing thoughts from entering your mind.

3. Continue to breathe for about fifteen minutes. Because the objective of meditation is to bring about a hypometabolic state, leading to body relaxation, do not use an alarm clock to remind you that the fifteen minutes have expired. The alarm will only trigger your stress response again, defeating the purpose of the exercise. It is fine to open your eyes once in a while to keep track of the time. But remember not to rush or anticipate the end of the fifteen minutes. This time has been set aside for meditation and you need to relax, take your time, and enjoy the exercise.

Which Technique is Best?

Each person reacts to stress in a different way. Therefore, the coping strategy used will depend mostly on the individual. It does not really matter which technique is used as long as it works. An individual may want to experiment with all of them to find out which works best. The person may also use a combination of two or more. All of the coping strategies discussed help to block out the stressor(s) and lead to mental and physical relaxation by diverting the attention to a different, nonthreatening action. Some of the techniques are easier to learn and may take less time per session.

Regardless of which technique is selected, when stress becomes a significant problem in life, the time spent performing stress management exercises is well worth the effort. People need to learn to "relax" and take time out for themselves. As noted earlier, it is not stress that makes people ill but, rather, the way in which they react to the particular stress-causing agent. Individuals who learn to be diligent and start taking control of themselves find out that they can enjoy a better, happier, and healthier life.

Bibliography

Andrasik, F., D. Coleman, and L. H. Epstein. "Biofeedback: Clinical and Research Considerations." In *Behavioral Medicine: Assessment and Treatment Strategies.* Edited by D. M. Doleys, R. L. Meredith, and A. R. Ciminero. New York: Plenum Press, 1982.

Blanchard, E. B., and L. H. Epstein. *A Biofeedback Primer.* Reading, MA: Addison-Wesley, 1978.

Blue Cross Association. *Stress.* Chicago: Association, 1974.

Brown, B. *New Mind, New Body.* New York: Harper & Row, 1974.

Chesney, M. A., J. R. Eagleston, and R. H. Roseman. "Type A Assessment and Intervention." In *Medical Psychology: Contributions to Behavioral Medicine.* Edited by C. K. Prokop and L. A. Bradley. New York: Academic Press, 1981.

Gauron, E. F. *Mental Training for Peak Performance.* Lansing, NY: Sport Science Associates, 1984.

Girdano, D., and G. Everly. *Controlling Stress and Tension: A Holistic Approach.* Englewood Cliffs, NJ: Prentice-Hall, 1986.

Greenberg, J. S. *Comprehensive Stress Management.* Dubuque, IA: Wm. C. Brown, 1983.

Kriegel, R. J., and M. H. Kriegel. *The C Zone: Peak Performance Under Stress.* Garden City, NY: Anchor Press/Doubleday, 1984.

Luthe, W. "Autogenic Training: Method, Research and Applications in Medicine." *American Journal of Psychotherapy* 17:174-195, 1963.

McKay, M., M. Davis, and P. Fanning. *Thoughts and Feelings: The Act of Cognitive Stress Intervention.* Richmond, CA: New Harbinger Publications, 1981.

Miller, L. H., and A. D. Smith. "Vulnerability Scale." Stress Audit, 1983.

Sarason, I. G., J. H. Johnson, and J. M. Siegel. "Assessing the Impact of Life Changes: Development of the Life Experiences Survey." *Journal of Consulting and Clinical Psychology* 46:932- 946, 1978.

Selye, H. *Stress Without Distress.* New York: Signet, 1974.

Selye, H. *The Stress of Life.* New York: McGraw-Hill, 1978.

Staff. "How Running Relieves Stress." *The Runner* 8(11):38-43, 82, 1986.

Turk, D. C., and R. D. Kerns. "Assessment in Health Psychology: A Cognitive-Behavioral Perspective." In *Measurement Strategies in Health Psychology,* edited by P. Karoly. New York: John Wiley & Sons, 1985.

Smoking Cessation

Tobacco has been used throughout the world for hundreds of years. Prior to the eighteenth century it was smoked primarily in the form of pipes or cigars. Cigarette smoking did not become popular until the mid-1800s, and its use started to increase dramatically at the turn of the century. In 1915, 18 billion cigarettes were consumed in the United States, as compared to 640 billion in 1981. Now more than 50 million Americans over the age of seventeen smoke an average of one and one-half packs of cigarettes per day.

The harmful effects of cigarette smoking and tobacco usage in general were not exactly known until the early 1960s, when researchers began to show a positive link between tobacco use and disease. In 1964, the United States Surgeon General issued the first major report presenting scientific evidence that cigarettes were indeed a major health hazard in our society.

Tobacco use in all forms is now considered a significant threat to life. Cigarette smoking is the largest preventable cause of illness and premature death in the United States. When considering all related deaths, smoking is responsible for more than 300,000 unnecessary deaths each year. There is a definite increase in death rates from heart disease, cancer, stroke, aortic aneurysm, chronic bronchitis, emphysema, and peptic ulcers. Maternal cigarette smoking has been linked to retarded fetal growth, increased risk for spontaneous abortion, and prenatal death. Smoking is also the most common cause of deaths and injuries from fire. The average life expectancy for a chronic smoker is seven years less than for a nonsmoker, and the death rate among chronic smokers during the most productive years of

life — between the ages of twenty-five and sixty-five — is twice that of the national average. Figure 10.1 shows the manifestations of emphysema.

According to American Heart Association estimates, 120,000 fatal heart attacks annually are attributed to smoking. Heart attack risk is 50 to 100 percent greater for smokers than nonsmokers. There is also an increased mortality rate following heart attacks, because they are usually more severe and the risk for deadly arrhythmias is much greater. Cigarette smoking affects the cardiovascular system by increasing heart rate, blood pressure, susceptibility to atherosclerosis, and blood clots. Evidence also indicates that it decreases high-density lipoprotein cholesterol, the "good" cholesterol that lessens the risk for heart disease. Finally, carbon monoxide in smoke decreases the oxygen delivery capacity of the blood to tissues of the body.

The American Cancer Society reports that 83 percent of lung cancer and 30 percent of all cancers result from smoking. It kills about 148,000

Figure 10.1. *Normal lung and diseased lung in emphysema*

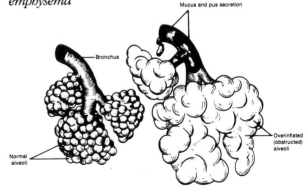

Figure 10.2. *Normal lung (left) and diseased lung (right). The white growth near the top is cancer; the dark appearance on the bottom half is emphysema*

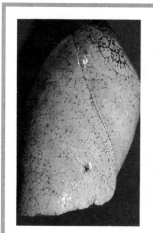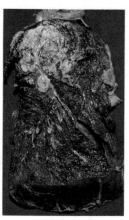

Reproduced by permission from "If You Smoke" slide show by Gordon Hewlett.

people each year. Lung cancer is the leading cancer killer; it is responsible for 30 percent of all cancer deaths. Although it is encouraging to note that over 50 percent of all cancers are now curable, the five-year survival rate for lung cancer is less than 10 percent. Tobacco usage also increases cancer risk of the oral cavity, larynx, esophagus, bladder, pancreas, and kidneys.

Even though many tobacco users often are aware of the health consequences of cigarette smoking, many fail to realize the risk of pipe smoking, cigar smoking, and tobacco chewing. As a group in general, the risk for heart disease and lung cancer is lower than for cigarette smokers. Nevertheless, blood nicotine levels in pipe and cigar smokers have been shown to approach those of cigarette smokers, because nicotine is absorbed through the membranes of the mouth. Therefore, there is still a higher risk for heart disease, as compared to nonsmokers. Cigarette smokers who substitute pipe or cigar smoking for cigarettes usually continue to inhale the smoke, which actually results in a greater amount of nicotine and tar being brought into the lungs. Consequently, the risk for disease is even greater if pipe or cigar smoke is inhaled. The risk and mortality rates for lip, mouth, and larynx cancer for pipe smoking, cigar smoking, or tobacco chewing are actually higher than for cigarette smoking.

The economical impact of cigarette smoking among American business and industry is also staggering. Companies pay in excess of $16 billion each year as a direct result of smoking in the workplace and another $37 billion in lost productivity and earnings because of illness, disability, and death. Heavy smokers have been shown to use the health care system, especially hospitals, over 50 percent more than nonsmokers. The yearly cost to a given company has been estimated between $624 and $4,611 per smoking employee. These costs include employee health care, absenteeism, additional health insurance, morbidity/disability and early mortality, on-the-job lost time, property damage/maintenance and depreciation, Workmen's Compensation, and involuntary smoking impact.

In spite of the fact that the ill effects of tobacco have been well-documented, not enough is being done to decrease and eradicate its use. Consider the following example. In the summer of 1985, over 1,500 people died around the world in major airplane accidents. These accidents resulted in a tremendous amount of worldwide media attention, and planes were grounded for safety reasons. Now imagine what the coverage and concern would be if 300,000 people each year died in the United States alone because of airplane accidents. People would not even consider flying anymore. Most individuals would think of it as a form of suicide.

Similarly, think of the public outrage if close to 300,000 Americans were to die annually in a meaningless war, or if a single nonprescription drug would cause over 138,000 cancer deaths and 120,000 fatal heart attacks. The American public would never tolerate such situations. We would probably mount a very intense fight to prevent these deaths. Yet, are we not committing a form of slow suicide by smoking cigarettes? Isn't tobacco actually a nonprescription drug available to almost anyone who wishes to smoke — killing in excess of 300,000 people each year?

We may ask ourselves: Why isn't there a greater campaign against all forms of tobacco use? There are primarily two reasons. First, it is extremely difficult to fight an industry that has as great a financial and political influence as the tobacco industry has in the United States. The tobacco industry produces 2.5 percent of the Gross National Product and has cleverly influenced elections by emphasizing the individual's right to smoke, avoiding the fact that so many people die because of its use. Second, tobacco had been socially accepted for so many years that many people just learned to live with it.

Also known is the fact that the biggest carcinogenic exposure in the workplace is cigarette smoke. For the first time, in the 1980s, however, cigarette smoking is no longer acceptable in many social circles. Nonsmokers and ex-smokers alike are fighting for their right to clean air and health. Estimates have indicated that if every smoker were to give up cigarettes, in one year alone sick time would be decreased by approximately 90 million days; there would be 280,000 fewer heart conditions and 1 million fewer cases of chronic bronchitis and emphysema; and total death rates from cardiovascular disease, cancer, and peptic ulcers would drastically decrease.

It is also interesting to note that many smokers are really unaware or simply do not care to realize how much cigarette smoke bothers nonsmokers. These smokers believe that it is not really that bad, and if they can put up with it, it should not bother nonsmokers that much. In most instances, they think that blowing the smoke off to the side is sufficient to get it out of the way. As a matter of fact, it is not enough. Smokers do not comprehend this until they quit and later find themselves in such situations. At times, ex-smokers are bothered even by someone else smoking several yards away and all of a sudden come to realize why cigarette smoke is so unpleasant and undesirable to most people.

WHY DO PEOPLE SMOKE?

In most instances, people begin to smoke without realizing the detrimental effects of tobacco on their health and life in general. Although people start to smoke for many different reasons, the three fundamental causes are peer pressure, the desire to appear "grown up," and rebellion against authority. Unfortunately, it takes only three packs of cigarettes to develop the physiological addiction, turning it into a "nasty habit" that has become the most widespread example of drug dependency in the country.

When tobacco leaves are burned, hot air and gases containing nicotine and tar (chemical compounds) are released in the smoke. Over 1,200 toxic chemicals have been found in tobacco smoke. Tar contains about thirty chemical compounds that are proven carcinogens. The drug nicotine has strong addictive properties. Within seconds of inhalation, nicotine affects the central nervous system and can act as both a tranquilizer and a stimulant. The stimulating effect produces strong physiological and psychological dependency. The addiction to nicotine is six to eight times greater than for alcohol and most likely greater than for some of the hard drugs currently used around the world.

The psychological dependency is developed over a longer period of time. Not only do people smoke to help themselves relax, but a certain amount of pleasure is also involved with the ritual of smoking. Smokers automatically associate many activities in daily life with cigarettes. Activities such as coffee drinking, alcohol drinking, social gatherings, a meal aftermath, talking on the telephone, driving, reading, and watching television can make habitual smokers crave cigarettes. In many cases, the social rituals of smoking are the most difficult to eliminate. This psychological dependency is so strong that even years after individuals have stopped smoking, they still crave cigarettes when they engage in some of the aforementioned activities.

Most people smoke for a variety of reasons. To find out why people smoke, a simple "Why-Do-You-Smoke Test" was developed by the National Clearinghouse for Smoking and Health (see Figure 10.3). The scores obtained on this test will give an indication on each of six factors that describe people's feelings when they smoke. The first three factors point out the positive feelings that people get from smoking. The fourth factor aids them in tension reduction and relaxation. The fifth shows their dependence on cigarettes. The last factor indicates habitual smoking or purely automatic smoking.

WHY-DO-YOU-SMOKE TEST

The "Why-Do-You-Smoke Test" contained in Figure 10.3 lists some statements people have made to describe what they get out of smoking cigarettes. Smokers should indicate how often they experience the feelings described in each statement when smoking by circling one number for each statement. It is important to answer every

Figure 10.3. *Why-Do-You-Smoke Test*

	Always	Fre-quently	Occa-sionally	Seldom	Never
A. I smoke cigarettes in order to keep myself from slowing down.	5	4	3	2	1
B. Handling a cigarette is part of the enjoyment of smoking it.	5	4	3	2	1
C. Smoking cigarettes is pleasant and relaxing.	5	4	3	2	1
D. I light up a cigarette when I feel angry about something.	5	4	3	2	1
E. When I have run out of cigarettes I find it almost unbearable until I can get them.	5	4	3	2	1
F. I smoke cigarettes automatically without even being aware of it.	5	4	3	2	1
G. I smoke cigarettes to stimulate me, to perk myself up.	5	4	3	2	1
H. Part of the enjoyment of smoking a cigarette comes from the steps I take to light up.	5	4	3	2	1
I. I find cigarettes pleasurable.	5	4	3	2	1
J. When I feel uncomfortable or upset about something, I light up a cigarette.	5	4	3	2	1
K. I am very much aware of the fact when I am not smoking a cigarette.	5	4	3	2	1
L. I light up a cigarette without realizing I still have one burning in the ashtray.	5	4	3	2	1
M. I smoke cigarettes to give me a "lift."	5	4	3	2	1
N. When I smoke a cigarette, part of the enjoyment is watching the smoke as I exhale it.	5	4	3	2	1
O. I want a cigarette most when I am comfortable and relaxed.	5	4	3	2	1
P. When I feel "blue" or want to take my mind off cares and worries, I smoke cigarettes.	5	4	3	2	1
Q. I get a real gnawing hunger for a cigarette when I haven't smoked for a while.	5	4	3	2	1
R. I've found a cigarette in my mouth and didn't remember putting it there.	5	4	3	2	1

Scoring Your Test:

Enter the numbers you have circled on the test questions in the spaces provided below, putting the number you have circled to question A on line A, to question B on line B, etc. Add the three scores on each line to get a total for each factor. For example, the sum of you scores over lines A, G, and M gives you your score on "Stimulation," lines B, H, and N give the score on "Handling," etc. Scores can vary from 3 to 15. Any score 11 and above is high; any score 7 and below is low.

A _____ + G _____ + M _____ = _____ Stimulation
B _____ + H _____ + N _____ = _____ Handling
C _____ + I _____ + O _____ = _____ Pleasure Relaxation
D _____ + J _____ + P _____ = _____ Crutch: Tension Reduction
E _____ + K _____ + Q _____ = _____ Craving: Psychological Addiction
F _____ + L _____ + R _____ = _____ Habit

From *A Self-Test for Smokers.* U.S. Department of Health and Human Services, 1983.

question. This test, as well as much of the remaining information in this chapter, is presented in the same format as it is given to smokers.

The "Why-Do-You-Smoke Test" examines reasons why you smoke. A score of 11 or above on any factor indicates that it is an important source of satisfaction for you. The higher you score (15 is the highest), the more important a particular factor is in your smoking and the more useful the discussion of that factor can be in your attempt to quit.

If you do not score high on any of the six factors, chances are that you do not smoke very much or have not been smoking for very many years. If so, giving up smoking — and staying off — should be fairly easy.

1. *Stimulation.* If you score high or fairly high on this factor, it means that you are one of those smokers who is stimulated by the cigarette. You feel that it helps wake you up, organize your energies, and keep you going. If you try to give up smoking, you may want a safe substitute — a brisk walk or moderate exercise, for example — whenever you feel the urge to smoke.

2. *Handling.* Handling things can be satisfying, but there are many ways to keep your hands busy without lighting up or playing with a cigarette. Why not toy with a pen or pencil? Or try doodling. Or play with a coin, a piece of jewelry, or some other harmless object.

3. *Accentuation of pleasure — pleasurable relaxation.* It is not always easy to find out whether you use cigarettes to feel good, that is get real, honest pleasure out of smoking or to keep from feeling bad (Factor 4). About two-thirds of smokers score high or fairly high on accentuation of pleasure, and about half of those also score as high or higher on reduction of negative feelings.

   Those who do get real pleasure out of smoking often find that an honest consideration of the harmful effects of their habit is enough to help them quit. They substitute social and physical activities and find that they do not seriously miss their cigarettes.

4. *Reduction of negative feelings, or "crutch."* Many smokers use the cigarette as a kind of crutch in moments of stress or discomfort. But the heavy smoker — the person who tries to handle severe personal problems by smoking many times a day — is apt to discover that cigarettes do not help in dealing with problems effectively.

   When it comes to quitting, this kind of smoker may find it easy to stop when everything is going well but may be tempted to start again in a time of crisis. Again, physical exertion or social activity may serve as a useful substitute for cigarettes, even in times of tension.

5. *"Craving" or dependence.* Quitting smoking is difficult for the person who scores high on this factor. For the addicted smoker, the craving for a cigarette begins to build up the moment the cigarette is put out, so tapering off is not likely to work. This smoker must go "cold turkey."

   If you are dependent on cigarettes, it may be helpful for you to smoke more than usual for a day or two, so that the taste for cigarettes is spoiled, and then isolate yourself completely from cigarettes until the craving is gone.

6. *Habit.* If you are smoking out of habit, you no longer get much satisfaction from your cigarettes. You just light them frequently without even realizing you are doing so. You may find it easy to quit and stay off if you can break the habitual patterns that you have built up. Cutting down gradually may be effective if you change the way you smoke the cigarettes and the conditions under which you smoked them. The key to success is becoming aware of each cigarette you smoke. This can be done by asking yourself, "Do I really want this cigarette?" You may be surprised at how many you do not want.

SMOKING CESSATION

Quitting cigarette smoking is no easy task. Only about 20 percent of smokers who try to quit for the first time each year succeed. The addictive properties of nicotine and smoke make it very difficult to quit. The American Psychiatric Association and the National Institute on Drug Abuse have indicated that nicotine is perhaps the most addictive drug known to man. Smokers develop tolerance to nicotine and smoke. They become dependent on both and experience physical and psychological withdrawal symptoms when they stop smoking. Although giving up smoking can be extremely difficult, cessation is by no means an impossible task.

Cigarette smoking is now a declining habit in the country. During the last several years there has been a gradual decrease among smokers of all ages with the exception of young women. Surveys have shown that between 75 and 90 percent of all smokers would like to quit.

Forty percent of the adult population — 53 percent of men and 32 percent women — smoked in 1964 when the U. S. Surgeon General first reported the link between smoking and increased risk for disease and mortality. By 1986, approximately 40 million Americans had given up cigarettes. An additional 2 million quit each year. A 1986 poll by the National Centers for Disease Control indicated that only 26.5 percent of adult Americans smoked — 29.5 percent of the men and 23.8 percent of the women. This percentage is the lowest ever reported, down from 37 percent in 1980 and 30.4 percent in 1985.

More than 95 percent of the successful ex-smokers have been able to do it on their own, either by quitting cold turkey or by using self-help kits available from organizations such as the American Cancer Society, the American Heart Association, and the American Lung Association. Only 3 percent of ex-smokers have done so as a result of formal cessation programs. Smoker's Information and Treatment Centers are commonly listed in the yellow pages of the telephone book.

DO-YOU-WANT-TO-QUIT TEST

The most important factor in quitting cigarette smoking is the person's sincere desire to do so. Some smokers can simply quit, but in most instances such is not the case. Those who can easily quit are primarily light or casual smokers. They realize that the pleasure of an occasional cigarette is not worth the added risk for disease and premature death. For heavy smokers, cessation will most likely be a difficult battle. Although many do not succeed the first time around, the odds of quitting are much greater for those who repeatedly try to stop.

To find out a smoker's preparedness to initiate a cessation program, the "Do-You-Want-To-Quit

Test" contained in Figure 10.4, also developed by the National Clearinghouse for Smoking and Health, will measure a person's attitude toward the four primary reasons why people want to quit smoking. The results will give an indication of whether the person is really ready to start the program.

On this test, the higher you score in any category, say health, the more important that reason is to you. A score of nine or above in one of these categories indicates that this is one of the most important reasons why you may want to quit.

1. *Health.* Knowing the harmful consequences of cigarettes, many people have stopped smoking and many others are considering it. If your score on the health factor is 9 or above, the health hazards of smoking may be enough to make you want to quit now.

   If your score on this factor is low (6 or less), look over the hazards of smoking. You may be lacking important information or may even have incorrect information. If so, health considerations are not playing the important role that they should in your decision to keep smoking or to quit.

2. *Example.* Some people stop smoking because they want to set a good example for others. Parents quit to make it easier for their children to resist starting to smoke, doctors to influence their patients, teachers to help their students, sports stars to set an example for their young fans, husbands to influence their wives, and vice versa.

   Such examples are an important influence on our behavior. Research shows that almost twice as many high school students smoke if both parents are smokers, as compared to those whose parents are nonsmokers or former smokers.

   If your score is low (6 or less), it may mean that you are not interested in giving up smoking in order to set an example for others. Perhaps you do not appreciate how important your example could be.

3. *Aesthetics* (the unpleasant aspects). People who score high (9 or above) in this category recognize and are disturbed by some of the unpleasant aspects of smoking. The smell of stale smoke on their clothing, bad breath, and stains on their fingers and teeth might be reason enough to consider breaking the habit.

Figure 10.4. *Do-You-Want-To-Quit Test.*

	Strongly Agree	Mildly Agree	Mildly Disagree	Strongly Disagree
A. Cigarette smoking might give me a serious illness.	4	3	2	1
B. My cigarette smoking sets a bad example for others.	4	3	2	1
C. I find cigarette smoking to be a messy kind of habit.	4	3	2	1
D. Controlling my cigarette smoking is a challenge to me.	4	3	2	1
E. Smoking causes shortness of breath.	4	3	2	1
F. If I quit smoking cigarettes, it might influence others to stop.	4	3	2	1
G. Cigarettes cause damage to clothing and other personal property.	4	3	2	1
H. Quitting smoking would show that I have willpower.	4	3	2	1
I. My cigarette smoking will have a harmful effect on my health.	4	3	2	1
J. My cigarette smoking influences others close to me to take up or continue smoking.	4	3	2	1
K. If I quit smoking, my sense of taste or smell will improve.	4	3	2	1
L. I do not like the idea of feeling dependent on smoking.	4	3	2	1

Scoring Your Test:

Write the number you have circled after each statement on the test in the corresponding space to the right. Add the scores on each line to get your totals. For example, the sum of your scores A, E, I gives you your score for the health factor. Scores can vary from 3 to 12. Any score of 9 or over is high; and score 6 or under is low.

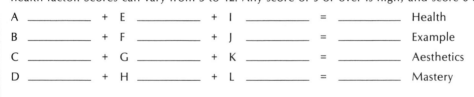

A _____ + E _____ + I _____ = _____ Health
B _____ + F _____ + J _____ = _____ Example
C _____ + G _____ + K _____ = _____ Aesthetics
D _____ + H _____ + L _____ = _____ Mastery

From *A Self-Test for Smokers.* U.S. Department of Health and Human Services, 1983.

4. *Mastery* (self-control). If you score 9 or above on this factor, you are bothered by the knowledge that you cannot control your desire to smoke. You are not your own master. Awareness of this challenge to your self-control may make you want to quit.

BREAKING THE HABIT

The following seven-step plan has been developed as a guide to help you quit smoking. The total program should be completed in four weeks or less. Steps one through four should take no longer than two weeks. A maximum of two additional weeks are allowed for the rest of the program.

Step One

The first step in breaking the habit is to decide positively that you want to quit. Avoid negative thoughts of how difficult this can be. Think positive. You can do it. Now prepare a list of the reasons why you smoke and why you want to quit (see Figure 10.5). Make several copies of the list and keep them in places where you commonly smoke. Review the reasons for quitting frequently,

Figure 10.5. *Reasons for smoking versus quitting*

Name: _____ Date: _____

Reasons for Smoking Cigarettes

1. _____
2. _____
3. _____
4. _____
5. _____
6. _____
7. _____
8. _____

Reasons for Quitting Cigarette Smoking

1. _____
2. _____
3. _____
4. _____
5. _____
6. _____
7. _____
8. _____

as this will motivate and psychologically prepare you for cessation. When the reasons for quitting outweigh the reasons for smoking, it will become a lot easier to quit. At this time you should also try to read as much information as possible on the detrimental effects of tobacco and the benefits of quitting.

Step Two

Initiate a personal diet and exercise program. About one-third of the people who quit smoking gain weight. This could be caused by one reason or a combination of several reasons: (a) food might become a substitute for cigarettes, (b) appetite may increase, and (c) basal metabolism may slow down. If the person initiates an exercise and weight control program prior to smoking cessation, weight gain should not be a problem. If anything, exercise and decreased body weight cause a greater awareness of healthy living and increase motivation for giving up cigarettes. Even if some weight is gained, the harmful effects of cigarette smoking are much more detrimental to human health than a few extra pounds of body weight. Experts have indicated that as far as the extra load on the heart is concerned, giving up one pack of cigarettes per day is the equivalent of losing between fifty and seventy-five pounds of excess body fat!

Step Three

Decide on the approach that you will use to stop smoking. You may quit cold turkey or gradually decrease the number of cigarettes smoked daily. Your decision should be based on the scores obtained on the "Why-Do-You-Smoke Test." If you scored 11 points or higher in either the "Crutch: Tension Reduction" or the "Craving: Psychological Addiction" categories, your best chance for success is quitting cold turkey. For any of the other four categories, you may choose either approach.

There is still argument as to which approach may be more effective. Quitting cold turkey may cause fewer withdrawal symptoms than gradually tapering off. When cutting down, the fewer the cigarettes smoked, the more important each one becomes. Therefore, there is a greater chance for relapse and returning to the original amount smoked. When the cutting down approach is used with a definite target date for quitting, however, the technique has been shown to be quite effective. Smokers who taper off without a target date for quitting are the most likely to relapse.

Step Four

For a few days, keep a daily log of your smoking habit. This will help you understand the situations under which you smoke. To assist you in doing so, make copies of Figure 10.6 or develop your own form. Keep this form with you, and every time you smoke, record the required information. You should keep track of the number of cigarettes smoked, time of day when smoked, event associated with smoking, the amount of cigarette smoked, and a rating of how badly you needed that cigarette. Rate each cigarette from 1 to 3. A 1 means desperately needed, a 2 means moderately needed, and a 3 means no real need.

This daily log will assist you in three ways. First, you will get to know your habit. Second, it will help you eliminate cigarettes that you really do not need. Third, it will aid you in finding positive substitutes for situations that trigger your desire to smoke.

Step Five

Set the target date for quitting. If you are going to taper off gradually, read the instructions under the cutting down section of this chapter before you proceed to Step 6. In setting the target date, choosing a special date may add a little extra incentive. An upcoming birthday, anniversary, vacation, graduation, and family reunion, are some examples of good dates to free yourself from smoking. Dates when you are going to be away from events that trigger your desire to smoke may be especially helpful. Once you have set the date, do not change it. Do not let anyone or anything interfere with this date. Let your friends and relatives know of your intentions and ask for their support. You may also consider asking someone else to quit with you. This way you can support each other in your efforts to stop.

Also, avoid anyone who will not support you in your effort to quit. It is unfortunate, but in many cases other people can be a prime obstacle when you are attempting to quit. Because many smokers can get quite "intolerable" when they first stop smoking, some friends and relatives prefer that the individual continue to smoke rather than make the extra effort and show increased patience for a few days.

Step Six

Stock up on low-calorie foods — carrots, broccoli, cauliflower, celery, popcorn (butter- and salt-free), fruits, sunflower seeds (in the shell), sugarless gum — and plenty of water. Keep such food handy on the day you stop and the first few days following cessation. Replace cigarettes with low-calorie foods when you want a cigarette.

Step Seven

On your quit day and the first few days thereafter, do not keep cigarettes handy. Stay away from friends and events that trigger your desire to smoke. Drink large amounts of water and fruit juices. An important factor in breaking the habit is to replace the old behavior with new behavior. You will need to replace smoking time with new, positive substitutes that will make smoking difficult or impossible.

When you desire a cigarette, take a few deep breaths and then occupy yourself by doing a number of things such as talking to someone else, washing your hands, brushing your teeth, eating a healthy snack, chewing on a straw, doing dishes, playing sports, going for a walk or bike ride, going swimming, and so on. Engage in activities that will necessitate the use of your hands. Try gardening, sewing, writing letters, drawing, doing household chores, or washing the car. Visit nonsmoking places such as libraries, museums, stores, theaters. Plan an outing or a trip away from home. Record your choice of activity or substitute under the "remarks/substitutes" column in Figure 10.6. All these activities have been shown to keep your mind away from cigarettes.

QUITTING COLD TURKEY

Many people have found that quitting all at once is the easiest way to do it. Most smokers have tried this approach at least once. Even though it may not work the first time, if they do not allow themselves to get discouraged, they eventually succeed. Many times after several attempts, all of a sudden they are able to overcome the habit without too much difficulty. On the average, as few as three smokeless days are sufficient to break the physiological addiction to nicotine. The psychological addiction may linger for years but will get weaker as time goes by.

CUTTING DOWN GRADUALLY

Tapering off cigarettes can be done in several ways. You may start by eliminating cigarettes that you do not necessarily need (those ranked as number 3 and 2 on your daily log); you can switch to a brand lower in nicotine/tar every couple of days; you can smoke less of each cigarette; or you can simply decrease the total number of cigarettes smoked each day.

Most people prefer using a combination of the four methods. When planning your strategy, it is important that you set a target date for quitting before you start cutting down. Remember — once the date is set, it is not to be changed. The total process until your quit date should not take longer than two weeks. You should reduce the total number of cigarettes smoked each day by 10 to 25 percent. As the number is decreased, be careful not to take more puffs or inhale more deeply as you smoke. This would offset the principle of cutting down.

As an aid in tapering off, make several copies of Figure 10.6 (by now you should have already completed the initial daily log of your smoking habit — see Step Four under "Breaking the Habit"). Start a new daily log, and every night review your data and set goals for the following day. You will have to decide which cigarettes will be easiest to give up, what brand you will smoke, the total number of cigarettes to be smoked, and how much of each you will smoke. You may also write down comments or note situations that you may want to avoid as well as any substitutes that you could use to help you in the program.

For example, if you always smoke with coffee, substitute juice for coffee. If you smoke while driving, arrange for a ride or take a bus to work. If you smoke with a given friend at lunch, avoid having lunch with that friend for a week or so. Continue using this log until you have completely stopped smoking.

LIFE AFTER CIGARETTES

When you first quit smoking, you can expect to experience a series of withdrawal symptoms. Among the physiological and psychological reactions that you will likely experience the first few days are a decrease in heart rate and blood pressure, headaches, gastrointestinal discomfort, changes in mood, irritability, aggressiveness, and difficulty in sleeping. The physiological addiction to nicotine is broken only three days following your last cigarette. As a result, you should not crave cigarettes as much on a regular basis.

For the habitual smoker, however, the psychological dependency could be the most difficult to break. The first few days may not be as hard as the first few months. Any of the activities in daily life — either stress or relaxation, joy or unhappiness — that have been associated with smoking may cause a relapse even months or at times years after cessation.

Ex-smokers should realize that even though some harm may have already been done, it is never too late to quit. The greatest early benefit is a decrease in the risk of sudden death. Furthermore, the risk for illness starts to decrease the moment you stop smoking. There will be a

Figure 10.6. *Daily cigarette smoking log*

Today's Date: _____ Quit Date: _____ Decision Date: _____

Cigarettes to be Smoked Today: _____ Brand: _____

No.	Time	Activity	Rating[a]	Amount Smoked[b]	Remarks/Substitutes
1.					
2.					
3.					
4.					
5.					
6.					
7.					
8.					
9.					
10.					
11.					
12.					
13.					
14.					
15.					
16.					
17.					
18.					
19.					
20.					

Additional comments, list of friends and/or activities to avoid

_____

_____

_____

_____

_____

_____

[a]Rating: 1 = desperately needed, 2 = moderately needed, 3 = no real need
[b]Amount Smoked: entire cigarette, two-thirds, half, etc.

decrease in sore throats, sores in the mouth, hoarseness, cigarette cough, and peptic ulcer risk. At the same time, there will be better blood circulation to the hands and feet, improved gastrointestinal function, and improved kidney and bladder function. In addition, everything will taste and smell better, you will have more energy, and you will experience a sense of freedom, pride, and well-being. You will no longer have to worry whether you have enough cigarettes to last you through a day, a party, a meeting, a weekend, a trip.

When you first quit and you think how tough it is and how miserable you feel because you cannot have a cigarette, try the opposite — think of the benefits and how great it is not to smoke! A final note of encouragement is that the ex-smoker's risk for heart disease approaches that of a lifetime nonsmoker ten years following cessation, and cancer fifteen years after cessation.

If you have been successful in quitting smoking, a lot of events can still trigger your urge to smoke. When confronted with such events, people might rationalize and think, "One will not hurt — I've been off for months (years in some cases)" or, "I can handle it; I'll just smoke today." This will not work! Before you know it, you will be back to the regular nasty habit. Therefore, be prepared to take action in those situations. Find adequate substitutes.

In addition to the many things that already have been discussed in this chapter, the list of tips given in Figure 10.7 should aid you in retraining yourself to live without cigarettes. You have to start thinking of yourself as a nonsmoker. There are no "buts." Remind yourself of how difficult it has been and how long it has taken you to get to this point. If you have come this far, you can certainly resist "but" small moments of temptation. It will get easier, not harder, as time goes on.

Bibliography

American Cancer Society. *Quitter's Guide: Seven-Day Plan to Help You Stop Smoking Cigarettes.* New York: ACS, 1978.

American Cancer Society. *Why Quit Quiz* (VHS tape). New York: ACS, 1979.

American Cancer Society. *Fifty Most Often Asked Questions About Smoking and Health . . . and the Answers.* New York: ACS, 1982.

American Cancer Society. *1986 Cancer Facts and Figures.* New York: ACS, 1986.

American Heart Association. *Smoking and Heart Disease.* Dallas: AHA, 1981.

American Heart Association. *The Good Life: A Guide to Becoming a Nonsmoker.* Dallas: AHA, 1984.

American Heart Association. *Heart at Work: Smoking Reduction Program-Coordinator's Guide.* Dallas: AHA, 1984.

American Heart Association. *How to Quit.* Dallas: AHA, 1984.

Carroll, C. R. *Drugs in Modern Society.* Dubuque, IA: Wm. C. Brown, 1985.

Channing, L. Bete Co. *Smoking and Your Heart.* South Deerfield, MA: Author, 1982.

Girdano, D. A., D. Dusek, and G. S. Everly. *Experiencing Health.* Englewood Cliffs, NJ: Prentice-Hall, 1985.

Halper, M. S. *How to Stop Smoking: A Preventive Medicine Institute/Strang Clinic Health Action Plan.* New York: Holt, Rinehart and Winston, 1980.

Hodgson, R. J., and P. Miller. *Self-watching: Addictions, Habits, Compulsions, What to Do.* New York: Facts on File, 1982.

National Cancer Institute. *Clearing the Air: A Guide to Quitting Smoking.* Bethesda, MD: NCI, 1979.

Public Health Service. *Smoking Tobacco and Health: A Fact Book.* Rockville, MD: U.S. Department of Health and Human Services, 1981.

Public Health Service. *Why People Smoke Cigarettes.* Rockville, MD: U.S. Department of Health and Human Services, 1982.

Public Health Service. *A Self-Test for Smokers.* Rockville, MD: U.S. Department of Health and Human Services, 1983.

Public Health Service. *Chronic Obstructive Lung Disease: A Report of the Surgeon General.* Rockville, MD: U.S. Department of Health and Human Services, 1984.

U. S. Office on Smoking and Health. *Smoking and Health: A Report of the Surgeon General.* Washington, DC: U.S. Department of Health, Education and Welfare, 1979.

Figure 10.7. *Tips for smoking cessation*

The following are various ways smokers have retrained themselves to live without cigarettes. Any one or several of these methods in combination might be helpful to you. Check the ones you like, and from these develop your own retraining program.

1. Before you quit smoking, try wrapping your cigarettes with a sheet of paper like a Christmas present. Every time you want a cigarette, unwrap the pack and write down what you are doing, how you feel, and how important this cigarette is to you. Do this for two weeks and you'll have cut down as well as developed new insights into your smoking.

2. If cigarettes give you an energy boost, try gum, modest exercise, a brisk walk, or a new hobby. Avoid eating new foods that are high in calories.

3. If cigarettes help you relax, instead try eating, drinking new beverages, or social activities within reasonable bounds.

4. When you crave cigarettes, you must quit suddenly. Try smoking an excess of cigarettes for a day or two before you quit so that the taste of cigarettes is spoiled. Or an opportune time to quit is when you are ill with a cold or influenza and have lost your taste for cigarettes.

5. On a 3" x 5" card, make a list of what you like and dislike about smoking. Add to it and read it daily.

6. Make up a short list of luxuries you have wanted or items you would like to purchase for a loved one. Next to each item write the cost. Now convert the cost to "packs of cigarettes." If you save the money each day from packs of cigarettes, you will be able to purchase these items. Use a special "piggy bank" for saving your money or start a Christmas Club account at your bank.

7. Never smoke after you get a craving for a cigarette until three minutes have passed since you got the urge. During those three minutes, change your thinking or activity. Telephone an ex-smoker or somebody you can talk to until the craving subsides.

8. Plan a memorable date for stopping. You might choose your vacation, New Year's Day, your birthday, a holiday, the birthday of your child, your anniversary. But don't make the date so distant that you lose momentum.

9. If you smoke under stress at work, pick a date for stopping when you will be away from your work.

10. Decide whether you are going to stop suddenly or gradually. If it is to be gradual, work out a tapering system so that you have intermediate goals on your way to an "I.Q." (I quit) day.

11. Don't store up cigarettes. Never buy a carton. Wait until one pack is finished before you buy another.

12. Never carry cigarettes about with you at home or at work. Keep your cigarettes as far from you as possible. Leave them with someone or lock them up.

13. Until you quit, make yourself a "smoking corner" that is far from anything interesting. If you like to smoke with others, always smoke alone. If you like to smoke alone, always smoke with others, preferably if they are nonsmokers. Never smoke while watching television.

14. Never carry matches or a lighter with you.

15. Put away your ashtrays or fill them with objects so they cannot be used for ashes. Plant flowers in them or fill them with walnuts. The latter will give you something to do with your hands.

16. Change your brand of cigarettes weekly so that you are always smoking a brand of lower tar and nicotine content than the week before.

17. Never say, "I quit smoking," because your resolution is broken if you have a cigarette. Better to say, "I don't want to smoke." This way you maintain your resolution even if you "accidentally" have a cigarette.

18. Try to help someone else quit smoking, particularly your spouse.

19. Always ask yourself, "Do I need this cigarette or is this just a reflex?"

(continued)

Figure 10.7. *Tips for smoking cessation (continued)*

20. Each day try to put off lighting your first cigarette.

21. Decide arbitrarily that you will smoke only on even- or odd-numbered hours of the clock.

22. Try going to bed early and rising a half hour earlier than usual to avoid hurrying through breakfast and rushing to work.

23. Keep your hands occupied. Try playing a musical instrument, knitting, or fiddling with hand puzzles.

24. Take a shower. You cannot smoke in the shower.

25. Brush your teeth frequently to get rid of the tobacco taste and stains.

26. If you have a sudden craving for a cigarette, take ten deep breaths, holding the last breath while you strike a match. Exhale slowly, blowing out the match. Pretend the match was a cigarette by crushing it out in an ashtray. Now immediately get busy on some work or activity.

27. Smoke only half a cigarette.

28. After you quit, start using your lungs. Increase your activities and indulge in moderate exercise, such as short walks before or after a meal.

29. Bet with someone that you can quit. Put the cigarette money in a jar each morning and forfeit it if you smoke. You keep the money if you don't smoke by the end of the week. Try to extend this period to a month.

30. If you gain weight because you are not smoking, wait until you get over the craving before you diet. Dieting is easier then.

31. If you are depressed or have physical symptoms that might be related to your smoking, relieve your mind by discussing this with your physician. It is easier to quit when you know your health status.

32. After you quit, visit your dentist and have your teeth cleaned to get rid of the tobacco stains.

33. If the cost of cigarettes is your motivation for quitting, purchase a money order equivalent to a year's supply of cigarettes and give it to a friend. If you smoke in the next year, he/she cashes the money order and keeps the money. If you don't smoke, he/she gives back the money order at the end of the year.

34. After you have quit, never face the confusion of craving a cigarette alone. Find someone you can call or visit at this critical time.

35. When you feel irritable or tense, shut your eyes and count backward from ten to zero as you imagine yourself descending a flight of stairs, or imagine that you are looking at the horizon as the sun sets in the West.

36. Get out of your old habits. Seek new activities or perform old activities in a new way. Don't rely on the old ways of solving problems. Do things differently.

37. If you are a "kitchen smoker" in the morning, volunteer your services to schools or nonprofit organizations to get you out of the house.

38. Stock up on light reading materials, crossword puzzles, and vacation brochures that you can read during your coffee breaks.

39. Frequent places where you can't smoke, such as libraries, buses, theatres, swimming pools, department stores, or just going to bed during the first weeks you are off cigarettes.

40. Give yourself time to think and get fit by walking one-half hour each day. If you have a dog, take the dog for a walk with you.

From *TIPS*. American Cancer Society, Texas Division, Inc., by permission.

Addictive Behavior And Prevention Of Sexually Transmitted Diseases

This chapter addresses two additional wellness components that may directly affect the well-being of students: (a) addiction and (b) prevention of sexually transmitted diseases (including AIDS). The discussion covers self-help and preventive approaches to these current wellness issues.

ADDICTION

When most people think of addiction, they probably think of dark and dirty alleys, an addict "shooting up" or a "junkie" passed out next to a garbage can after an evening bout with alcohol. Jacquelyn Small, psychotherapist and author, defines addiction as a problem of imbalance or unease within the body and mind. There are many types of addiction, including food, television, work, compulsive shopping, even exercise, and, most seriously, chemical dependency (e.g., tobacco, coffee, alcohol, cocaine, heroin, marijuana, prescription drugs). Some addictive behaviors are worse than others.

People can become addicted to food. They eat to release stress, relieve boredom, or reward themselves for every small personal achievement. A great number of people are addicted to television. Estimates indicate that the average adult in the United States spends seven hours per day watching television.

Other individuals become so addicted to their jobs that all they think about is work. Although work may start out as an enjoyable leisure activity, when it totally consumes a person's life, work can become an unhealthy behavior. If you find

that you are readily irritated, moody, grouchy, constantly tired, not as alert as you used to be, or make more mistakes than usual, you are probably becoming a workaholic and need to slow down or take time off work.

Exercise has enhanced the health and quality of life of millions of people, but for a very small group of individuals, exercise can become an obsessive behavior with potential addictive and overuse properties. Compulsive exercisers often express feelings of guilt and discomfort after missing a day's workout. These individuals continue to exercise even during periods of injury and sickness that require proper rest for adequate recovery. People who exceed the recommended guidelines for fitness development and maintenance (see Chapters 2, 3, and 4) are exercising for reasons other than health, including addictive behavior.

Caffeine addiction can also produce undesirable side effects. Caffeine doses in excess of 200 to 500 mg can produce an abnormally rapid heart rate, abnormal heart rhythms, increased blood pressure, birth defects, increased body temperature, and increased secretion of gastric acids leading to stomach problems. It may also induce symptoms of anxiety, depression, nervousness, and dizziness. The caffeine content of various drinks differs depending upon the product. The content of 6 ounces of coffee, for instance, varies from 65 mg for instant coffee to as high as 180 mg for drip coffee. Soft drinks, mainly colas, range in caffeine content from 30 to 60 mg per 12-ounce can.

The previous examples, as well as more serious forms of chemical dependency, are by no means the only types of addiction; they only illustrate addictive behaviors. Other examples are gambling, pornography, sex, people, and places. Although all forms of addiction are unhealthy, this chapter focuses on three of the most serious, self-destructive forms of addiction in our society: marijuana, cocaine, and alcohol (addiction to cigarette smoking and tobacco in general has already been discussed in detail in Chapter 10).

DRUGS AND DEPENDENCE

Approximately 60 percent of the world's production of illegal drugs is consumed in the United States. Each year Americans spend over $100 billion on illegal drugs — an amount that surpasses the total taken in from all crops by United States farmers. According to the U.S. Department of Education, today's drugs are stronger, more addictive, and pose a greater risk than ever before. Drugs lead to physical and psychological dependence. With regular use, they integrate into the body's chemistry, increasing drug tolerance and forcing the user to constantly increase the dosage to obtain similar results. Drug abuse leads to serious health problems. Furthermore, over half of all adolescent suicides are drug-related.

Marijuana

Marijuana (pot or grass, as it is commonly referred to) is the most widely used illegal drug in the United States. Estimates indicate that 64 percent of Americans between the ages of eighteen and twenty-five and 23 percent of those twenty-six and older have smoked marijuana. Approximately 20 million people in the country regularly use marijuana. This psychoactive drug is prepared from a mixture of crushed leaves, flowers, small branches, stems, and seeds from the hemp plant, Cannabis Sativa.

Marijuana in small doses has a sedative effect, whereas larger doses produce physical and psychic changes. Earlier studies in the 1960s indicated that the potential effects of marijuana were exaggerated and that the drug was relatively harmless. The drug as it is used today, however, is as much as ten times stronger than when the initial studies were conducted. Ninety percent of research today shows marijuana to be a dangerous and harmful drug.

The major and most active psychoactive and mind-altering ingredient of marijuana is thought to be delta-9-tetrahydrocannabinol (THC). In the 1960s, THC content in marijuana ranged from .02 to 2 percent. Users called the latter "real good grass." Today's THC content averages 4 to 6 percent, although it has been reported as high as 20 percent. The THC content in sinsemilla, a seedless variety of high-potency marijuana grown from the seedless female cannabis plant, is approximately 8 percent.

THC reaches the brain within 30 seconds of inhalation of marijuana smoke, and the psychic and physical changes reach their peak in about two or three minutes. THC is then metabolized in the liver to waste metabolites, but 30 percent of it remains in the body one week after marijuana was first smoked. In fact, studies indicate that thirty days or longer are required to completely eliminate THC following an initial dose of the drug. For regular users the drug will always remain in the system.

Some of the short-term effects of marijuana include tachycardia (increased heart rate, sometimes as high as 180 beats per minute), dryness of the mouth, reddening of the eyes, increased appetite, decrease in coordination and tracking (following a moving stimulus), difficulty in concentration, intermittent confusion, impairment of short-term memory and continuity of speech, and interference with the physical and mental learning process during periods of intoxication.

Another common effect of marijuana use is the amotivational syndrome, characterized by loss of motivation, dullness, apathy, and no interest in the future. This syndrome persists even after periods of intoxication, but it usually disappears a few weeks after the individual stops using the drug.

Long-term harmful effects include atrophy of the brain, leading to irreversible brain damage, decreased resistance to infectious diseases, chronic bronchitis, lung cancer (may contain as much as 50 percent more cancer-producing hydrocarbons than cigarette smoke), and possible sterility and impotence.

One of the most common myths about marijuana use is that it does not lead to addiction. Ample scientific evidence clearly shows that regular marijuana users do develop physical and psychological dependence. Similar to cigarette smoking, when regular users go without the drug, they crave the substance, experience changes in mood, irritability, and nervousness, and develop an obsession to get more "pot."

Cocaine

Similar to marijuana, cocaine was thought for many years to be a relatively harmless drug. This misconception came to an abrupt halt in 1986 when two well-known athletes, Len Bias (basketball) and Don Rogers (football), died suddenly following a cocaine overdose. Estimates indicate that between four and eight million Americans use cocaine, 96 percent of whom had previously used marijuana.

Cocaine (2-beta-carbomethoxy-3-betabenozoxytropane) is the primary psychoactive ingredient derived from coca plant leaves. Over the years it has been given several different names, including coke, C, snow, blow, toot, flake, Peruvian lady, white girl, and happy dust. The drug is commonly sniffed or snorted, but it can be smoked or injected. Cocaine is an expensive drug. Some users pay in excess of $2000 per ounce. Cocaine used in medical therapy sells for about $100 per ounce. Because of the high cost, cocaine is viewed as a luxury drug. Many users are well-educated, affluent, upwardly mobile professionals who are otherwise law-abiding citizens.

Cocaine has become the fastest growing drug problem in the United States. About 5,000 people try cocaine for the first time each day. The addiction begins with a desire to get high, often at social gatherings, with the assurance that occasional use is harmless. About one in five will continue to use the drug now and then, and for some of them it is the beginning of a lifetime nightmare.

The popularity of cocaine is based on the almost universal guarantee that the user will enter an immediate state of euphoria and well-being. When cocaine is snorted, it is quickly absorbed through the mucous membranes of the nose into the bloodstream. The drug is usually arranged in fine powder lines one to two inches long. Each line results in about thirty minutes of central and autonomic nervous system stimulation. The drug seems to help relieve fatigue and increase energy levels, as well as decrease the need for appetite and sleep. Following this

stimulation comes a "crash," a state of physiological and psychological depression, often leaving the user with the desire to get more. This can lead to a constant craving for the drug. Researchers indicate that addiction becomes a lifetime illness, and, similar to alcoholism, the individual recovers only through complete abstinence from the drug. A single pitfall frequently results in renewed addiction.

Light to moderate use of cocaine is commonly associated with feelings of pleasure and well-being. Sustained cocaine snorting can lead to a constant runny nose, nasal congestion and inflammation, and perforation of the nasal septum. Long-term consequences of cocaine use in general are a loss of appetite, digestive disorders, weight loss, malnutrition, insomnia, confusion, anxiety, and cocaine psychosis. The latter is characterized by paranoia and hallucinations. In a particular type of hallucination, referred to as "formication" or "coke bugs," the chronic user perceives imaginary insects or snakes crawling on or underneath the skin.

High doses of cocaine can cause nervousness, dizziness, blurred vision, vomiting, tremors, seizures, high blood pressure, strokes, angina, and cardiac arrhythmias. Freebase (a purer, more potent smokable form of cocaine) users increase their risk for lung disease, and intravenous users are at risk for hepatitis, AIDS, and other infectious diseases. Large overdoses of cocaine can lead to sudden death as a result of respiratory paralysis, cardiac arrhythmias, and severe convulsions. Some individuals may lack an enzyme used in metabolizing cocaine, and as little as two to three lines of cocaine may be fatal. Chronic users who constantly crave the drug often turn to crime, including murder, to sustain their habit. Some users view suicide as the only solution to this sad syndrome.

Alcohol

Drinking alcohol has been a socially acceptable behavior for centuries. Alcohol is frequently consumed at parties, ceremonies, dinners, sport contests, the establishment of kingdoms or governments, and the signing of peace treaties. Alcohol has also been used for medical reasons as a mild sedative or as a pain killer for surgery.

For a short period of fourteen years, from 1920 to 1933, by constitutional amendment, the sale and use of alcohol were declared illegal in the United States. This amendment was repealed because both drinkers and nondrinkers questioned the right of the government to pass judgment on individual moral standards. In addition, the country experienced a tremendous growth in organized crime to smuggle and illegally sell alcohol.

The alcohol contained in drinks is known as ethyl alcohol, a depressant drug that affects the brain and slows down central nervous system activity. As with most drugs that affect the brain, it has strong addictive properties and therefore can be easily abused. In fact, alcohol is one of the most significant health-related drug problems in the United States today. Estimates indicate that seven in ten adults, or over 100 million Americans eighteen years and older, are drinkers. Approximately 10 million of them will experience a drinking problem, including alcoholism, in their lifetime. Another 3 million teenagers are thought to have a drinking problem.

The addiction to alcohol develops slowly. Most people believe that they are in control of their drinking habits and do not realize that they have a problem until they become alcoholics — when they develop a physical and emotional dependence on the drug, characterized by excessive use and constant preoccupation with drinking. Alcohol abuse, in turn, leads to mental, emotional, physical, and social problems.

Alcohol intake reduces peripheral vision, decreases visual and hearing acuity, decreases reaction time, impairs concentration and motor performance (including increased swaying and impaired judgment of distance and speed of moving objects), decreases fear, increases risk-taking behaviors, increases urination, and induces sleep. A single large dose of alcohol may also decrease sexual function. One of the most unpleasant, dangerous, and life-threatening effects of drinking is the synergistic action of alcohol when combined with other drugs, particularly central nervous system depressants. The effects of mixing alcohol with another drug can be much greater than the sum of two drug actions by themselves. Within the range of individual differences as to how the body will react to a combination of alcohol and other drugs, the effects range from loss of consciousness to death.

Long-term effects of alcohol abuse are serious and often life-threatening. Some of these detrimental effects are cirrhosis of the liver (scarring of the liver, which is often fatal); increased risk for oral, esophageal, and liver cancer; cardiomyopathy (a disease that affects the heart muscle); elevated blood pressure; increased risk for strokes; inflammation of the esophagus, stomach, small intestine, and pancreas; stomach ulcers; sexual impotence; malnutrition; brain cell damage leading to loss of memory; psychosis; depression; and hallucinations.

HOW TO CUT DOWN YOUR DRINKING

To find out if drinking is a problem in your life, refer to the questionnaire "Alcohol Abuse: Are You Drinking Too Much?" contained in Figure 11.1. If you give two or more "yes" answers on this questionnaire, you may be jeopardizing your health through excessive consumption of alcohol. Now is the time to start limiting your intake of alcohol. For many people who are determined to control the problem, it is not that hard to do. The first and most important step is to want to cut down. If you want to cut down but find you cannot, you had better accept the probability that alcohol is becoming a serious problem for you, and you should seek guidance from your physician or from an organization such as Alcoholics Anonymous. The next few suggestions may also help you cut down alcohol intake.

1. Set reasonable limits for yourself. Decide not to exceed a certain number of drinks on a given occasion, and stick to your decision. No more than two beers or two cocktails a day is a reasonable limit. You have proven to yourself that you can control your drinking if you set such a target and regularly do not exceed it.

2. Learn to say no. Many people have "just one more" drink because others in the group are having one or because someone puts pressure on them, not because they really want a drink. When you reach the sensible limit you have set for yourself, politely but firmly refuse to exceed it. If you are being the generous host, pour yourself a glass of water

Figure 11.1. *Alcohol abuse: Are you drinking too much?*

1. When you are holding an empty glass at a party, do you always actively look for a refill instead of waiting to be offered one?
2. If given the chance, do you frequently pour out a more generous drink for yourself than seems to be the "going" amount for others?
3. Do you often have a drink or two when you are alone, either at home or in a bar?
4. Is your drinking ever the direct cause of a family quarrel, or do quarrels often seem to occur, if only by coincidence, after you have had a drink or two?
5. Do you feel that you must have a drink at a specific time every day — right after work, for instance?
6. When worried or under unusual stress, do you almost automatically take a stiff drink to "settle your nerves?"
7. Are you untruthful about how much you have had to drink when questioned on the subject?
8. Does drinking ever cause you to take time off work, or to miss scheduled meetings or appointments?
9. Do you feel physically deprived if you cannot have at least one drink every day?
10. Do you sometimes crave a drink in the morning?
11. Do you sometimes have "mornings after" when you cannot remember what happened the night before?

Evaluation

You should regard a "yes" answer to any one of the above questions as a warning sign. Do not increase your consumption of alcohol. Two "yes" answers suggest that you may already be becoming dependent on alcohol. Three or more "yes" answers indicate that you may have a serious problem, and you should get professional help.

*Reproduced by permission from *Family Medical Guide* by The American Medical Association. New York: Random House, 1982.

or juice "on the rocks." Nobody will notice the difference.

3. Drink slowly. Never gulp down a drink. Choose your drinks for their flavor, not their "kick," and savor the taste of each sip.

4. Dilute your drinks. If you prefer cocktails to beer, try having long drinks. Instead of downing your gin or whiskey neat or nearly so, drink it diluted with a mixer such as tonic, water, or soda water, in a tall glass. That way you can enjoy the flavor as well as the act of drinking, but it will take longer to finish each drink. Also, you can make your two-drink limit last all evening or switch to the mixer by itself.

5. Do not drink on your own. Make a point of confining your drinking to social gatherings. It is sometimes hard to resist the urge to pour yourself a relaxing drink at the end of a hard day, but many formerly heavy drinkers have found that a cup of coffee or a soft drink satisfies the need as well as alcohol did, and that it was just a habit. What may help you really unwind, even with no drink at all, is a comfortable chair, loosened clothing, and perhaps a soothing record, a television program, or a good book to read.

TREATMENT OF ADDICTION

Treatment of drug addiction (including alcohol) is seldom accomplished without professional guidance and support. Of course the initial step is to recognize that you have a problem. The questionnaire given in Figure 12.2 can help you recognize possible addictive behavior in yourself (or in someone you know). If the answers to more than half of these questions are positive, you may have a problem and should speak to your doctor or contact the local mental/health clinic for a referral (see the Yellow Pages in your phone book).

Figure 11.2. *Addictive Behavior Questionnaire: Could You Be An Addict?*

Directions

The following test, designed by Dr. Lawrence J. Hatterer, is not a way to diagnose whether you are in the early, middle, or chronic stage of addictive disease. It is merely meant to help you understand addictive behavior better so you can recognize it in yourself or perhaps in people you know.

1. I am a person of excesses. I can't regulate what I do for pleasure, and often use a substance or indulge in an activity heavily, in order to get high.
2. I am an extremely self-involved person. People tell me that I am into myself too much.
3. I am compulsive. I must have what I want when I want it, regardless of the consequences.
4. I am excessively dependent on or independent of others.
5. I am preoccupied. I spend a lot of time thinking or fantasizing about a particular activity or substance. Also, I will work my day around doing it or go to pains to make sure it's available.
6. I deny that I do this and lie about it to others who ask me.
7. I have been involved in this behavior for at least one year.
8. I've told myself I could easily stop, even though I've shown no signs of slowing down.
9. Once I start indulging in this behavior or substance, I find I have trouble stopping.
10. One or more members of my family are also involved in some kind of excessive behavior or substance abuse.
11. I find I gravitate mostly toward people who have the same behavior or take the same substance as I do.
12. I seem to be developing a tolerance to the behavior or substance. I have had a need to steadily increase the amounts I take or the time I spend doing it.
13. I have found that my excessive use of highs has, in fact, only made my problems worse.
14. If someone tries to keep me from obtaining the substance or practicing the activity, I get angry and reject or abuse them.
15. I experience withdrawal symptoms if I cannot indulge in the substance or activity.
16. This has gotten in the way of my functioning. I have missed something important — days at work, time with my friends, family, children — because of it.
17. The substance/activity is destroying my home life. I know I am hurting those closest to me.
18. I have failed in many goals in life, lost money, given up many social and occupational contacts, all because of my excessive behavior.
19. I have tried to stop or cut down on my excesses but have been unsuccessful.
20. I have physically endangered myself or others in accidents that were a direct result of my excessive behavior.

Evaluation

If you answer "yes" to one-half or more of the questions, you may have a problem with addictive disease and should seek immediate professional help. For a referral, contact your local mental health clinic (look in the Yellow Pages) or speak to your doctor.

SEXUALLY TRANSMITTED DISEASES*

Sexually transmitted diseases (STDs) have become an epidemic of national proportions in the United States. There are now over twenty-five known STDs, some of which are still incurable. According to the Centers for Disease Control in Atlanta, in 1986 more than 10 million new people were infected with STDs. These included 4.6 million cases of chlamydia, 1.8 million of gonorrhea, 1 million of genital warts, half a million of herpes, 90,000 of syphilis, and — attracting most of the attention because of its life-threatening potential — 15,000 new cases of Acquired Immune Deficiency Syndrome (AIDS). The American Social Health Association indicates that 25 percent of all Americans will acquire at least one STD in their lifetime.

Chlamydia

Chlamydia, a bacterial infection that can cause significant damage to the reproductive system, may occur without symptoms. The disease is considered to be a major factor in male and female infertility. Because of its asymptomatic condition, victims frequently don't even know that they are infected. When symptoms do occur, they tend to mimic other STDs; therefore, the disease can often be mistreated. The Centers for Disease Control indicate that about 20 percent of all college students are infected with chlamydia. The disease can be effectively treated with oral antibiotics, but successful treatment will not reverse any damage that has already occurred to the reproductive system.

Gonorrhea

One of the oldest STDs is gonorrhea. This disease is also caused by a bacterial infection. If left untreated, it can lead to pelvic inflammation in women, infertility, widespread bacterial infection, heart damage, arthritis in men and women, and blindness in children born to infected women. Gonorrhea is successfully treated with penicillin and other antibiotics.

---

* Adapted with permission from Hafen, B. Q., A. L. Thygerson, and K. J. Frandsen. *Behavioral Guidelines for Health & Wellness.* Englewood, CO: Morton Publishing, 1988.

Genital Warts

Genital warts, caused by a viral infection, appear anywhere from a month and a half to eight months following exposure. Genital warts may be flat or raised. They are usually found on the penis, around the vulva, and the vagina, but can also be found in the mouth, throat, rectum, on the cervix, or around the anus.

Health problems associated with genital warts include an increased risk of cervical cancer and enlargement and spread of the warts leading to obstruction of the urethra, vagina, and anus. Babies born to infected mothers commonly develop warts over their bodies; therefore, Cesarean sections are recommended in such cases. Treatment requires complete removal of all warts; it can be accomplished by freezing them with liquid nitrogen, dissolving them with chemicals, or removing them with electrosurgery or laser surgery.

Herpes

Herpes is also caused by a viral infection (herpes simplex virus types I and II), and no known cure is yet available for the disease. Herpes is characterized by the appearance of sores on the mouth, genitals, rectum, or other parts of the body. The symptoms usually disappear within a few weeks, causing some individuals to believe that they are cured. Nevertheless, herpes is presently incurable, and these victims do remain infected. Repeated outbreaks are common. The disease is very contagious and can be transmitted through simple finger contact from the mouth to the genitals. Victims are most contagious when outbreaks occur. In conjunction with the appearance of sores, victims usually experience mild fever, swollen glands, and headaches.

Syphilis

Another common type of STD, also caused by bacterial infection, is syphilis. Approximately three weeks following infection, a painless sore appears where the bacteria entered the body. This sore disappears on its own in a few weeks. If untreated, additional sores may appear within six months of the initial outbreak, but these will again disappear by themselves. A latent stage, during which the victim is not contagious, may last up to thirty years, leading the victim to believe that he/she is healed.

During the last stage of the disease, some people will suffer from paralysis, crippling, blindness, heart disease, brain damage, insanity, and even death. One of the oldest STDs known, syphilis used to kill its victims prior to the discovery of penicillin and other antibiotics now used in its treatment.

AIDS

AIDS is the most frightening of all STDs because it has no known cure, and few victims have survived the disease. Anywhere from 1.5 to 4 million Americans are thought to carry the HIV or AIDS virus. This virus attacks cells, weakening their immune system. Although there is much debate as to how many carriers will actually get AIDS, it is thought that one-third to one-half of them will develop the disease. Even if the person doesn't develop AIDS, he/she can pass the virus on to others who could easily develop the disease (including pregnant women to their unborn babies).

Government estimates indicate that by the year 1991 over 270,000 Americans will have been diagnosed with AIDS and about 60,000 will die that year alone from the disease. Unless an appropriate cure is found, the outlook is even worse. By the year 2,000 more than 200,000 people are projected to die from AIDS, making it the third leading cause of death behind cardiovascular disease and cancer.

Based on 1986 estimates, almost all of the AIDS cases have occurred in the following groups of people:

- Gay and bisexual men: 66 percent
- Heterosexual intravenous drug users: 17 percent
- Gay and bisexual men who abuse intravenous drugs: 8 percent
- Heterosexual sex partners of the above groups: 4 percent
- Hemophiliacs and people who have had blood transfusions: 3 percent

As shown by the previous estimates, high-risk individuals for AIDS are primarily homosexual males with multiple sexual partners and intravenous drug users, but health experts believe that in future years the disease may become just as common among heterosexuals. The virus is transmitted through blood and semen during sexual intercourse or by using hypodermic needles previously used by an infected individual.

Small concentrations of the virus have also been found in saliva and teardrops. The AIDS virus, however, cannot live long outside the human body. Unlike some people think, AIDS cannot be caught by spending time or shaking hands with an infected person, or from a toilet seat, dishes, or silverware used by an AIDS patient, or using a towel or clothes from a person with AIDS, or from donating blood.

Once a person becomes infected with the AIDS virus, there will be an incubation period ranging from a few months to six years during which no symptoms appear. The virus weakens and incapacitates the immune system, leaving the victim vulnerable to all types of infectious diseases and certain types of cancer. Initial symptoms of the disease include unexplained weight loss, constant fatigue, mild fever, swollen lymph glands, diarrhea, and sore throats. Advanced symptoms include loss of appetite, skin diseases, night sweats, and deterioration of the mucous membranes.

The AIDS virus itself doesn't kill; rather, the ineffectiveness of the immune system in dealing with the various illnesses is what leads to death. Most of these illnesses are usually harmless and rare among the general population but prove to be fatal to the AIDS patient. The two most common fatal conditions seen in AIDS victims are pneumocystis carinii pneumonia (a parasitic infection of the lungs) and kaposis sarcoma (a certain type of skin cancer). The AIDS virus may also attack the nervous system, leading to brain and spinal cord damage.

Although several drugs are being tested to treat and slow down the disease process, there is no known cure for AIDS. Furthermore, the possibility of developing a vaccine in the near future is very slim. The best advice at this point is a preventive approach.

Guidelines for the Prevention Of Sexually Transmitted Diseases

With all the grim news about STDs, there is also some very good news: There are things you can do to prevent their spread, and precautions you can take to keep yourself from becoming a victim.

The facts are in: The best prevention technique is a mutually monogamous sexual relationship. This means that you have sexual relationships with only one person, who has sexual relationships only with you. That one behavior, says Dr. James Mason, director of the Centers for Disease Control in Atlanta, will almost completely remove you from any risk of developing a STD.

What about those who do not have — or do not desire — a monogamous relationship? Still other things can be done to lower the risk of developing sexually transmitted diseases in general:

1. Know your partner. The days are gone when anonymous bathhouse or singles bars sex is safe. You should limit your sexual relationships or you should be able to reassure your partner that you are infection-free, and you deserve the same right from your partner.

2. Limit the number of sexual partners you have. Having one partner lowers your chance of infection. The greater your number of partners, the greater your chance of infection.

3. If you are sexually promiscuous, consider having periodic checkups from your physician. It is easy to get exposed to a STD by a person who does not have any symptoms and who is unaware of the infection. Sexually promiscuous men and women between the ages of fifteen and thirty-five are considered to be in a particularly high-risk group for developing STDs.

4. Use "barrier" methods of contraception to help prevent the spread of disease. Condoms, diaphragms, the contraceptive sponge, and spermicidal suppositories, foams, and jellies can all help prevent the spread of STDs; spermicidal agents may help act as a disinfectant as well. Many physicians are especially encouraging promiscuous teenagers to use condoms; traditionally, teenagers do not use any birth-control methods at all, and they remain at high risk for STDs.

5. Be responsible enough to abstain from sexual activity if you know that you have an infection. Go to a physician or clinic for appropriate treatment, and ask your doctor when it will be safe to resume sexual activity. Abstain until it is safe.

6. Urinate immediately following sexual intercourse. Although this is not a foolproof method, it may help (especially among men) flush bacteria and viruses from the urinary tract.

7. Wash thoroughly immediately following sexual activity; though washing with hot soapy water will not provide a guaranteed measure of safety against STDs, such washing can prevent you from spreading certain germs on your fingers and may wash away bacteria and viruses that have not yet entered the body.

8. If you suspect that your partner is infected, ask. He/she may not even be aware of the infection, so look for signs of infection, such as sores, redness, inflammations, a rash, growths, warts, or discharge. If you are unsure, abstain.

9. Consider abstaining from sexual relations if you have any kind of an illness or disease, even a common cold. Any kind of illness makes you more susceptible to other illnesses, and lowered immunity can make you extra vulnerable to STDs. The same holds true for times when you are under extreme stress, when you are fatigued, and when you are overworked. Drugs and alcohol can also lower your resistance to disease.

10. Wear loose-fitting clothes made of natural fibers; tight-fitting clothing made of synthetic fibers (especially underwear and nylon pantyhose) can create conditions that encourage the growth of bacteria and can actually aggravate STDs.

AIDS: Risk Reduction

Observance of the following precautions, which are based upon reports and recommendations from the U.S. Public Health Service, can help reduce your risk of getting AIDS.

1. Avoid having multiple and anonymous sexual partners.

2. Don't have sexual contact (this includes open-mouthed or French kissing, because

the AIDS virus may be present in saliva; it should be noted, however, that there is no evidence that AIDS has been transmitted in this way) with anyone who has symptoms of AIDS or who is a member of a high-risk group for AIDS.

3. Avoid sexual contact with anyone who has had sex with persons at risk for getting AIDS.

4. Don't have sex with prostitutes.

5. If you do have sex with someone who might be infected with the AIDS virus or whose history is unknown to you, avoid exchange of body fluids and receptive anal intercourse. Unless you know with absolute certainty that your partner is not infected, a condom should be used during each sexual act, from start to finish, to help prevent contact with the AIDS virus. Use of a spermicidal agent may also provide some protection.

6. Don't share toothbrushes, razors, or other implements that could become contaminated with blood, with anyone who is, or who might be, infected with the AIDS virus.

7. Exercise caution regarding procedures, such as acupuncture, tattooing, and ear piercing, in which needles or other unsterile instruments may be used repeatedly to pierce the skin or mucous membranes. Such procedures are safe if proper sterilization methods are employed or disposable needles are used. Before undergoing such procedures, ask what precautions are being taken.

8. If you are planning to undergo artificial insemination, insist on frozen sperm obtained from a laboratory that tests all donors for infection with the AIDS virus. Test donors twice before the sperm is used — once at the time of donation and again a few months later.

9. If you know that you will be having surgery in the near future, and you are able, consider donating blood for your own use. This will eliminate completely the already small risk of contracting AIDS through a blood transfusion. It will also eliminate the more substantial risk of contracting other bloodborne diseases, such as hepatitis, from a transfusion.

IN CONCLUSION

Keep in mind that the achievement of total well-being is a process and you have to put forth a constant effort to achieve and maintain a higher quality of life. Positive lifestyle habits take time to develop, especially if they are to take the place of negative behaviors that are a threat to health and life itself. To develop positive lifestyle habits, you need to surround yourself with a good, healthy environment and plan ahead to take appropriate action when you are confronted with situations that may lead to self-destructive behaviors. If you are applying most of the principles outlined in this textbook, you are probably already practicing several new health-enhancing behaviors. These should be carried on throughout life to help you in your quest for wellness.

Bibliography

American Medical Association. *Family Medical Guide*. New York: Random House, 1982.

Carroll, C. R. *Drugs in Modern Society*. Dubuque, IA: Wm. C. Brown Publishers, 1985.

Channing L. Bete Co. *About AIDS and Shooting Drugs*. South Deerfield, MA: Author, 1986.

Gordon, E. and E. Golanty. *Health & Wellness*. Boston: Jones and Bartlett Publishers, 1985.

Hafen, B. Q., A. L. Thygerson, and K. J. Frandsen. *Behavioral Guidelines for Health & Wellness*. Englewood, CO: Morton Publishing, 1988.

Institute for Aerobics Research. "Addiction." *Aerobic News*. Dallas: Institute, July 1987.

Charting Your Future Path To Wellness

Throughout this textbook you have had an opportunity to assess various components of fitness and wellness. You should now take the time to evaluate how well you achieved your own objectives. Ideally, if time allows, and if facilities and technicians are available, you should reassess the health-related components of physical fitness. If you are unable to reassess these components, subjectively determine how well you accomplished your objectives using the form provided in Appendix A, Figure A.1.

BEHAVIORAL OBJECTIVES FOR THE FUTURE

Now that you are about to finish this course, you will be faced with a new challenge: a lifetime commitment to fitness and wellness. It is a lot easier to adhere to a program while you are in a structured setting, but from now on you will be on your own. Realizing that you may not have achieved all of your objectives during this course, or perhaps you need to reach beyond your current achievements, a final assignment should be conducted to help you chart your personal wellness program for the future.

To complete this assignment, you should use the Wellness Guide given in Figure 12.1. This guide provides a list of various wellness components, each illustrating a scale from 5 to 1. A 5 indicates a low or poor rating; a 1 indicates an excellent or "wellness" rating for that particular component. Using the Wellness Guide, rate yourself for each component according to the following instructions:

1. Color in red a number from 5 to 1 to indicate where you stood on each component at the beginning of the semester. For example, if at the start of this course, you rated poor in cardiovascular endurance, you would color the number 5 in red.

2. Color in blue a second number from 5 to 1 to indicate where you stand on each component at the present time. If your level of cardiovascular endurance improved to average by the end of the semester, color the number 3 in blue. If you were not able to work on a given component, simply color in blue on top of the previous red.

3. Select one or two components that you intend to work on in the next two months. It takes time to develop new behavior patterns, and trying to do too much at once will most likely decrease your chances for success. In addition, start with components in which you think you will have a high chance for success. Next, color in yellow the intended objective (number) to accomplish by the end of this period. If your objective in the next two months is to achieve a "good" level of cardiovascular endurance, color the number 2 in yellow. Once you achieve this level, you may later color the number 1, also in yellow, to indicate your next objective.

Once you have determined the component(s) that you will work on in the next two months, you should write specific behavioral objectives that will help you accomplish your goal(s). As you write (using Figure 12.2) and work on these objectives, keep in mind the following guidelines:

1. Objectives can be both general and specific. The general objective is the ultimate goal that you intend to achieve; the specific objectives are the necessary steps required to reach this general objective. For example, a general objective could be to achieve ideal body weight. Several specific objectives could be: (a) to lose an average of one pound (or one fat percentage point) per week, (b) to monitor body weight prior to breakfast every morning, (c) to assess body composition every two weeks, (d) to decrease fat intake to less than 30 percent of total calories, (e) to eliminate all pastries from the diet during this time, and (f) to exercise in the appropriate target zone for thirty minutes, five times per week.

2. Whenever possible, objectives (general and specific) should be measurable. To simply state "to lose weight" is not measurable. In the previous general objective, "ideal body weight" implies lowering your body weight (fat) to the ideal percent body fat standards given in Chapter 5 (Table 5.6). If this person was a nineteen-year-old female, ideal fat percent would be 17 percent. To be more descriptive, you could reword your general objective as follows: To reduce body weight until 17 percent body fat is achieved. The sample specific objectives given above in number 1 are also measurable. For instance, you can easily determine whether you are losing one pound per week, you can conduct a nutrient analysis to assess the average fat intake, or you can monitor your weekly exercise sessions to make sure that this specific objective is being met.

3. Objectives must be realistic. If you currently weigh 170 pounds and your target weight at 17 percent is 120 pounds, it would be unsound, if not impossible, to implement a weight loss program to lose fifty pounds in two months. Such a program would not allow implementation of adequate behavior modification techniques and ensure weight maintenance at the target weight.

4. Objectives can be either short-term or long-term. If the general objective is to achieve ideal body weight and you are fifty pounds overweight, it would be a lot easier to set a general short-term objective of losing ten pounds and to write specific objectives to accomplish this goal. In this manner, the task will not seem as overwhelming and will be easier to accomplish.

5. Set a specified date by which you plan to achieve your objective. To simply state "I will lose weight" is not time-specific enough to accomplish the objective. It is a lot easier to work on a task if a deadline is established.

6. Educate yourself with regard to the objective that you plan to work on. You cannot lose weight if you do not know the principles that govern weight loss and maintenance. This is the reason why only three in ten individuals achieve the target weight loss and only one in those three is able to keep it off thereafter.

7. Think positive and reward yourself for your accomplishments. As difficult as some tasks may seem, "if there is a will, there is a way." If you prepare an adequate plan of action according to these guidelines, there is no reason why you shouldn't achieve your objective. Also remember to reward yourself for your accomplishments. Buy yourself new clothing, exercise shoes, or something special that you have wanted for some time.

8. Seek environmental support. It becomes very difficult to lose weight if meal planning and cooking are shared with other roommates who enjoy foods that are high in fat and refined carbohydrates. This can be even worse if they also have a weight problem and do not desire or have the willpower to lose weight. Surround yourself with people who will help and encourage you along the way. If necessary, plan and prepare your own meals.

9. Recognize that there will be obstacles. It is almost inevitable that you will make mistakes. Making mistakes is human and does not indicate failure. Failure comes only to those who give up. Use your mistakes and learn from them by preparing a plan that will

Figure 12.1. *Wellness guide*

Name: _____ Course: _____ Section: _____ Date: _____

Wellness Components	Rating					TOTAL WELLBEING
Cardiovascular Endurance	⑤	④	③	②	①	△
Muscular Strength/Endurance	⑤	④	③	②	①	△
Muscular Flexibility	⑤	④	③	②	①	△
Body Composition	⑤	④	③	②	①	△
Nutrition	⑤	④	③	②	①	△
Cardiovascular Disease Risk Reduction	⑤	④	③	②	①	△
Cancer Prevention	⑤	④	③	②	①	△
Stress Management	⑤	④	③	②	①	△
Tobacco use	⑤	④	③	②	①	△
Control of Addictive Behaviors*	⑤	④	③	②	①	△
Sexuality*	⑤	④	③	②	①	△
Accident Prevention and Personal Safety	⑤	④	③	②	①	△
Health Education	⑤	④	③	②	①	△

*These two components are personal, and you are not required to reveal this information. If you think that counseling is necessary, you are encouraged to seek professional help.

help you get around self-defeating behaviors in the future.

10. Monitor your progress regularly. There will be times when the specific objectives are not being met. In such cases you will have to evaluate your objectives and perhaps make changes in the general or specific objectives, or both. Also recognize that there are individual differences and that you may not be able to progress as fast as someone else. Be flexible with yourself and reconsider your plan of action.

THE FITNESS/WELLNESS EXPERIENCE AND A CHALLENGE FOR THE FUTURE

The content of this textbook has been written with the intent of providing you with the information and experiences necessary to implement your personal lifetime fitness and wellness program. If you have read and successfully completed all of the assignments in this course, including your regular exercise program, you should be convinced of the value of exercise and healthy lifestyle habits in the achievement of a new quality of life.

For most people who engage in a personal fitness and wellness program, this new quality of life is experienced after only a few weeks of training and practicing healthy lifestyle patterns. In some instances, however — especially for individuals who have led a poor lifestyle for a long time — it may take a few months before positive habits are established and feelings of well-being are experienced. But in the end everyone who applies the principles of fitness and wellness will reap the desired benefits. Perhaps this new quality of life was best explained by Dr. George Sheehan, cardiologist and runner, when he wrote:

For every runner who tours the world running marathons, there are thousands who run to hear the leaves and listen to the rain, and look to the day when it is all suddenly as easy as a bird in flight. For them, sport is not a test but a therapy, not a trial but a reward, not a question but an answer.

As pointed out earlier, the real challenge will come now that you are about to finish this course. To make the transition from a classroom setting to a lifetime commitment to fitness and wellness easier, remember to enjoy yourself and have fun along the way. Implement your program based on your interests and what you enjoy doing most. If such is the case, adhering to your new lifestyle will not be difficult.

Hopefully, the activities that you have conducted over the last few weeks or months have helped you develop positive "addictions" that will carry on throughout life. If you truly experience the feelings expressed by Dr. Sheehan, there will be no looking back. But if you don't get there, it will be difficult to know what it is like. Improving the quality and most likely the longevity of your life is now in your hands. For some it may require persistence and commitment, but *only you can take control of your lifestyle and thereby reap the benefits of wellness.*

Bibliography

Hoeger, W. W. K. *Principles and Laboratories for Physical Fitness & Wellness.* Englewood, CO: Morton Publishing, 1988.

Human Relations Media. "What is Fitness?" *Dynamics of Fitness: The Body in Action.* Pleasantville, NY: Author, 1980.

Kemper, D. W., J. Giuffre, and G. Drabinski. *Pathways: A Success Guide for a Healthy Life.* Boise, ID: Healthwise, 1985.

Figure 12.2. *Short-term wellness objectives*

Indicate below one or two general objectives that you will work on in the next couple of months, and write specific objectives that you will use to accomplish each general objective (you may not have eight specific objectives; write only as many as you need).

General Objective: _____

Specific Objectives:

1. _____

2. _____

3. _____

4. _____

5. _____

6. _____

7. _____

8. _____

General Objective: _____

Specific Objectives:

1. _____

2. _____

3. _____

4. _____

5. _____

6. _____

7. _____

8. _____

Physical Fitness and Wellness Profile*

* Fill out the enclosed profile as you obtain the results for each fitness and wellness component. You should attempt to determine the fitness components (cardiovascular endurance, muscular strength/endurance, muscular flexibility, and body composition) during the first two or three weeks of the semester so that you may proceed with your exercise program. After determining each component, discuss the objectives to be accomplished and the date of completion with your instructor.

Name: _____   Course: _____   Section: _____   Date: _____

| Item | Pre-Assessment | | | Objective[a] | Post-Assessment | | |
	Date	Test Results	Classification		Date	Test Results	Classification
Cardiovascular Endurance							
Muscular Strength							
Muscular Flexibility							
Body Composition							
Cardiovascular Risk							
Cancer Risk							
Lung							
Colon-Rectum							
Skin							
Breast[b]							
Cervical[b]							
Endometrial[b]							
Prostate[c]							
Testicular[c]							
Pancreatic							
Kidney & Bladder							
Esophageal & Stomach							
Ovarian[b]							
Thyroid							
Leukemia							
Lymphomas							
Stress							
Life Exp. Survey							
Vulnerability Scale							
Tobacco Use[d]							

Instructor's Signature: _____   Student's Signature: _____

[a] Indicate specific objective and date of completion.
[b] Women only.
[c] Men only.
[d] For test results indicate type and amount smoked, for classification indicate smoker, ex-smoker, non-smoker.

Nutrient Analysis

- Nutritive Value of Selected Foods
- Dietary Analysis Forms
- Recommended Dietary Allowances

Table B.1.
Nutritive Value of Selected Foods

Code	Food	Amount	Weight gm	Calories	Protein gm	Fat gm	Sat. Fat gm	Cholesterol mg	Carbohydrate gm	Calcium mg	Iron mg	Sodium mg	Vit A I.U.	Vit B₁ mg	Vit B₂ mg	Niacin mg	Vit C mg
001.	All-Bran cereal	1/4 c	21	53	3.0	.4	0.1	0	16	17	3.4	242	947	0.28	0.33	3.8	11
002.	Almond Joy, candy bar	1.5 oz.	42	227	2.5	12	10.2	0	28	3	1.2	0	0	0.00	0.00	0.0	0
003.	Almonds, shelled	1/4 c	36	213	6.6	19	1.4	0	9	83	1.7	2	0	0.09	0.33	1.3	0
004.	Apple, raw, unpared	1 med	150	80	0.3	1	0.0	0	20	10	0.4	1	120	0.04	0.03	0.1	6
005.	Apple juice, canned or bottled	1/2 c	124	59	0.1	0	0.0	0	15	8	0.7	1	0	0.01	0.03	0.1	1
006.	Apple pie	1 piece (3½")	118	302	2.6	13	3.5	0	45	9	0.4	355	40	0.02	0.02	0.5	1
007.	Applesauce, canned, sweetened	1/2 c	128	116	0.3	0	0.0	0	31	5	0.7	3	50	0.02	0.01	0.0	2
008.	Apricots, raw	3 (12 per lb)	114	55	1.1	0	0.0	0	14	18	0.5	1	2,890	0.06	0.04	0.6	11
009.	Apricots, canned, heavy syrup	3 halves; 1¾ tbsp liq.	85	73	0.5	0	0.0	0	19	9	0.3	1	1,480	0.02	0.02	0.3	3
010.	Apricots, dried, sulfured, uncooked	10 med halves	35	91	1.8	0	0.0	0	23	23	1.9	9	3,820	0.00	0.06	1.2	4
011.	Asparagus, cooked green spears	4 med	60	12	1.3	0	0.0	0	2	13	0.4	1	540	0.10	0.11	0.8	16
012.	Avocado, raw	1/2 med	120	185	2.4	19	3.2	0	7	11	.6	4	310	0.12	0.22	1.7	15
013.	Bacon, cooked, drained	2 slices	15	86	3.8	8	2.7	30	1	2	0.5	153	0	0.08	0.05	0.8	0
014.	Bacon/lettuce/tomato sandw.	1	130	327	11.6	19	4.7	21	31	84	2.5	661	426	0.42	0.28	4.1	12
015.	Banana, nut bread	1 slice	50	169	3.0	8	1.5	33	22	18	0.9	172	49	0.09	0.09	0.8	1
016.	Banana, raw	1 sm (7¼")	140	81	1.0	0	0.0	0	21	8	0.7	1	180	0.05	0.06	0.7	10
017.	Beans, green snap, cooked	1/2 c	65	16	1.0	0	0.0	0	3	32	0.4	4	340	0.05	0.06	0.3	8
018.	Beans, lentils	1/4 c	50	53	3.9	0	0.0	0	10	12	1.0	0	10	0.03	0.04	0.4	0
019.	Beans, lima (Fordhook), froz., cooked	1/2 c	85	84	6.0	0	0.0	0	17	40	2.1	1	240	0.15	0.08	1.1	15
020.	Beans, red kidney, cooked	1 c	185	218	14.4	1	0.0	0	40	70	4.4	6	10	0.20	0.11	1.3	0
021.	Beans, refried	1/2 c	145	148	9.0	1	0.2	0	25	71	2.6	614	0	0.07	0.08	0.7	9
022.	Bean sprouts, mung, raw	1/2 c	52	18	2.0	0	0.0	0	4	10	0.7	3	10	0.07	0.07	0.4	10
023.	Beef-chuck, cooked,	3 oz.	85	212	25.0	12	7.8	80	0	11	3.1	43	20	0.05	0.19	3.8	0
024.	Beef, corned canned	3 oz.	85	163	21.0	10	8.0	70	0	22	5.0	802	0	0.02	0.27	3.9	0
025.	Beef, ground, lean	3 oz.	85	186	23.3	10	5.0	81	0	10	3.0	57	20	0.08	0.20	5.1	0
026.	Beef, meatloaf	1 piece	111	246	20.0	15	6.1	125	5.6	37	2.4	434	181	0.08	0.23	4.1	1
027.	Beef, round steak, cooked, trimmed	3 oz.	85	222	24.3	13	6.0	77	0	10	3.0	60	20	0.07	0.20	4.8	0
028.	Beef, rump roast	3 oz.	85	177	24.7	9	4.0	80	0	10	3.1	61	10	0.06	0.19	4.4	0
029.	Beef, sirloin, cooked	3 oz.	85	329	19.6	27	13.0	77	0	9	2.5	48	50	0.05	0.15	4.0	0
030.	Beef, T-bone steak	3 oz.	85	401	16.7	37	15.6	66	0	7	2.2	40	23	0.07	0.14	3.5	0
031.	Beef, thin/sliced	3 oz.	85	105	18.5	3	1.1	36	0	11	1.8	1,409	0	0.07	0.16	4.5	0
032.	Beer	12 fl. oz.	360	151	1.1	0	0.0	0	14	18	0.0	25	0	0.01	0.11	2.2	0
033.	Beets, red, canned, drained	1/2 c	80	32	0.8	0	0.0	0	8	15	0.6	164	15	0.01	0.02	0.1	2

(continued)

Table B.1.
Nutritive Value of Selected Foods (continued)

Code	Food	Amount	Weight gm	Calories	Protein gm	Fat gm	Sat. Fat gm	Cholesterol mg	Carbohydrate gm	Calcium mg	Iron mg	Sodium mg	Vit A I.U.	Vit B₁ mg	Vit B₂ mg	Niacin mg	Vit C mg
034.	Beet greens, cooked	1/2 c	73	13	1.3	0	0.0	0	2	72	1.4	55	3,700	0.05	0.11	0.2	11
035.	Biscuits, baking powder, made from mix	1 med	35	114	2.5	6	1.1	0	18	60	0.8	272	0	0.06	0.06	0.7	0
036.	Blueberries, fresh cultivated	1/2 c	73	45	0.5	0	0.0	0	11	10	0.8	1	75	0.02	0.05	0.4	10
037.	Blueberry pie	1 piece (3½")	158	380	4.0	17	4.0	0	55	26	2.1	423	140	0.17	0.14	1.7	6
038.	Bologna	1 slice (1 oz.)	28	86	3.4	8	3.0	15	0	2	0.5	369	0	0.05	0.06	0.7	0
039.	Bouillon, broth	1 cube	4	5	.8	1	0.0	0	0	0	0.0	960	0	0.00	0.00	0.0	0
040.	Bran Cereal	1/2 c	30	72	3.8	1	0.0	0	22	25	3.0	247	2,000	1.00	0.80	3.0	20
041.	Brandy	1 oz.	28	69	0.0	0	0.0	0	11	0	0.0	1	0	0.00	0.00	0.0	0
042.	Bread, Corn	1 slice	78	161	5.8	6	0.1	0	23	94	0.9	490	120	0.10	0.15	0.5	1
043.	Bread, cracked wheat	1 slice	25	65	2.3	1	0.2	0	12	16	0.7	106	0	0.10	0.10	0.8	0
044.	Bread, French enriched	1 slice	35	102	3.2	1	0.2	0	19	15	0.8	203	0	0.10	0.08	0.9	0
045.	Bread, rye (American)	1 slice	25	61	2.3	0	0.0	0	13	19	0.4	139	0	0.05	0.02	0.4	0
046.	Bread, white enriched	1 slice	25	68	2.2	1	0.2	0	13	21	0.6	127	0	0.06	0.05	0.6	0
047.	Bread, whole wheat	1 slice	25	61	2.6	1	0.6	0	12	25	0.8	132	0	0.06	0.03	0.7	0
048.	Broccoli, raw	1 sm stalk	114	38	4.1	0	0.0	0	7	117	1.3	17	2,835	0.10	0.23	0.9	125
049.	Broccoli, cooked drained	1 sm stalk	140	36	4.3	0	0.0	0	6	123	1.1	14	3,500	0.13	0.28	1.1	126
050.	Brownies, with nuts	1	20	95	1.3	6	1.4	18	11	9	0.4	51	20	0.05	0.05	0.3	0
051.	Brussels sprouts, froz., cooked drained	1/2 c	78	28	3.2	0	0.0	0	5	25	0.8	8	405	0.06	0.11	0.5	63
052.	Bulgur, wheat	1 c	135	227	8.4	1	0.0	0	47	27	1.8	809	0	0.07	0.04	3.2	0
053.	Burrito, bean	1	166	307	12.5	9.5	3.6	14	45	173	2.4	983	283	0.25	0.22	2.3	5
054.	Burrito, combination, Taco Bell	1	175	404	21.0	16	0.0	0	43	91	3.7	300	1,666	0.34	0.31	4.6	15
055.	Butter	1 tsp	5	36	0.0	4	0.4	12	0	1	0.0	46	160	0.00	0.00	0.0	0
056.	Buttermilk, cultured	1 c	245	88	8.8	0	1.3	5	12	296	0.1	319	10	0.10	0.44	0.2	2
057.	Cabbage, raw chopped	1/2 c	45	11	0.6	0	0.0	0	3	22	0.2	9	60	0.03	0.03	0.2	21
058.	Cabbage, boiled, drained	1/2 c	85	16	0.9	0	0.0	0	3	36	0.3	10	100	0.02	0.02	0.1	21
059.	Cake, angel food, plain	1 piece	60	161	4.3	0	0.0	0	36	5	0.1	170	0	0.01	0.08	0.1	0
060.	Cake, devil's food, iced	1 piece	99	365	4.5	16	5.0	68	55	69	1.0	233	160	0.02	0.10	0.2	0
061.	Candy, hard	1 oz.	28	109	0.0	0	0.0	0	28	6	0.5	9	0	0.00	0.00	0.0	0
062.	Cantaloupe	1/4 melon 5" diam.	239	35	2.0	0	0.0	0	10	20	0.8	17	4,620	0.06	0.04	0.6	45
063.	Caramel (candy, plain or choc.)	1 oz.	28	113	1.1	3	1.6	0	22	42	0.4	64	0	0.01	0.05	0.1	0
064.	Carrots, raw	1 carrot 7½" long	81	30	0.8	0	0.0	0	7	27	0.5	34	7,930	0.04	0.04	0.4	6
065.	Carrots, cooked, drained	1/2 c	73	23	0.7	0	0.0	0	5	24	0.5	10	7,615	0.04	0.04	0.4	5
066.	Cashew-roasted-unsalted	2 oz.	57	326	9.2	27	5.4	0	16	23	2.3	10	0	0.24	0.10	1.0	0
067.	Cauliflower, cooked, drained	1/2 c	63	14	1.5	0	0.0	0	3	13	0.5	6	40	0.06	0.05	0.4	35
068.	Celery, green, raw, long	1 outer stalk 8"	40	7	0.4	0	0	0	2	16	0.1	50	110	0.01	0.01	0.1	4
069.	Champagne	4 oz.	113	87	0.2	0	0	0	2	6	0.4	7	0	0.00	0.01	0.1	0

No.	Food	Amount															
070.	Cheerios cereal	1 c	23	89	3.4	1	.2	0	16	3.6	38	246	949	0.32	0.32	4.0	12
071.	Cheese, American	1 oz. slice	28	100	6.0	8	5.6	27	1	0.1	188	307	343	0.01	0.10	0.0	0
072.	Cheese, blue	1 oz.	28	100	6.0	8	5.3	25	0	0.1	89	510	204	0.01	0.11	0.3	0
073.	Cheese, cheddar	1 oz.	28	114	7.0	9	6.0	30	4	0.2	204	171	300	0.01	0.11	0.0	0
074.	Cheese, cottage, 2%	1/2 c	113	103	15.5	2	1.4	10	3	0.2	78	459	79	0.03	0.21	0.2	0
075.	Cheese, cottage, creamed	½ cup	105	112	14.0	5	6.4	15	1	0.3	99	241	180	0.03	0.26	0.1	0
076.	Cheese, creamed	1 oz.	28	99	6.0	8	3.0	31	7	0.3	167	71	320	0.02	0.14	0.0	0
077.	Cheese, souffle	1 portion	110	240	10.9	19	9.5	189	29	1.1	221	400	880	0.06	0.26	0.2	2
078.	Cheeseburger, McDonalds	1	115	321	15.2	16	6.7	40	24	2.9	170	736	353	0.30	0.24	4.4	4
079.	Cheesecake	1 piece (3½")	85	257	4.6	16	9.0	150	12	0.4	48	189	216	0.03	0.11	0.4	41
080.	Cherries	10	75	47	0.9	0	0.0	0	45	0.3	15	8	450	0.20	0.24	1.6	1
081.	Cherry Pie	1 piece (3½")	118	308	3.1	13	5.0	137	0	0.4	17	355	40	0.02	0.02	0.5	0
082.	Chicken breast/roast w/skin	1	98	193	29.2	8	2.1	83	0	1.0	14	69	91	0.07	0.12	12.5	0
083.	Chicken, drumstick Kentucky Fried		54	136	14.0	8	2.2	73	2	0.9	20	320	30	0.04	0.12	2.7	0
084.	Chicken, drumstick, roasted	1	52	112	14.1	6	1.6	48	0	0.7	6	47	52	0.04	0.11	3.1	0
085.	Chicken McNuggets	6	111	329	19.5	21	5.2	64	15	1.3	11	521	92	0.16	0.14	7.7	2
086.	Chicken, patty sandwich	1	157	436	24.8	23	6.1	68	34	1.9	44	2,732	47	0.3	0.26	9.2	4
087.	Chicken, wing, Kentucky Fried	1	45	151	11.0	10	2.9	70	4	0.6	0	300	0	0.03	0.07	0.0	0
088.	Chicken, roast, light meat without skin	3 oz.	85	141	27.0	3	0.4	45	0	1.2	10	54	51	0.03	0.09	9.9	0
089.	Chicken, roast, dark meat without skin	3 oz.	85	149	24.0	5	0.8	50	0	1.5	11	54	127	0.06	0.19	4.7	0
090.	Chili con carne	1 c	255	339	19.1	16	5.8	28	31	4.3	82	1,354	150	0.08	0.18	3.3	8
091.	Chocolate cake w/icing	1 piece	69	235	3.0	8	3.6	37	40	1.4	41	181	100	0.07	0.10	0.6	0
092.	Chocolate fudge	1 oz.	28	115	0.6	3	2.1	1	21	0.3	22	54	0	0.01	0.03	0.1	0
093.	Chocolate, M&M's, plain	1 oz.	28	140	1.9	6	3.3	0	19	0.5	47	24	30	0.01	0.07	0.2	0
094.	Chocolate, M&M's w/peanuts	1 oz.	28	145	3.2	7	3.2	0	16	0.4	35	17	15	0.02	0.05	0.9	0
095.	Chocolate, milk	1 oz.	28	147	2.0	9	3.6	5	16	0.3	65	27	80	0.02	0.10	0.1	0
096.	Chocolate, milk w/almonds	1 oz.	28	150	2.9	10	4.4	5	15	0.6	61	23	30	0.03	0.13	0.3	0
097.	Chocolate, Milky way bar	1 oz.	28	128	1.4	4	3.0	7	20	0.2	40	65	41	0.01	0.07	0.1	0
098.	Chocolate, Snickers bar	1 oz.	28	138	3.0	6	3.0	0	17	0.2	32	70	9	0.01	0.05	0.1	0
099.	Clam, canned drained	3 oz.	85	83	13.0	7	0.2	50	2	3.5	46	750	93	0.01	0.09	0.9	9
100.	Clam chowder (north east)	1 c	248	163	9.5	7	3.0	22	16	1.5	187	992	160	0.07	0.24	1.0	4
101.	Cocoa, hot, with whole milk	1 c	250	218	9.1	9	6.1	33	26	0.8	298	123	318	0.10	0.44	0.4	2
102.	Cocoa, plain, dry	1 tbsp	5	14	0.9	1	0.0	0	3	0.6	7	0	0	0.01	0.02	0.1	0
103.	Coconut, shredded, packed	½ c	65	225	2.3	23	20.0	0	6	1.1	8	165	0	0.03	0.01	0.3	2
104.	Cod, cooked	3 oz.	85	144	24.3	4	1.5	60	0	0.9	27	63	150	0.06	0.09	2.7	0
105.	Coffee	¾ cup	180	1	0.0	0	0.0	0	0	0.2	1	2	0	0.00	0.00	0.1	0
106.	Coffee cake	1 piece	72	230	4.5	7	2.5	47	38	1.2	44	310	120	0.14	0.15	1.3	0
107.	Cola	12 oz.	369	144	0.0	17	0.0	0	37	0.0	27	30	0	0.00	0.00	0.0	0
108.	Coleslaw	1 c	120	173	1.6	6	1.0	5	6	0.5	53	144	190	0.06	0.06	0.4	35
109.	Collards, leaves without stems, cooked, drained	½ c	95	32	3.4	1	2.0	0	5	0.8	178	28	7,410	0.01	0.19	1.2	72
110.	Cookies, chocolate chip homemade	2 2¼" diam.	20	103	1.0	6	1.7	14	12	0.4	7	70	20	0.02	0.02	0.2	0

(continued)

Table B.1.
Nutritive Value of Selected Foods (continued)

Code	Food	Amount	Weight gm	Calories	Protein gm	Fat gm	Sat. Fat gm	Cholesterol mg	Carbohydrate gm	Calcium mg	Iron mg	Sodium mg	Vit A I.U.	Vit B$_1$ mg	Vit B$_2$ mg	Niacin mg	Vit C mg
111.	Cookies, oatmeal raisin	2 2" diam.	26	122	1.5	5	1.3	1	18	9	.6	74	20	0.04	0.04	0.5	0
112.	Cookies, vanilla	5 1¾" diam.	20	93	1.0	3	0.8	10	15	8	0.1	50	25	0.00	0.01	0.0	0
113.	Corn, boiled on cob	1 ear 5" long	140	70	2.5	1	0.0	0	16	2	0.5	1	310	0.09	0.08	1.1	7
114.	Corn, canned, drained	1/2 c	83	70	2.2	1	0.0	0	16	4	0.4	195	290	0.03	0.04	0.8	4
115.	Corn chips	1 oz.	28	155	2.0	9	1.8	0	16	35	0.5	233	110	0.04	0.05	0.4	1
116.	Cornflakes	1 c	25	97	2.0	0	0.0	0	21	3	0.6	251	180	0.29	0.55	2.9	9
117.	Cornmeal, degermed, yellow, enriched cooked	1/2 c	120	60	1.3	0	0.0	0	13	1	0.5	264	70	0.07	0.05	0.6	0
118.	Crackers, graham	2 squares	14	55	1.1	1	0.3	0	10	6	0.2	95	0	0.01	0.03	0.2	0
119.	Crackers, Ritz	1	3	15	0.2	1	0.2	0	2	3	0.1	30	0	0.01	0.01	0.1	0
120.	Crackers, saltines	4 squares	11	48	1.0	1	0.3	0	8	2	0.1	123	0	0.00	0.00	0.1	0
121.	Crackers, Soda	1	3	13	0.3	0	0.1	0	2	1	0.1	39	0	0.02	0.01	0.1	0
122.	Crackers, Triscuits	1	5	23	0.4	1	0.3	0	3	0	0.0	0	0	0.00	0.00	0.0	0
123.	Crackers, Wheat Thins	1	2	9	0.2	0	0.1	0	1	1	0.1	17	0	0.01	0.01	0.1	0
124.	Cream, light coffee or table	1 tbsp	15	20	0.5	2	0.5	5	1	16	0.1	7	70	0.00	0.02	0.0	0
125.	Cream, heavy whipping	1 tbsp	15	53	0.3	6	1.3	12	1	11	0.0	5	230	0.00	0.02	0.0	0
126.	Croissant		57	235	4.7	12	4.0	13	27	20	2.1	452	50	0.17	0.13	1.3	0
127.	Croissants (Sara Lee)	1 roll	18	59	1.6	2	0.3	0	8	22	0.6	105	0	0.14	0.09	0.8	0
128.	Cucumbers, raw pared	9 sm slices	28	4	0.3	0	0.0	0	1	7	0.3	2	70	0.01	0.01	0.1	3
129.	Dates hydrated	5	46	110	0.9	0	0.0	0	29	24	1.2	1	20	0.04	0.04	0.9	0
130.	Doughnuts, plain		42	164	1.9	8	2.0	19	22	17	0.6	210	30	0.07	0.07	0.5	0
131.	Dressing, blue cheese	1 tbsp	15	77	0.7	8	1.9	4	1	12	0.0	8	32	0.00	0.02	0.0	0
132.	Dressing, French	1 tbsp	16	83	0.1	9	1.4	0	1	2	0.1	184	0	0.00	0.00	0.0	0
133.	Dressing, Italian	1 tbsp	15	69	0.1	9	1.3	0	2	1	0.0	73	29	0.00	0.00	0.0	0
134.	Dressing, ranch style	1 tbsp	15	54	0.4	6	0.9	6	1	15	0.0	65	36	0.01	0.02	0.0	0
135.	Eggs, hard cooked	1 large	50	72	6.0	5	1.8	250	1	24	1.0	54	520	0.05	0.13	0.0	0
136.	Egg, fried with butter	1	46	95	5.4	6	2.4	278	1	28	0.9	113	320	0.04	0.13	0.0	0
137.	Egg McMuffin	1	138	327	18.5	15	5.9	259	31	226	2.9	885	591	0.47	0.44	3.8	1
138.	Egg salad sandwich	1	111	325	10.0	19	3.9	215	28	95	2.5	461	242	0.29	0.29	2.1	0
139.	Eggs, White	1 large	33	17	3.6	0	0.0	0	0	3	0.0	48	0	0.00	0.09	0.0	0
140.	Enchilada, beef	1	200	487	21.8	23	8.8	63	26	425	2.9	262	595	0.02	0.27	3.5	5
141.	Enchilada, cheese	1	230	632	25.3	34	17.6	82	31	876	2.6	596	1,672	0.13	0.40	1.2	15
142.	Farina, enriched, quick cooking, cooked	1/2 c	123	51	1.6	0	0.0	0	11	5	6.0	176	0	0.06	0.03	0.5	0
143.	Figs, dried	1 large	21	60	1.0	0	0.0	0	15	26	0.6	1	20	0.16	0.17	3.9	0
144.	Filet of Fish, McDonald's	1	131	402	15.0	23	7.9	43	34	105	1.8	709	152	0.28	0.28	3.9	4
145.	Fish, sticks	2	56	140	12.0	6	1.6	52	8	22	0.6	106	40	0.06	0.10	1.2	0
146.	Flounder	3 oz.	85	171	25.5	7	1.0	60	0	21	1.2	201	0	0.06	0.06	2.1	3
147.	Flour, all purpose enriched	1 c	125	455	13.0	1	0.0	0	95	20	3.6	3	0	0.55	0.33	4.4	0
148.	Flour, whole wheat	1 c	120	400	16.0	2	0.0	0	85	49	4.0	4	0	0.66	0.14	5.2	0

No.	Food	Amount														
149.	Frankfurters, cooked	1	57	176	7.0	16	5.6	45	1	4	1.1	627	0	0.09	0.11	1.5	0
150.	Frankfurter, turkey/cooked	1	45	102	6.4	8	2.7	39	1	58	0.8	454	60	0.04	0.08	1.7	0
151.	Fruit cocktail	1 c	245	91	1.0	0	0.0	0	24	22	1.0	12	370	0.05	0.02	1.2	5
152.	Ginger ale	12 oz.	366	113	0.0	0	0.0	0	29	0	0.0	45	0	0.00	0.00	0.0	0
153.	Granola, Nature Valley	1/2 c	57	252	5.8	10	7.0	0	38	36	1.9	116	41	0.20	0.10	0.4	0
154.	Grapefruit, raw white	1/2 med	301	56	1.0	0	0.0	0	15	22	0.5	1	10	0.05	0.03	0.3	52
155.	Grapefruit, juice unsweetened canned	1/2 c	124	50	0.6	0	0.0	0	12	11	0.2	2	10	0.05	0.03	0.3	46
156.	Grapes, raw seedless European	10 grapes	50	34	0.3	0	0.0	0	9	6	0.2	2	50	0.03	0.03	0.2	2
157.	Grape juice, unsweetened bottled	1/2 c	127	84	0.3	0	0.0	0	21	14	0.4	3	0	0.05	0.03	0.3	0
158.	Gravy, beef, homemade	1 tbsp	17	19	0.3	2	1.0	1	1	1	0.1	49	0	0.01	0.01	0.1	0
159.	Haddock, fried (dipped in egg, milk, bread crumbs)	3 oz.	85	141	17.0	5	1.0	54	5	33	0.9	150	0	0.03	0.06	2.7	3
160.	Halibut, broiled with butter or margarine	3 oz.	85	144	21.0	6	2.1	55	0	15	0.6	114	570	0.03	0.06	7.2	1
161.	Ham (cured pork)	3 oz.	85	318	20.0	26	9.4	77	0	9	2.6	48	0	0.43	0.20	3.8	0
162.	Ham, lunch meat	1 slice	28	37	5.5	1	0.5	13	.3	2	0.2	405	0	0.26	0.06	1.4	7
163.	Hamburger, Big Mac	1	204	581	25.1	36	12.0	85	40	207	5.0	999	388	0.49	0.39	7.3	3
164.	Hamburger, McDonald's	1	99	257	13.0	9	3.7	26	30	63	3.0	526	231	0.23	0.23	5.1	2
165.	Honey	1 tbsp	21	64	0.0	0	0.0	0	17	1	0.1	1	0	0.00	0.01	0.1	0
166.	Ice cream, vanilla	1/2 c	67	135	3.0	7	4.4	27	14	97	0.1	42	295	0.03	0.14	0.1	1
167.	Ice cream cone	1 small	115	185	4.3	5	2.2	24	30	183	0.1	109	218	0.06	0.36	0.4	1
168.	Ice cream cone, Dairy Queen	medium	142	230	6.0	7	4.6	15	35	200	0.0	150	300	0.09	0.26	0.0	0
169.	Ice cream, hot fudge sund.	1	164	357	7.0	11	5.4	27	58	215	0.6	170	233	0.07	0.31	1.1	2
170.	Ice milk, vanilla	1/2 c	61	100	3.0	3	1.8	13	15	102	0.1	45	140	0.04	0.15	0.1	1
171.	Inst. breakfast/whole milk	1 c	281	280	15.0	8	5.1	33	34	301	8.0	286	2,057	0.39	0.46	5.2	29
172.	Jams or preserves	1 tbsp	7	18	0.0	0	0.0	0	5	1	0.1	1	1	0.00	0.00	0.0	0
173.	Jelly	1 tbsp	18	49	0.0	0	0.0	0	13	4	0.3	3	0	0.00	0.01	0.0	1
174.	Kale, fresh cooked, drained	1/2 c	55	22	2.5	0	0.0	0	3	103	0.9	24	4,565	0.06	0.10	0.9	51
175.	Kool Aid, with sugar	1 c	240	100	0.0	0	0.0	0	25	9	0.0	0	0	0.00	0.00	0.0	6
176.	Lamb leg, roast, trimmed	3 oz.	85	237	22.0	16	7.3	60	0	9	1.4	53	0	0.13	0.23	4.7	0
177.	Lasagna, homemade	1 piece	220	357	23.6	18	8.3	50	27	413	2.8	703	1,008	0.19	0.30	3.3	6
178.	Lemon juice, fresh	1 tbsp	15	4	0.1	0	0.0	0	1	1	0.0	1	1	0.00	0.00	0.0	7
179.	Lemonade (concentrate)	12 oz.	340	137	0.2	0	0.1	0	36	6	0.6	3	73	0.02	0.00	0.1	13
180.	Lentils, cooked	1/2 c	100	106	8.0	0	0.0	0	19	25	2.1	0	20	0.07	0.07	0.6	0
181.	Lettuce, crisp head	1 c sm chunks	75	10	0.7	0	0.0	0	2	15	0.4	7	250	0.05	0.06	0.2	5
182.	Lettuce, cos or romaine	1 c chopped	55	10	0.7	0	0.0	0	2	37	0.8	5	1,050	0.08	0.04	0.2	10
183.	Liver, beef, fried	1 slice 3 oz.	85	195	22.0	9	2.5	345	5	9	7.5	156	45,390	0.22	3.56	14.0	23
184.	Liverwurst, fresh	1 slice 1 oz.	28	87	5.0	7	3.5	50	1	3	1.5	0	1,800	0.06	0.37	1.6	0
185.	Lobster	1 c	145	138	27.0	2	1.0	293	1	94	1.2	305	0	0.15	0.10	0.0	0
186.	Macaroni, enriched cooked	1/2 c	70	78	2.4	0	0.0	0	16	6	0.7	1	0	0.10	0.06	0.8	0
187.	Macaroni and cheese	1/2 c	100	215	8.2	11	4.0	21	20	181	0.9	543	430	0.10	0.20	0.9	0
188.	Maple syrup	3 tbsp.	60	150	0.0	0	0.0	0	39	99	0.7	9	0	0.10	0.00	0.7	0
189.	Margarine	1 tsp	5	34	0.0	4	0.7	2	0	1	0.0	46	160	0.00	0.00	0.0	0

(continued)

Table B.1.
Nutritive Value of Selected Foods (continued)

Code	Food	Amount	Weight gm	Calories	Protein gm	Fat gm	Sat. Fat gm	Cholesterol mg	Carbohydrate gm	Calcium mg	Iron mg	Sodium mg	Vit A I.U.	Vit B₁ mg	Vit B₂ mg	Niacin mg	Vit C mg
190.	Matzo	1 piece	30	117	3.0	0	0.0	0	25	*	*	0	*	*	*	*	*
191.	Mayonnaise	1 tsp	5	36	0.0	4	0.7	3	0	1	0.0	28	13	0.00	0.00	0.0	0
192.	Milk, evaporated whole	1/2 c	126	172	9.0	10	5.8	40	13	329	0.2	149	405	0.05	0.43	0.2	2
193.	Milk, lowfat (2% fat)	1 c	246	145	10.0	5	3.1	5	15	352	0.1	150	200	0.10	0.52	0.2	2
194.	Milk shake, chocolate	1 (10 fluid oz.)	340	433	11.5	13	7.8	45	70	383	1.1	328	312	0.20	0.83	0.5	0
195.	Milk shake, strawberry	1 (10 fluid oz.)	340	383	11.4	10	6.0	37	64	384	0.4	281	408	0.15	0.66	0.6	3
196.	Milk shake, vanilla (McDonald's)	1	289	323	10.0	8	5.1	29	52	346	0.2	250	346	0.12	0.66	0.6	3
197.	Milk skim	1 c	245	88	9.0	0	0.3	5	12	296	0.1	126	10	0.09	0.44	0.2	2
198.	Milk, whole (3.5% fat)	1 c	244	159	9.0	9	5.1	34	12	288	0.1	120	350	0.07	0.40	0.2	2
199.	Molasses, medium	1 tbsp	20	50	0.0	0	0.0	0	13	33	0.9	3	0	0.01	0.01	0.0	0
200.	Muffin, blueberry		45	135	3.0	5	1.5	19	20	54	0.9	198	40	0.10	0.11	0.9	1
201.	Muffin, bran		45	125	3.0	6	1.4	24	19	60	1.4	189	230	0.11	0.13	1.3	3
202.	Muffin, cornmeal		45	145	3.0	5	1.5	23	21	66	.9	169	80	0.11	0.11	0.9	0
203.	Muffin, English w/butter		63	186	5.0	5	2.3	15	30	117	1.5	310	164	0.28	0.49	2.6	1
204.	Mushrooms, fresh cultivated	1/2 c sliced	35	12	1.0	0	0.0	0	2	4	0.5	4	0	0.04	0.12	2.4	1
205.	Mustard greens, cooked drained	1/2 c	70	16	1.7	0	0.0	0	3	96	1.2	13	4,060	0.05	0.10	0.4	33
206.	Noodles, egg, enriched cooked	1/2 c	80	100	3.3	1	0.0	0	19	8	0.7	2	55	0.11	0.07	1.0	0
207.	Nuts, Brazil	1 oz. (6-8 nuts)	28	185	4.1	19	4.8	0	3	53	1.0	0	0	0.27	0.03	0.5	0
208.	Nuts, pecans	1 oz.	28	195	2.6	20	1.4	0	4	21	0.7	0	40	0.24	0.04	0.3	1
209.	Nuts, walnuts	1 oz. (14 halves)	28	185	4.2	18	1.0	0	5	28	0.9	1	10	0.09	0.04	0.3	1
210.	Oatmeal, quick, cooked	1/2 c	120	66	2.4	1	0.2	0	12	11	0.7	262	0	0.10	0.03	0.1	0
211.	Oil, soybean	1 tsp.	5	44	0.0	5	2.0	0	0	0	0.0	0	0	0.00	0.00	0.0	0
212.	Okra, cooked drained	1/2 c	80	23	1.6	0	0.0	0	5	74	0.4	2	390	0.11	0.15	0.7	16
213.	Olives, black ripe	10 extra large	55	61	0.5	7	1.0	0	1	40	0.8	385	30	0.00	0.00	0.0	0
214.	Onions, mature cooked, drained	1/2 c sliced	105	31	1.3	0	0.0	0	7	25	0.4	8	40	0.03	0.03	0.2	8
215.	Onion rings, fried	3	30	122	1.6	8	2.3	0	11	9	0.5	113	68	0.08	0.04	1.1	0
216.	Onion rings (Brazier) Dairy Queen	1 serving	85	360	6.0	17	6.0	15	33	20	0.4	125	0	0.09	0.00	0.4	2
217.	Orange, raw (medium skin)	1 med	180	64	1.3	0	0.0	0	16	54	0.5	1	260	0.13	0.05	0.5	66
218.	Orange juice, froz. reconstituted	1/2 c	125	61	0.9	0	0.0	0	15	13	0.1	1	270	0.12	0.02	0.5	60
219.	Oysters, raw Eastern	1/2 c (6-9 med)	120	79	10.0	2	1.3	60	4	113	6.6	145	370	0.17	0.22	3.0	0
220.	Pancakes	1 6" diam x 1/2" thick	73	169	5.2	5	1.0	36	25	74	0.9	310	90	0.12	0.16	0.9	0
221.	Papaya, raw	1/2 med	227	60	0.9	0	0.0	0	15	31	0.5	5	2,660	0.06	0.06	0.5	85
222.	Parsnips, cooked	1 large 9" long	160	106	2.4	1	0.0	0	24	72	1.0	13	50	0.11	0.13	0.2	16
223.	Peaches, raw, peeled	1 2¾" diam.	175	58	0.9	0	0.0	0	15	14	0.8	2	2,030	0.03	0.08	1.5	11

No.	Food	Serving	Wt (g)	Cal	Prot	Fat	Sat. Fat	Chol	Carb	Ca	Fe	Na	Vit A	Thiamin	Ribo	Niacin	Vit C
224.	Peaches, canned, heavy syrup	1 half 2⅛ tbsp liq.	96	75	0.4	0	0.0	0	19	4	0.3	2	410	0.01	0.02	0.6	3
225.	Peanut butter	2 tbsp	32	188	8.0	16	1.0	0	6	18	0.6	194	0	0.04	0.04	4.8	0
226.	Peanut butter/jam sandwich	1	100	340	11.4	14	2.6	0	45	87	2.3	414	1	0.32	0.22	5.3	0
227.	Peanuts, roasted	1 oz.	28	166	7.0	14	1.0	0	5	21	0.6	119	0	0.09	0.04	4.9	0
228.	Pears, Bartlett, raw	1 pear	180	100	1.1	1	0.0	0	25	13	0.5	2	30	0.03	0.07	0.2	7
229.	Pears, canned, heavy syrup	1 half 2¼ tbsp liq.	103	78	0.2	0	0.0	0	20	5	0.2	1	0	0.01	0.02	0.1	1
230.	Peas, frozen, cooked drained	1/2 c	80	55	4.1	0	0.0	0	10	15	1.5	92	480	0.22	0.07	1.4	11
231.	Peas, early, canned, drained	1/2 c	85	75	4.0	0	0.0	0	14	22	1.6	200	585	0.08	0.05	0.7	7
232.	Peppers, sweet, raw	1 pepper 3¼"x3" diam.	200	36	2.0	0	0.0	0	8	15	1.1	21	690	0.13	0.13	0.8	210
233.	Pickles, dill	1 large 4" long	135	15	0.9	0	0.0	0	3	35	1.4	1,928	140	0.00	0.03	0.0	8
234.	Pickles, sweet	1 large 3" long	35	51	0.2	0	0.0	0	13	4	0.4	0	30	0.00	0.01	0.0	2
235.	Pineapple, raw	1/2 c diced	78	41	0.3	0	0.0	0	11	13	0.4	1	55	0.07	0.03	0.2	13
236.	Pineapple, canned, heavy syrup	1/2 c	128	95	0.4	0	0.0	0	25	14	0.4	2	65	0.10	0.03	0.3	9
237.	Pizza, Cheese, Thin 'n Crispy, Pizza Hut	1/2 10" pie	*	450	25.0	15	7.0	125	54	450	4.5	1,200	750	0.30	0.51	5.0	1
238.	Pizza, Cheese, Thick 'n Chewy, Pizza Hut	1/2 10" pie	*	560	34.0	14	6.0	110	71	500	5.4	1,100	1,000	0.68	0.68	7.0	1
239.	Plums, Japanese and hybrid, raw	1 plum 2⅛" diam.	70	32	0.3	0	0.0	0	8	8	0.3	1	160	0.02	0.02	0.3	4
240.	Popcorn, cooked/oil	1 c	11	55	0.9	3	0.5	0	6	3	0.3	86	20	0.01	0.02	0.1	0
241.	Popcorn, popped, plain, large kernel	1 c	6	12	0.8	0	0.0	0	5	1	0.2	0	0	0.00	0.01	0.1	0
242.	Pork, roast, trimmed	2 slices 3 oz.	85	179	24.0	8	2.2	65	0	11	3.1	863	0	0.55	0.22	4.3	0
243.	Pork, sausage, cooked	1 sm link	17	72	2.8	6	2.1	13	1	0	0.3	221	0	0.00	0.00	0.0	0
244.	Potato, baked in skin	1 potato 2 1/3x4¼"	202	145	4.0	0	0.0	0	33	14	1.1	6	0	0.15	0.07	2.7	31
245.	Potato chips	10 chips	20	114	1.1	8	2.1	0	10	8	0.4	150	0	0.04	0.01	1.0	3
246.	Potato, French fried long	10 strips 3½–4"	78	214	3.4	10	1.7	0	28	12	1.0	5	0	0.10	0.06	2.4	16
247.	Potato, mashed, milk added	1/2 c	105	69	2.2	1	0.4	8	14	25	0.4	316	20	0.09	0.06	1.1	11
248.	Potato salad w/eggs/mayo	1/2 c	125	179	3.4	10	7.8	85	14	24	0.8	662	262	0.10	0.08	1.1	12
249.	Potatoes, hash brown	1/2 c	78	170	2.5	9	3.5	0	22	12	1.2	27	0	0.09	0.02	1.9	5
250.	Pound cake	1 piece	30	120	2.0	5	1.0	32	15	20	0.5	98	200	0.05	0.06	0.5	0
251.	Pretzel, thin, twists	1 oz.	28	113	2.8	1	0.3	0	23	8	0.6	456	0	0.09	0.07	1.2	0
252.	Prunes, dried "softenized" without pits	5 prunes	61	137	1.1	0	0.0	0	36	26	0.1	4	860	0.05	0.09	0.9	2
253.	Prune juice, canned or bottled	1/2 c	128	99	0.5	0	0.0	0	24	18	5.3	3	0	0.02	0.02	0.5	3
254.	Pumpkin Pie	1 (3½")	114	241	4.6	13	3.0	70	28	58	0.6	244	2,810	0.03	0.11	0.6	0
255.	Quiche, Lorraine	1 piece	242	825	18.0	66	31.9	392	40	290	1.9	898	2,250	0.15	0.44	1.7	1
256.	Raisins, unbleached, seedless	1 oz.	28	82	0.7	1	0.0	0	22	18	1.0	8	10	0.03	0.02	0.1	0
257.	Rice, brown, cooked	1/2 c	96	116	2.5	0	0	0	25	12	0.5	275	0	0.09	0.02	1.3	0
258.	Rice Crispies (Kellogg's)	3/4 c	22	85	1.4	0	0.0	0	19	3	1.4	255	971	0.30	0.30	3.8	11
259.	Rice, white enriched, cooked	1/2 c	103	113	2.1	0	0.0	0	25	11	0.9	384	0	0.12	0.01	1.1	0
260.	Rueben sandwich	1	237	488	28.7	28	10.4	85	30	364	5.3	1,685	461	0.25	0.44	3.9	12
261.	Salami, dry	1 oz.	28	128	7.0	11	1.6	24	0	4	1.0	349	0	0.10	0.07	1.5	0

(continued)

Table B.1.
Nutritive Value of Selected Foods (continued)

Code	Food	Amount	Weight gm	Calories	Pro-tein gm	Fat gm	Sat. Fat gm	Cho-les-terol mg	Car-bohy-drate gm	Cal-cium mg	Iron mg	Sodium mg	Vit A I.U.	Vit B$_1$ mg	Vit B$_2$ mg	Niacin mg	Vit C mg
262.	Salmon, broiled with butter or margarine	3 oz.	85	156	23.0	6	2.2	53	0	0	0.9	99	150	0.15	0.06	8.4	0
263.	Salmon, canned Chinook	3 oz.	85	179	16.6	12	0.8	30	0	131	0.7	105	197	0.03	0.01	6.2	0
264.	Sardines, canned drained	1 oz.	28	58	7.0	3	1.0	20	0	124	0.8	233	60	0.01	0.06	1.5	0
265.	Sauerkraut, canned	1/2 c	118	21	1.2	0	0.0	0	5	43	0.6	878	60	0.04	0.05	0.3	17
266.	Sherbet	1/2 c	97	135	1.1	2	1.3	7	29	52	0.2	44	92	0.02	0.04	0.1	2
267.	Shredded Wheat-large bisc.	1	19	65	2.1	2	0.0	0	11	8	0.6	1	0	0.06	0.05	0.9	0
268.	Shrimp, boiled	3 oz.	85	99	18.0	1	0.1	128	1	99	2.7	1	60	0.00	0.03	1.5	0
269.	Soda pop, diet	12 oz.	340	2	0	0	0.0	0	0	13	0.1	31	0	0.00	0.00	0.0	0
270.	Soup, chicken, cream	1 c	248	191	7.5	12	4.6	27	15	180	0.7	1,046	710	0.07	0.26	0.9	1
271.	Soup, chicken noodle	1 c	241	75	4.0	2	.7	7	9	17	0.8	900	711	0.05	0.06	1.4	0
272.	Soup, cream of mushroom condensed, prepared with equal volume of milk	1 c	245	216	7.0	14	5.4	15	16	191	0.5	955	250	0.05	0.34	0.7	1
273.	Soup, split pea, condensed, prepared with equal volume of water	1 c	245	145	9.0	3	1.1	0	21	29	1.5	941	440	0.25	0.15	1.5	1
274.	Soup, tomato, condensed, prepared with equal volume of water	1 c	245	88	2.0	3	0.5	0	16	15	0.7	970	1,000	0.05	0.05	1.2	12
275.	Soup, tomato with milk	1 c	248	160	6.0	6	2.9	17	22	159	1.8	932	850	0.13	0.25	1.5	68
276.	Soup, vegetable beef, condensed, prepared with equal volume of water	1 c	245	78	5.0	2	0.0	0	10	12	0.7	1,046	2,700	0.05	0.05	1.0	0
277.	Sour cream	1/2 c	115	247	3.6	24	16.3	51	5	134	0.1	62	910	0.04	0.17	0.1	1
278.	Spaghetti, in tomato sauce with cheese	1 c	250	260	8.8	9	2.0	10	37	80	2.3	955	1,080	0.25	0.18	2.3	13
279.	Spaghetti, with meatballs and tomato sauce	1 c	248	332	18.6	11.7	3.0	75	39	124	3.7	1,009	1,590	0.25	0.30	4.0	22
280.	Spareribs, cooked	3 oz.	85	377	17.8	33	12.0	73	0	8	2.2	31	0	0.37	0.18	2.9	0
281.	Spinach, raw, chopped	1 c	55	14	1.8	0	0.0	0	2	51	1.7	39	4,460	0.06	0.11	0.3	28
282.	Spinach, canned, drained	1/2 c	103	25	2.3	1	0.0	0	4	121	2.6	242	8,200	0.02	0.12	0.3	15
283.	Spinach, froz., cooked, drained	1/2 c	103	24	3.1	0	0.0	0	4	116	2.2	54	8,100	0.07	0.16	0.4	20
284.	squash, summer, cooked	1/2 c	90	13	0.8	0	0.0	0	3	23	0.4	1	350	0.05	0.07	0.7	9
285.	Squash, winter, baked mashed	1/2 c	103	70	1.9	0	0.0	0	18	41	1.0	1	6,560	0.05	0.14	0.7	8
286.	Strawberries, raw	1 c	149	55	1.0	1	0.0	0	13	31	1.5	1	90	0.04	0.10	0.9	88
287.	Stuffing, bread, prepared	1/2 c	70	250	4.6	15	3.1	0	25	46	1.1	627	455	0.09	0.10	1.3	0
288.	Sundae, choc. Dairy Queen	medium	184	300	6.0	7	4.9	79	53	200	1.1	175	300	0.06	0.26	0.0	0
289.	Sugar, brown granulated	1 tsp	5	17	0.0	0	0.0	0	5	4	0.1	0	0	0.00	0.00	0.1	0
290.	Sugar, white granulated	1 tsp	4	15	0.0	0	0.0	0	4	0	0.0	0	0	0.00	0.00	0.0	0
291.	Sweet potato, baked	1 potato 5" long	146	161	2.4	1	0.0	0	37	46	1.0	14	9,230	0.10	0.08	0.8	25

292.	Syrup (maple)	1 tbsp	20	50	0.0	0	0.0	0	13	33	0.2	3	0	0.00	0.00	0.0	0
293.	Taco, Taco Bell	1	83	186	15.0	8	0.0	0	14	120	2.4	79	120	0.09	0.16	2.9	0
294.	Tangerine	1 med 2⅜" diam.	116	39	0.7	0	0.0	0	10	34	0.3	2	360	0.05	0.02	0.1	27
295.	Tea, brewed	3/4 c	180	0	0.0	0	0.0	0	0	0	0.0	0	0	0.00	0.00	0.0	0
296.	Tomato juice, canned	1 c	244	42	1.9	0	0.1	0	10	22	1.4	881	1,357	0.12	0.08	1.6	45
297.	Tomato sauce (catsup)	1 tbsp	15	16	0.3	0	0.0	0	4	3	0.1	156	105	0.01	0.01	0.2	2
298.	Tomatoes, raw	1 tomato 3½ oz.	100	20	1.0	0	0.0	0	4	12	0.5	3	820	0.05	0.04	0.6	21
299.	Tomatoes, canned	½ c	121	26	1.2	0	0.0	0	5	7	0.6	157	1,085	0.06	0.04	0.9	21
300.	Tortilla chips	1 oz.	28	139	2.2	8	1.1	0	17	82	1.0	140	7	0.01	0.02	0.2	0
301.	Tortillas, corn, lime	1 6" diam.	30	63	1.5	1	0.0	0	14	60	0.9	0	6	0.04	0.02	0.3	0
302.	Tortilla, flour	1	35	105	2.6	3	.4	0	19	21	0.5	134	0	0.13	0.08	1.2	0
303.	Tostada	1	148	200	9.2	8	.3	14	25	167	1.8	200	445	0.06	0.13	.8	6
304.	Tuna, canned, oil pack, drained	3 oz.	85	167	25.0	7	1.7	60	0	7	1.6	0	70	0.04	0.10	10.1	0
305.	Tuna, canned, water pack, solids and liquid	3½ oz.	99	126	27.7	1	0.0	55	0	16	1.6	161	0	0.00	0.10	13.2	0
306.	Turkey, roast (light and dark mixed)	3 oz.	85	162	27.0	5	1.5	73	0	7	1.5	111	0	0.04	0.15	6.5	0
307.	Turnip, cooked, drained	½ c cubed	78	18	0.6	0	0.0	0	4	27	0.3	27	0	0.03	0.04	0.3	17
308.	Turnip greens, cooked drained	½ c	73	19	2.1	0	0.0	0	3	98	1.3	14	5,695	0.04	0.08	0.4	16
309.	Veal, cooked loin	3 oz.	85	199	22.0	11	4.0	90	0	9	2.7	55	0	0.06	0.21	4.6	0
310.	Vegetables, mixed, cooked	1 c	182	116	5.8	0	0.0	0	24	46	2.4	348	4,505	0.02	0.13	2.0	15
311.	Watermelon	1 c diced	160	42	0.8	0	0.0	0	10	11	0.8	2	940	0.05	0.05	0.3	11
312.	Wheat germ, plain toasted	1 tbsp	6	23	1.8	1	0.0	0	3	3	0.5	0	10	0.11	0.05	0.3	1
313.	Whiskey, gin, rum, vodka 90 proof	1½ oz (jigger)	42	110	0	0	0.0	0	0	0	0.0	0	0	0.00	0.00	0.0	0
314.	White cake, choc. icing	1 piece	71	268	3.5	11	3.7	2	40	35	0.3	162	40	0.19	0.14	1.6	0
315.	Whole wheat cereal, cooked	½ c	123	55	2.2	1	0.0	0	12	9	0.06	260	0	0.08	0.03	0.8	0
316.	Whole wheat flakes, ready-to-eat	1 c	30	106	3.1	1	0.0	0	24	12	2.0	310	1,410	0.35	0.42	3.5	11
317.	Whopper, Burger King	1	*	606	29.0	32	10.5	100	51	37	6.0	909	641	0.02	0.03	5.2	13
318.	Wine, dry table 12% alc.	3½ fl. oz.	102	87	0.1	0	0.0	0	4	9	0.4	5	0	0.00	0.01	0.1	0
319.	Wine, red dry 18.8% alc.	2 fl. oz.	59	81	0.1	0	0.0	0	5	5	0.0	4	0	0.01	0.02	0.2	0
320.	Yeast, brewers	1 tbsp	8	23	3.1	0	0.0	0	3	17	1.4	10	0	1.25	0.34	3.0	0
321.	Yogurt, fruit	1 c	227	231	9.9	2	1.6	10	43	345	0.2	125	104	0.08	0.40	0.2	2
322.	Yogurt, plain low fat	1 8-oz. container	226	113	7.7	4	2.3	15	12	271	0.1	115	150	0.09	0.41	0.2	2

"0" represents both less than 1 and 0

List of foods expanded from the original publication of 228 foods contained in Lifetime Physical Fitness & Wellness: A Personalized Program, Morton Publishing Company, 1986. All new food items have been reproduced with permission from the Food Processor nutrient analysis software by Esha Research, P.O. Box 13028, Salem, Oregon, 97309.

Original list adapted from:
Nutritive Value of American Foods in Common Units. Agriculture Handbook No. 456. U.S. Dept. of Agriculture. Washington, D.C. November 1975.

Young, E. A., E. H. Brennan, and C. L. Irving, Guest Eds. Perspectives on Fast Foods. Public Health Currents, 19(1), 1979, Published by Ross Laboratories, Columbus, OH.

Dennison, D. The Dine System: the Nutrition Plan For Better Health. C. V. Mosby Comp. St. Louis, Mo, 1982.

Pennington, S. A. T. and H. N. Church. Food Values of Portions Commonly Used. Harper and Row Publishers, New York, 1985.

Kullman, D. A. ABC Milligram Cholesterol Diet Guide. Merit Publications, Inc. North Miami Beach, Florida 1978.

Figure B.1. *Dietary analysis form*

Date: _____

Foods	Amount	Calories	Protein (gm)	Fat (total) (gm)	Sat. Fat (gm)	Chol-esterol (mg)	Carbo-hydrates (gm)	Cal-cium (mg)	Iron (mg)	Sodium (mg)	Vit. A (I.U.)	Vit. B₁ (mg)	Vit B₂ (mg)	Nia-cin (mg)	Vit. C (mg)
Totals															

Figure B.1. *Dietary analysis form (continued)*

Date: _____

Foods	Amount	Calories	Protein (gm)	Fat (total) (gm)	Sat. Fat (gm)	Chol-esterol (mg)	Carbo-hydrates (gm)	Cal-cium (mg)	Iron (mg)	Sodium (mg)	Vit. A (I.U.)	Vit. B₁ (mg)	Vit B₂ (mg)	Nia-cin (mg)	Vit. C (mg)
Totals															

Figure B.1. *Dietary analysis form (continued)*

Date: _____

Foods	Amount	Calories	Protein (gm)	Fat (total) (gm)	Sat. Fat (gm)	Chol- esterol (mg)	Carbo- hydrates (gm)	Cal- cium (mg)	Iron (mg)	Sodium (mg)	Vit. A (I.U.)	Vit. B₁ (mg)	Vit B₂ (mg)	Nia- cin (mg)	Vit. C (mg)
Totals															

Figure B.2. *Three-day nutrient analysis*

Name: _____

Day	Calories	Protein (gm)	Fat (gm)	Sat. Fat (gm)	Choles-terol (mg)	Carbo-hydrates (gm)	Calcium (mg)	Iron (mg)	Sodium (mg)	Vit. A (I.U.)	Vit. B$_1$ (mg)	Vit. B$_2$ (mg)	Niacin (mg)	Vit. C (mg)
One														
Two														
Three														
Totals														
Average[a]														
Percentages[b]														

Recommended Dietary Allowances

	Calories	Protein (gm)	Fat (gm)	Sat. Fat (gm)	Choles-terol (mg)	Carbo-hydrates (gm)	Calcium (mg)	Iron (mg)	Sodium (mg)	Vit. A (I.U.)	Vit. B$_1$ (mg)	Vit. B$_2$ (mg)	Niacin (mg)	Vit. C (mg)
Men 15-18 yrs.	See below[c]	See below[d]	<30%[e]	<10%[e]	<300[e]	50%>[e]	1,200	18	3,000[e]	5,000	1.4	1.7	18	60
Men 19-22 yrs.			<30%	<10%	<300	50%>	800	10	3,000	5,000	1.5	1.7	19	60
Men 23-50 yrs.			<30%	<10%	<300	50%>	800	10	3,000	5,000	1.4	1.6	18	60
Women 15-18 yrs.			<30%	<10%	<300	50%>	1,200	18	3,000	4,000	1.1	1.3	14	60
Women 19-22 yrs.			<30%	<10%	<300	50%>	800	18	3,000	4,000	1.1	1.3	14	60
Women 23-50 yrs.			<30%	<10%	<300	50%>	800	18	3,000	4,000	1.0	1.2	13	60
Pregnant			<30%	<10%	<300	50%>	+400	See below[f]	3,000	5,000	+0.4	+0.3	+2	+20
Lactating			<30%	<10%	<300	50%>	+400		3,000	6,000	+0.5	+0.5	+5	+40

[a] Divide totals by 3 or number of days assessed.
[b] Percentages: Protein and Carbohydrates = multiply average by 4 and divide by average calories, Fat and Saturated Fat = multiply average by 9 and divide by average calories.
[c] Use Table 6.3 (Chapter 6) for all categories.
[d] Protein intake should be .8 grams per kilogram of body weight. Pregnant women should consume an additional 30 grams of daily protein, while lactating women should have an extra 20 grams.
[e] Based on recommendations by nutrition experts.
[f] Add 30 to 60 mg of supplemental iron during and three months after pregnancy.

Figure B.3. *Daily nutrient intake form for computer software use (make additional copies as necessary)*

Date: _____

Name: _____ Age: _____ Weight: _____

Sex: Male—M, Female—F (Pregnant—P, Lactating—L, Neither—N)

Activity Rating: Sedentary (limited physical activity) = 1
Moderate physical activity = 2
Hard labor (strenuous physical activity) = 3

Number of days to be analyzed: _____ Day: _____

No.	Code*	Food	Amount
1			
2			
3			
4			
5			
6			
7			
8			
9			
10			
11			
12			
13			
14			
15			
16			
17			
18			
19			
20			
21			
22			
23			
24			
25			
26			
27			
28			
29			
30			
31			

*When done, to advance to the next day or end, type 0 (zero).

A P P E N D I X   C

Health Protection Plan
For Environmental Hazards,
Crime Prevention, and Personal Safety*

* Questionnaire published by the Preventive Medicine/Strang Clinic, New York, 1982. Reproduced with permission.

Personal Environment In addition to environmental

problems in the community at large there are also important problems in our own immediate environment that affect our health, well-being, and comfort. These are problems we can control and improve ourselves.
The following self-assessment relates to environmental hazards dealing with water, wastes, noise and air pollution in our everyday lives.
All "no" answers are a cue to ACTION.

Concerning AIR POLLUTION, do you...?	YES	NO
...Know the optimal conditions for temperature, humidity and air movement in your home?	○	○
...Change the air filters once a year in your air conditioners or forced air heating systems?	○	○
...Are your work areas ventilated so that fumes and dusts do not accumulate?	○	○
...Do your throat or nasal passages feel moist and clear in the morning (not dry or stuffy)?	○	○
...Know what to do when the weather report says the quality of the air is unsatisfactory?	○	○
...Know what a "killer smog" is?	○	○
...If you smoke, do you avoid smoking in a bedroom or areas where children play?	○	○

RISK FACTORS:

- *Bronchitis, asthma, emphysema, and heart disease are all aggravated by air pollution.*
- *Chronic exposure to dusts of metal or wood are risk factors for cancer of the respiratory passages.*
- *Children of cigarette smokers have a higher than usual incidence of respiratory infections.*
- *Many so-called allergies of the sinuses and upper respiratory tract are really due to air pollution.*

AWARENESS COUNTS:

- **The optimal air comfort levels are 66-68°F temperature, 30-40% humidity, and air movement at 20-50 feet per minute. Lower humidity will lead to dryness of the respiratory passages, increase skin evaporation and make your home feel colder than it is.**
- **When the air quality is reported as "unsatisfactory" people with heart and lung disease should stay indoors.**
- **"Killer smog" refers to trapped air which cannot rise, with no available dispersing breeze, which accumulates industrial, auto and heating combustion products into a suffocating density. This may be fatal to those with cardiopulmonary disease, and uncomfortable for everyone.**

Concerning WATER...?	YES	NO
...Have you checked your home drinking water in the last year for clarity, color and taste?	○	○
...If you shake up a glass of tap water does it remain clear (not foamy or frothy)?	○	○
...Do you have a screen filter on your water tap?	○	○
...Do you check restaurant water and ice for clarity and cleanliness?	○	○
...Do you know the common water-borne diseases?	○	○
...Do you know what kind of water purification tablets are best for traveling?	○	○
...Do you take care when traveling in developing countries or in unsettled areas to drink bottled water, or coffee, tea, or soup made with boiling water, and to avoid ice cubes?	○	○
...Do you think all wilderness water is safe?	○	○
...Do you know what source of water is almost always safe to drink?	○	○

Concerning WASTE...?	YES	NO
...Do you place ordinary kitchen waste in plastic bags for disposal?	○	○
...Do you know what kinds of wastes require special handling?	○	○
...Are your garbage cans free from bad odors?	○	○
...Is your sink or toilet bowl free from bad odors or back up of waste water in your drain?	○	○
...If you live in a home with a septic tank do you know its location?	○	○
...Do you know the last time the septic tank was cleaned?	○	○

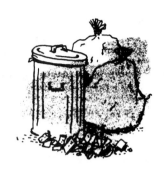

RISK FACTORS: WATER AND WASTE

- *Diseases associated with water and waste include: typhoid fever, cholera, hepatitis, poliomyelitis, E. coli dysentery and amoebic dysentery.*
- *Very hard water containing large amounts of magnesium can cause diarrhea in children. It is difficult to wash with, and will cause deposits in water pipes.*
- *Chlorine is commonly used for water purification. An excess is harmful since it may be converted into chloroform, a toxic chemical.*
- *The presence of water supplies in proximity to industrial plants is a cause for concern since there are many instances of toxic chemicals leaking into local water supplies in this country.*

AWARENESS COUNTS: WATER

- All water taps should have screen filters to trap particulate material which may accidentally enter the water supply. These should be removed and cleaned regularly.
- Frothy water is due to detergents leaking into the water supply and this can cause intestinal upsets.
- Cloudy water may be due only to rusty pipes and while it may stain kitchen utensils it is not harmful; but turbid water with an odor may be due to seepage of sewage or industrial wastes into the water supply and this can be dangerous to health. Every state has a water supply agency that can give you information on the condition of your local water supply. However, if your water comes from a well, no one is checking it for purity. You must take the initiative and find out from the state agency how this can be done.
- The best type of water purification tablets is the iodine-releasing variety rather than the chlorine type. These are obtainable from your local pharmacy. Use these only if traveling in an area where bottled water is not available.
- Not all wilderness water is pure. It may come from springs which have toxic chemicals, or be contaminated by animal use upstream. If purified water is not available, the safest water to drink is rain water. (Make sure it is stored in a clean container.)

AWARENESS COUNTS: WASTE

- Plastic bags for disposal of ordinary wastes have the advantage of keeping your garbage containers, indoor and outdoor, clean and free of odors. This helps prevent fly, roach, and rodent infestation, and the accidental contamination of food.
- Aerosol cans, solvents, and fuels should not be placed in plastic bags, and should not be disposed of with household wastes because of the hazards of fire and explosion; your local waste disposal service should be contacted regarding special handling.
- Bad odors or backup of waste water into your sink, tub, or toilet is a serious matter since this is untreated sewage and poses a health hazard. There may be an obstruction in the sewage system; check with your plumber first. If you have a septic tank, it may have to be cleaned. The frequency of cleaning of septic tanks depends on size and use. Three to four years of regular use is an average duration of time before cleaning is necessary.
- It's important to know the location of your septic tank and also those of your neighbors in relationship to your well water supply. There should be a distance of 100 feet between the septic tank and well. Your board of health can give you additional information about specific conditions in your area.

Concerning NOISE…?	YES	NO
…Do you know how to tell if you are in an environment which could damage your hearing?	◯	◯
…Do you know that permanent hearing loss can occur with a single exposure to a painfully loud noise?	◯	◯
…Are you aware of the other effects on your health that noise can have other than hearing loss?	◯	◯
…Do you know the accidents that can occur due to noise causing "warning concealment"?	◯	◯
…Are you aware of "slow reaction time" as a noise associated danger?	◯	◯
… Do you know what age group is especially susceptible to noise induced hearing loss?	◯	◯

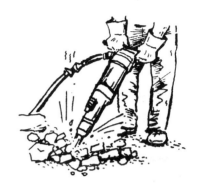

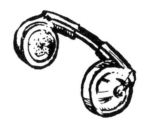

RISK FACTORS:

NOISE

- *Noise hazards can lead not only to permanent hearing damage, but it has been established that noise can cause personality disorders, increase aggressive behavior and have an aggravating effect on headaches, hypertension, and peptic ulcers. It also lowers work efficiency and interferes with sleep patterns.*

AWARENESS COUNTS:

- *If you are in a noisy environment several hours a day where you have to raise your voice to be heard, you are in an area of potential danger for hearing loss. Noise that is painfully loud, such as pneumatic hammers or amplified rock music, has the greatest potential to damage hearing.*

- *The age group in which there is particular susceptibility to hearing loss is adolescence.*

- *It is particularly important to sleep in a quiet environment; use rugs, drapes, double windows, and finally ear plugs if necessary, to obliterate disturbing sound. (Cotton makes a poor plug unless saturated with wax or vaseline. Sponge plastic ear plugs are better.)*

- *Pleasant background music can sometimes be used to mask disturbing sounds. However, background noise can conceal safety warnings, or lead to slow reaction time and thus contribute to accidents.*

FOLLOW-THROUGH

For information on all environmental hazards, write to:

The U.S. Environmental Protection Agency
Office of Public Affairs (A-107) Washington, D.C. 20460

For information about noise hazards, write to:

The National Information Center for Quiet
P.O. Box 57171 Washington, D.C. 20037

Crime Prevention

Through your own efforts, you can learn to reduce the opportunity and temptation for the criminal by accepting the responsibility to do everything possible for the protection of your personal well being and property.
All "no" answers are a cue to ACTION.

To protect yourself, do you...?	YES	NO
...Always us a peephole or chain lock to identify your visitor?	○	○
...Watch out for suspicious people or cars in your neighborhood?	○	○
...Make an effort to get better acquainted with your neighbors, especially if you live in a large apartment building?	○	○
...Avoid resisting the orders of a robber or purse snatcher?	○	○
...List only your last name and initials in the phone directory and on the mailbox?	○	○
...Always lock your doors during the day, even if you are at home?	○	○
...Leave lights on doors you will be using when you return after dark?	○	○
...Always have your key in your hand when you return home so you can open the door immediately?	○	○

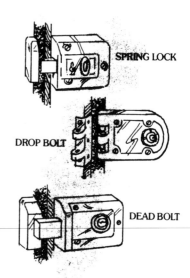

SPRING LOCK

DROP BOLT

DEAD BOLT

RISK FACTORS:
PROTECTING YOURSELF

- *Women alone and the elderly are at highest risk at being victims of crime.*

- *People who are disabled are more vulnerable to crime.*

- *Certain areas of every large city are high crime areas and should be avoided if possible.*

AWARENESS COUNTS:

- **List only your last name and initial in the phone directory and on the mailbox, particularly if you are a woman living alone.**
- **Always have your key ready when you return home.**
- **Always ask a visitor to identify himself before you let him in.**
- **Use automatic timers to turn on lights, radio, etc.**
- **If a window or lock has been forced or broken while you were out, use a neighbor's phone to call the police and wait outside until they arrive.**
- **Be cautious of unidentified phone callers. Hang up immediately if the caller will not identify himself.**
- **When traveling about at night, try to have a companion with you.**
- **Remember to ask for identification *before* you let repairmen, meter readers, or any other stranger into your home.**

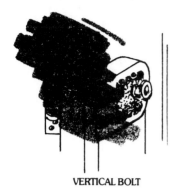

VERTICAL BOLT

To protect yourself, do you…?	YES	NO
…Make specal plans for your home when you are away on vacation?	○	○
…Avoid leaving a key under the doormat or in any accessible area?	○	○
…Have you made sure that your door (s) have sturdy locks?	○	○
…Check all windows and doors regularly for security?	○	○
…Stop newspaper and milk deliveries when you go on vacation?	○	○
…Keep especially valuable items in a safety deposit box away from home?	○	○

RISK FACTORS:

PROTECTING YOUR HOME

- Those at higher risk of home crime are people who leave their homes unattended for long periods of time and those who are nighttime travellers.
- Most crime takes place under cover of darkness.
- Letting mail and newspapers accumulate at your door announces the vulnerability of your home.

AWARENESS COUNTS:

- **Keep your doors locked at all times.**
- **Have lights on an automatic timer while you are away.**
- **An alarm system is a useful crime deterrent.**
- **Make sure windows are secured.**
- **Make sure doorways and hallways are well lighted.**
- **Leave a radio on (a radio uses little electricity and gives the impression that your home is occupied).**

About Locks: Doors should be equipped with either a drop-bolt or dead-bolt lock. Do not use spring locks on any outside door. Spring locks work simply by closing the door and can be easily opened with a plastic card. Drop-bolt or dead-bolt locks can only be unlocked with a key.

FOLLOW-THROUGH

Check with your local police department about joining the Operation Identification Program. You are provided with a sticker to display on your home and your valuable property is engraved with a non-removable code number. The police have a registered list of this property and statistics show that burglars avoid such homes because marked items are difficult to dispose of. Many police departments have crime prevention units and will give you personal advice.

Many states make available the Federal Crime Insurance Program – it provides federal crime insurance against burglary and robbery losses – rates depend upon the crime rate in the area where your home is located. For more information write to:

Federal Crime Insurance, P.O. Box 11033
Washington, D.C. 20014 Toll Free (800) 638-8780

Review your homeowner's insurance coverage to make sure you have adequate coverage.

Personal Safety

While not all accidents are preventable, many are. Failure to take simple precautionary measures increases the risk of an avoidable accident. See if you can identify safety problem areas. All "yes" answers are a cue to Action.

Concerning PERSONAL SAFETY,	YES	NO
...Have you had any accidents in the past years which could have been prevented?	◯	◯
...If yes, where did this occur? at home?	◯	◯
in your automobile?	◯	◯
at work?	◯	◯

To ensure your SAFETY AT HOME,	YES	NO
...Do you fail to go through your dwelling, room by room, deliberately looking for safety hazards once a year?	◯	◯
Does your dwelling have fewer than two means of escape in the event of an emergency?	◯	◯

	YES	NO
...If you smoke, do you ever smoke in bed?	◯	◯
...Do you fail to keep a first aid kit, smoke alarm and fire extinguisher at home?	◯	◯
...Are there loose electrical wiring or fixtures around your home?	◯	◯
...Are carpets put down without non-skid backings?	◯	◯
...Are poisons and pills in areas within reach of pre-school children?	◯	◯

In the BATHROOM, do you fail to...	YES	NO
...Check the temperature of bath or shower water with your hand first?	◯	◯
...Make sure electrical appliances are never used near water?	◯	◯
...Use non-skid paste-ons or rubber mats for bathtub and shower surfaces?	◯	◯

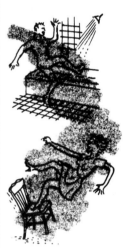

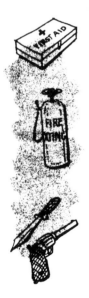

In the KITCHEN, do you fail to...	YES	NO
...Store knives with points away from the hand, or in special holders?	◯	◯
...Keep curtains away from the cooking range?	◯	◯
...Keep electrical appliances away from water?	◯	◯
...Keep floors clean of grease and dirt?	◯	◯
...Are you currently exposed to any of the material listed below?	◯	◯
dust (such as wood, leather, heavy metals, dyestuff)?	◯	◯
petroleum products?	◯	◯
radiation?	◯	◯
solvents?	◯	◯
...If yes to any of the above...was your exposure usually indoors?	◯	◯

	YES	NO
...Did your exposure occur for an equivalent of at least one eight hour day per week for a period of five years?	◯	◯
...If yes to dust, chemicals or petroleum products, was your skin or clothing regularly contacted by these materials?	◯	◯

To ensure your SAFETY IN YOUR AUTOMOBILE, do you...?	YES	NO
...Neglect to <u>always</u> fasten your seat belts?	◯	◯
...Ever drink alcoholic beverages before driving?	◯	◯
...Drive even when you are sleepy?	◯	◯
...Drive more than <u>40%</u> of the time in the dark?	◯	◯
...Have you received more than <u>one</u> moving traffic violation this past year?	◯	◯
...Have you had more than <u>one</u> accident this past year?	◯	◯

RISK FACTORS: PERSONAL SAFETY

- *Accidents are the leading cause of death among those under 44 years old.*
- *Accidents are the fourth most common cause of death in this country ranking behind heart disease, cancer and stroke.*

AWARENESS COUNTS:

- **It is especially important that potential problem areas at home, on the road, and at work be identified so that you can create a relatively accident free environment. Improving your accident-prone behavior is the only way to decrease your risk of accidents.**
- **Your home or apartment should be regularly checked for safety hazards:** ■ Slippery stairways ■ Unfastened carpets ■ Faulty fixtures or outlets ■ Store poisons, firearms in safe place ■ Have safety guard rails on upper level windows ■ Place smoke detectors in strategic areas ■ Have emergency numbers posted by the phone ■ Fire strikes more than 1,500 homes every day.
- **Automobile accidents take more lives each year than any other type of accident or illness. Many of these can be prevented:** ■ Make sure your car is in safe running condition, especially brakes and tires ■ Wear seat belts at <u>all</u> times. ■ Never drive while drinking. ■ Never drive while sleepy. ■ Always lock your car.

To ensure your SAFETY AT WORK,	YES	NO
...Does your place of work fail to have regular safety checks?	○	○
...Does your place of work fail to have regular emergency drills such as fire drills?	○	○
...Does your place of work fail to have a current fire emergency plan?	○	○
...Does your place of work fail to have rules governing the use of machinery and protective equipment?	○	○
...Have you ever worked at a job where you were exposed to: asbestos? ○○ chemicals? ○○ coal dust? ○○		

RISK FACTORS:

SAFETY AT WORK

- *13,000 accidental deaths per year occur on the job and over 2 million people are disabled or injured.*
- *Almost 30 billion dollars per year and about 25 million work days are lost due to accidents at work.*

AWARENESS COUNTS:

- **Know where fire extinguishers are located.**
- **Is there a fire emergency plan in your office?**
- **Know the mandatory safety standards which apply to your business or industry.**
- **Use all protective clothing required.**
- **Know the names and hazards of <u>all</u> materials you are exposed to.**

FOLLOW-THROUGH

For information regarding safety procedures and requirements <u>on the job</u> write to:
The U.S. Department of Labor, Washington, D.C. 20212
Or get in touch with the Department of Labor office in your region. Or write to:
The National Institute for Occupational Safety and Health, Post Office Building, Cincinnati, Ohio 45202
For information regarding the safety of consumer products, write to:
U.S. Consumer Product Safety Commission Office of Washington, D.C. 20207
For information regarding all kinds of accidents, write to:
The National Safety Council, 444 N. Michigan Avenue, Chicago, Illinois 60611

Preventive Medicine Institute/Strang Clinic   55 East 34 Street • New York, N.Y. 10016 • (212) 683-1000

Blood Pressure Assessment

BLOOD PRESSURE ASSESSMENT *

Blood pressure is assessed with the use of a sphygmomanometer and a stethoscope. The sphygmomanometer consists of an inflatable bladder contained within a cuff, and a mercury gravity manometer or an aneroid manometer from which the pressure is read. The appropriate size cuff must be selected in order to get accurate readings. The size is determined by the width of the inflatable bladder, which should be about 40 percent of the circumference of the mid-point of the arm.

The measurement of blood pressure is usually done in the sitting position with the forearm and the manometer at the same level as the heart. Initially the pressure should be recorded from each arm, with subsequent pressures recorded from the arm with the highest reading. The cuff should be applied approximately one inch above the natural crease of the elbow with the center of the bladder applied directly over the inner arm. The stethoscope should be applied firmly, but with little pressure, over the brachial artery on the inside of the elbow. The arm should be slightly flexed and placed on a flat surface. The bladder can be inflated while feeling the radial pulse to about 30 to 40 mmHg above the disappearance of the pulse. Avoid overinflating the cuff, as such may cause blood vessel spasm, resulting in higher blood pressure readings. The pressure should be released at a rate of two mmHg/second. As the pressure is released, systolic blood pressure is determined at the point where the first pulse sound is heard. The diastolic pressure is determined at the

point where the pulse sound disappears. The recordings should be made to the nearest two mmHg (even numbers) and expressed as systolic over diastolic pressure, i.e., 124/80. The person measuring the pressure should also note whether the pressure was recorded from the left or the right arm.

In some cases the loudness of the pulse sounds decreases in intensity (point of muffling of sounds) and can still be heard at a lower pressure (50 or 40 mmHg) or even all the way down to zero. In this situation the diastolic pressure is recorded at the point where there is a clear/definite change in the loudness of the sound (also referred to as fourth phase), and at complete disappearance of the sound (fifth phase), i.e., 120/78/60 or 120/82/0.

A final consideration when measuring blood pressure is that several readings by different people or at different times of the day should be taken to establish true blood pressure values. One single reading may not be an accurate value, since many factors can affect blood pressure. Excitement, nervousness, food, smoking, pain, temperature, physical activity, etc. can all significantly alter the pressure. Whenever possible, blood pressure readings should be taken in a quiet, comfortable room, following a few minutes of rest in the recording position. When more than one reading is taken, the bladder should be completely deflated to avoid venous congestion in the forearm and at least one minute should be allowed before the next reading is made.

*Reference: Recommendations for Human Blood Pressure Determination by Sphygmomanometers. American Heart Association, 1980.

Figure D.1. *Blood pressure recording form*

Name: _____ Course: _____ Section: _____ Date: _____

Date	Arm	Blood Pressure	Recorder's Name

Index